Autoimmune Hepatitis

Autoimmune Hepatitis

Edited by

Mikio Nishioka

Kagawa University School of Medicine, Kagawa, Japan

Gotaro Toda

and

Mikio Zeniya

Jikei University School of Medicine, Tokyo, Japan

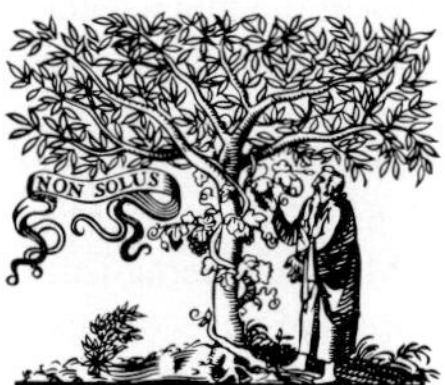

1994

ELSEVIER

AMSTERDAM·LONDON·NEW YORK·TOKYO

ELSEVIER SCIENCE B.V.
Sara Burgerhartstraat 25
P.O. Box 211, 1000 AE Amsterdam, the Netherlands

Library of Congress Cataloging in Publication Data

Autoimmune hepatitis / edited by Mikio Nishioka, Gotaro Toda, and
    Mikio Zeniya.
        p.   cm.
    Includes bibliographical references and index.
    ISBN 0-444-88196-4 (alk. paper)
    1. Chronic active hepatitis.   2. Liver—Immunology.   I. Nishioka,
Mikio, 1936–   . II. Toda, Gotaro.   III. Zeniya, Mikio.
    [DNLM: 1. Hepatitis, Chronic Active.   2. Autoimmune Diseases.   WC
536 A939 1994]
RC848.C4A88   1994
616.3′623—dc20
DNLM/DLC
for Library of Congress   93-41919
                                                                        CIP

ISBN: 0 444 88196 4

Foreword

More than thirty-five years have passed since Waldenström reported the first liver disease related to immune mechanisms. In Japan, the first symposium on autoimmune hepatitis, in which I reported the antigenicity of liver microsomal fractions, was in 1962. Since then research on autoimmune hepatitis has steadily advanced and with recent developments in molecular and cellular biology the last five years have witnessed tremendous advances in the diagnosis and pathogenesis of this disease. It seems timely that this book, the first monograph concerned with autoimmune hepatitis, is edited by three Japanese scientists. The book provides a great deal of modern knowledge about autoimmune hepatitis that will be of value to hepatologists, and results from a close cooperation of distinguished individuals who are major contributors to the recent developments world-wide in the field of immunology in hepatology.

Each chapter in this book represents a fusion of ideas from both clinical and experimental viewpoints. I hope that the cooperation shown in the pages that follow will continue, and am sure that this book will encourage young researchers interested in liver immunology.

Haruo Kameda
President of the Tokyo Hospital, Tokyo

Preface

In the last few years there have been many creative and exciting developments in hepatitis research.

The discovery of the HCV genome is an epoch-making development which has opened up liver research to molecular and cellular biological techniques. In particular, recombinant techniques and the clinical application of the polymerase chain reaction have made a tremendous impact upon the further understanding of the pathogenesis of not only viral hepatitis but also of autoimmune hepatitis. The development of diagnostic methods for HCV infection provided us with the existence of a characteristic group of patients with chronic active hepatitis in whom corticosteroid, not interferon, is effective in interrupting hepatitis. Moreover, identification of HCV opened another interesting research field of liver immunology. HCV infection was shown to induce the production of an autoantibody. GOR antibody, the epitope of which was partially homologous to the HCV polyprotein. In patients with type II autoimmune hepatitis characterized by liver-kidney microsomal antibody type I (LKM-1), a high incidence of HCV infection was reported.

Immunologic studies have also advanced, but at a somewhat slower pace due to the unavailability of suitable tissue culture and animal models. HLA restriction is a great barrier to the analysis of the immune reaction in the course of hepatitis. Nevertheless, thanks to the continuous efforts of a tenacious group of immunologists, most of whom have contributed to this book, much has been clarified in the last few years.

This book summarizes the present knowledge of autoimmune hepatitis and represents the first monograph on this characteristic subject including the first historical review and the clinical status in both the East and West of autoimmune hepatitis. We hope that it will be a landmark in the field and that it will encourage research in the areas of immunology and hepatology.

If the reader discovers that some chapters fit equally well in two or more sections of the book, this belongs to the editors' responsibility. No book is easy to compile and the editors would like to thank all of the contributors who made the editors' task that much easier and wrote their chapters in a cooperative spirit, which hopefully will continue.

Mikio Nishioka
Gotaro Toda
Mikio Zeniya

Contents

3. Clinical characteristics of autoimmune hepatitis in Japan
Y. Ohta and M. Onji   45

4. Hepatitis C virus in type 1 autoimmune hepatitis
G. Toda, M. Zeniya, Y. Aizawa and H. Watanabe   55

5. Autoimmunity in hepatitis virus infection
K. Sakaguchi, H. Kawamoto, A. Takaki, H. Shimomura and T. Tsuji .   69

III. Pathology of Autoimmune Hepatitis **83**

6. Pathology of autoimmune hepatitis and related diseases
Y. Nakanuma, K. Harada, A. Nonomura, E. Matsushita and M. Unoura   85

7. Histopathology of autoimmune hepatitis

H.P. Dienes and F. Autschbach

IV. Autoantibodies in Autoimmune Hepatitis

8. Anti-asialoglycoprotein receptor antibodies

B.M. McFarlane and I.G. McFarlane

18. Treatment of autoimmune hepatitis in Japan

T. Kuroki, T. Monna and S. Yamamoto 305

VIII. Recent Aspects of Autoimmune Hepatitis 317

19. Recent aspects of autoimmune hepatitis

M. Nishioka and S.A. Morshed 319

xvi   *Contents*

Section I

Historical Overview

Autoimmune Hepatitis
Edited by M. Nishioka, G. Toda and M. Zeniya
© *1994, Elsevier Science B.V. All rights reserved*

Chapter 1

The history of autoimmune hepatitis

Ian R. Mackay[1] and Brian D. Tait[2]

[1]*Centre for Molecular Biology and Medicine, Monash University, Clayton 3168, Victoria (Australia)*
and [2]*Tissue Typing Laboratory, Royal Melbourne Hospital, Parkville 3050, Victoria (Australia)*

1. Introduction

This history of chronic active hepatitis (CAH) spans 50 years, from 1940 to 1990. The autoimmune type of CAH (AI-CAH) was unsuspected before the 1950s. In fact, until the 1970s, there was no clear perception of heterogeneity within the general rubric of CAH, either by pathologists or clinicians, and the general adjectival usage 'autoimmune' in relation to CAH can be dated as late as the 1980s.

In the *1940s*, the term 'chronic active hepatitis' was first used to describe a disease that represented a delayed or failed recovery from a presumed acute infectious hepatitis. In the *1950s*, CAH became more particularly applied to an insidious chronic liver disease occurring in young women with unusual immunological accompaniments, and the proposal arose that a newly recognized cause of disease, autoimmunity, might be applicable to such cases. Hence the term 'lupoid hepatitis' was coined to ascribe clinical relationships between this disease and systemic lupus erythematosus (SLE) and to introduce the notion of an autoimmune pathogenesis, which then seemed applicable to SLE. In the *1960s*, the newly introduced technique of immunofluorescence was applied to the serological identification of various types of autoimmune disease, including CAH and, in that decade, many reports substantiated the reality of lupoid hepatitis, and long-term immune-suppressive treatment appeared beneficial. In the *1970s*, it was recognized that the generic category of CAH subsumed various histologically similar subtypes with, particularly, an autoimmune subtype (archetypal CAH) and a viral (hepatitis B virus (HBV)) subtype. Also, studies were published on the association with autoimmune CAH of major histocompatibility (MHC) alleles, HLA-Al and -B8. In the *1980s*, interest developed in an earlier described

3

(1973) second type of autoimmune CAH (type 2), with different clinical features
and an association with liver–kidney microsomal autoantibodies. Also, the role
of a newly identified hepatitis virus (hepatitis C virus (HCV)), in CAH became
appreciated.

2. The clinical aspects

2.1. Introductory comments

Knowledge 50 years ago on diffuse liver disease was very different from that
available today. Acute hepatitis was known to be a transmissible disease,
although the identity of the infectious agents was unknown. Cirrhosis of the liver
was, of course, well known, but types, causes and pathogenesis were poorly
delineated. Text-books of that era referred to 'portal' (or Laennec) cirrhosis and
'biliary' cirrhosis, with the connotations that *portal* causes could be attributed to
the portal venous inflow from the gut, e.g., toxins such as alcohol, or *biliary* causes
to disease of the biliary tract, such as, ascending infections.

Pathologists had a dominant influence on concepts of cirrhosis, since different
nodular patterns could be distinguished morphologically. The usual pattern was
that of small (1 cm or less) evenly sized nodules, as in the typical portal
micronodular cirrhosis. However, in a less frequently occurring type, there were
much larger and unevenly sized nodules, macronodular cirrhosis, suggestive of
an episode or episodes of massive necrosis and parenchymal collapse with
nodular regeneration. A further interpretation for macronodular cirrhosis, based
on clinical inferences, was that this pattern could be a sequel to a non-healing
infectious hepatitis, hence designated as 'post-hepatitic' cirrhosis.

2.2. The 1940–1950 decade

In the late 1940s, there was a further attempt to synthesize pathogenesis and
morphology by use of the terms 'trophopathic' and 'toxipathic' cirrhosis which
differentiated liver disease primarily attributable to nutritional disorders or toxic
insults.

In summary, in the early 1940s, the known or suspected aetiologies for cirrhosis
of the liver (CAH was not written about at that time) were alcohol abuse,
nutritional deficiency, toxins, metal overload, and biliary obstruction, with
a suspected infectious basis related to the agent that caused acute infectious
hepatitis. In the 1940s, autoimmunity was scarcely recognized as a cause of
disease, although autoantibodies to various tissues including liver were recognized as an accompaniment of tissue damage due to infectious agents.

Knowledge on chronic hepatitis developed during the 1940s from several
sources. First, epidemiological studies and follow-up observations on cases of

epidemic hepatitis, particularly on soldiers during the 1939–1945 World War, stimulated interest in states of delayed recovery from viral hepatitis. Second, needle biopsy of the liver was introduced. Third, technical laboratory advances in protein chemistry allowed for the identification of a raised globulin level in serum which became recognized as a marker of CAH and, more particularly, as a marker of cases attributable to autoimmunity.

Clinical aspects of late sequelae of acute hepatitis among troops in the Mediterranean theatre in World War II were reported by Barker et al. (1945) and Capps (1948). Cases of chronic hepatitis, defined as non-recovery after 4 months, were specified as 'active' if symptoms were present, and as 'inactive' if symptoms were absent, but there were laboratory-defined abnormalities. This was the origin of the designation 'CAH'. Capps (1948) reported that of observed cases of viral hepatitis with jaundice, 'active' hepatitis was present after 4 months in 10% and after 1 year in 3%. In contemporary studies from the Rockefeller Institute on 400 cases of clinically diagnosed viral hepatitis, there were 2% that had not recovered after 2 years (Kunkel et al., 1947; Kunkel and Labby, 1950). An analysis of 68 cases of acute viral hepatitis by Liebowitz (1950) disclosed 7 (11%) that progressed to 'chronic active hepatitis' over periods of observation of 6–24 months after the onset of the initial acute attack. However, these 7 cases were not truly typical of acute viral hepatitis of early adult life, since their average age was 47 years, and two were 'alcoholic'; in two cases, a liver biopsy showed cirrhosis in one and fatty infiltration in the other.

Biochemical studies on blood came into use in the 1940s as empirical diagnostic markers for chronic hepatitis. These depended essentially upon reciprocal alterations in the levels of serum albumin and serum globulins that occurred as a result of liver dysfunction and inflammation. We can recall the attention given in earlier years to the 'albumin–globulin ratio'. There was a decrease in serum albumin due to parenchymal loss, but more striking was the increase in level of serum globulins. The technique of moving boundary electrophoresis of serum showed that the serum globulin increase was mainly accounted for by raised levels of γ-globulin in the blood, in cases of chronic hepatitis and cirrhosis of the liver. Reference to these earlier studies, together with an electrophoretic pattern showing extreme hypergammaglobulinaemia in cirrhosis of the liver, are cited in an earlier review by Mackay (1975). In the 1940–1960 era, serological tests depending on altered serum globulin levels were used extensively by clinicians, e.g., the cephalin flocculation and thymol turbidity tests, and a procedure was developed to equate one of the turbidometric procedures (zinc sulphate) with actual levels of serum γ-globulin (Weiden, 1953), although the true significance of the increase in γ-globulin was not appreciated at the time.

Thus, in summary, a disease entity known as CAH was described in the 1940s as a late sequel to a presumed acute viral hepatitis. There is no clear indication among the descriptions at that time of a disease resembling the CAH of the 1950s, although the description in the monograph by Himsworth (1947) best approaches this. He alluded to 'the form of subacute hepatitis which appears to arise as such, without the patient ever having had an acute illness suggestive of liver disease… jaundice being absent or so faint as to pass unnoticed… the condition affects women more often than men… the patient may date her present illness from an acute infection, such as cystitis or bronchitis, some 1 or 2 years previously… since then she has never felt really well… rheumatic pains, without evidence of articular damage are often noticed… or she may delay attending until the condition has passed into the next stage of post necrotic scarring… a particular problem is why do nearly all cases of sub-acute massive necrosis inevitably progress… ?'.

2.3. *The 1950–1960 decade*

The year 1950 is reasonably cited as the time of recognition of what is presently recognized as AI-CAH, as judged by the conference report of Waldenström (1950) and the abstract of Kunkel et al. (1951) as the archetypal descriptions. However, as an earlier pointer, Wood and colleagues (1948) in Australia described 12 cases, mostly children or young adults, with active hepatitis for more than 4 months, splenomegaly, raised serum globulin levels, and recurrences of jaundice. They wrote in 1948 that a 'progressive destructive lesion in the liver appeared to be present… the cause of this progression is unknown… virus remains in the liver throughout the course of the disease… its activities are accelerated, causing a flare-up in the symptoms, or progressive changes may be due to the production of tissue-destroying antibodies provoked by the original infection'.

The description by Waldenström (1950) from Sweden, captures the clinical presentation of cases of CAH that were beginning to be recognized at that time in adolescent females, marked by endocrine features including spider naevi, acne and amenorrhoea, and an increase in γ-globulin attributed to infection with a persisting virus. 'Dazu kommt bei fast allen Fällen das Auftreten von sog. Sternchen (Naevi aranei) und bei den Mädchen auch eine besondere Tendenz zur schweren Akneeruption. Eine langdauernde Amennorrhöe ist charakteristisch, die wahrscheinlich anovulatorisch ist… Es ist damit möglich, dass in der Zukunft eine Anzahl von diesen Fällen mit Acth. gebessert werden können… Die zweite Frage, ob die nachgewiesene Erhöhung des Gammaglobulins als Zeichen eines chronischen Immunisierungsprozesses aufzufassen ist, verdient meines Erachtens grösste Aufmerksamkeit… Die Atiologie dieser chronischen Leberleiden ist – wei wir alle wissen – immer noch unbekannt. Es werden toxische, infektiöse und Nahrungsfaktoren als Urasche angenommen… Es scheint sehr wohl möglich, dass die gammaglobulinvermehrung als Symptom einer Immunisierung gegen das im Körper verbleibende Virus aufzufassen ist'.

Kunkel and Labby (1950) in the U.S.A., at the same time reported on cases of cirrhosis of the liver that seemed attributable to a past infectious hepatitis, noting in such cases a pronounced hyperglobulinaemia. This report was followed by the abstract of Kunkel et al. (1951) which vividly depicts the presentation, as seen in the 1950s, of CAH in the following terms. 'Total proteins ranged from 9–13 per cent... this rise was due entirely to gamma globulin increase... eleven of these twelve patients were females... the maximum age was 32... onset of disease was insidious... course was prolonged and either stationary or downhill... frequently marked by periods of high fever, arthralgia, and arthritis... remarkable degree of plasma cell infiltration in the liver... which diminished during the course of disease... the etiology of the syndrome remains unknown'. This prompted the further observation by Zimmerman et al. (1951) of extreme hyperglobulinaemia (87 g/l) in a 36-year-old man with chronic liver disease and slowly developing jaundice in whom the liver histology was interpreted as 'subacute necrosis'. These authors made the interesting remark that 'the initial injury causes an alteration in liver protein, which stimulates the formation of anti-liver antibodies. These newly formed antibodies produce more liver injury, thus releasing more altered liver protein, which again contributes to the vicious circle of continuing necrosis'.

The studies in Melbourne on cases of young women with chronic hepatitis and hyperglobulinaemia continued and cases were described by Saint et al. (1953) as 'active chronic infectious hepatitis'. Their report noted 'fairly well defined clinical features, a highly characteristic pattern of biochemical tests including hypergammaglobulinaemia, and a histological picture which seems to indicate active chronic inflammatory changes... in many cases an initial history of contact or even a history of typical acute infectious hepatitis was lacking... but little doubt existed that the liver disease was due to infection with a virus'. This report followed the nomenclature used in the earlier descriptions by Capps (1948) of 'active' and 'inactive' chronic hepatitis, except that Saint et al. (1953) used histological (biopsy) criteria to draw the distinction between 'active' and 'inactive'. The 'active chronic' cases were, of course, clinically the more prominent. For some years, 'active chronic hepatitis' and 'chronic active hepatitis' became used interchangeably, although the earlier used version, 'chronic active', eventually prevailed.

These studies on 'active chronic hepatitis' led to a key observation in 1955. One of the patients in this category, a female aged 34 years, complained of arthralgia, a symptom also described by Kunkel et al. (1951). This and other features prompted testing for lupus erythematosus (LE) cells in the blood. The LE cell was a recently recognized diagnostic marker for SLE and, by that time, was becoming recognized as a result of degradation of nuclear material by a circulating antibody. A positive test in this patient with CAH led to the case report by Joske and King (1955). They commented that the liver biopsy showed the typical picture of an active chronic viral hepatitis, including cellular infiltration with lymphocytes and plasma cells and fibroblastic activity, and that 'fairly numerous' LE cells were demonstrable in the blood. Moreover it was noted that cortisone produced a dramatic improvement in her arthralgia. The authors recalled that a previous case had been reported by Leoni (1954) in which LE cells had been detected in the ascitic fluid from a patient with hepatic cirrhosis. The interest by F.M. Burnet in the paper of Joske and King (1955) is reflected by his thoughts in the discussion to that paper: 'we suggest that the LE cell and related phenomena might be based either: (1) on an abnormality of the antibody-producing mechanism... or (2) on changes in red or white cells or their constituents... which modify their characteristic "self markers"'.

The next clue to the cause of CAH was derived in Melbourne serendipitously in 1956 when D.C. Gajdusek, a sabbatical visitor in Burnet's laboratory, was developing a complement fixation (CF) reaction as a serological diagnosis for infectious hepatitis. The 'antigen' was a liver homogenate from a patient who had died from acute hepatitis, on the premise that this liver would contain hepatitis virus proteins. Since CAH was then thought to be related to a persisting viral infection in the liver, sera from the Melbourne case were tested by the CF procedure, as well as cases of acute viral hepatitis. The outcome was that whereas sera from cases of acute viral hepatitis were only weakly if at all reactive, sera from cases of CAH were strongly reactive (Gajdusek, 1958; Mackay and Gajdusek, 1958; Mackay and Larkin, 1958). Reactivity was clearly unrelated to antibodies to hepatitis virus for two reasons: (1) sera from cases of primary biliary cirrhosis and SLE were strongly reactive; and (2) reactivity in the CF test was independent of virus-infected liver, since normal liver and most other mammalian tissues were reactive, with liver and kidney more particularly so. The reaction was called the autoimmune complement fixation (AICF) test. The AICF reaction yielded a further finding of interest, this being that the serum of a patient with a lymphoproliferative disease and macroglobulinaemia reacted for tissue antibodies to an extremely high titre (Mackay, 1959). This observation proved critical to the formulation of Burnet's clonal selection theory of acquired immunity, and the concept of 'forbidden' clones as a theoretical explanation for autoimmune reactions.

The strongly positive reactions with the AICF test in CAH, and particularly in the initial case in which LE cells were demonstrable, pointed further to an autoimmune component to this disease, and stimulated a search for further cases showing a positive LE cell test. The ready identification of several such cases led to a reappraisal of the syndrome in which the multisystem features of the disease were emphasized and a relationship to SLE was proposed: the term 'lupoid hepatitis' was therefore introduced (Mackay et al., 1956). Thus, CAH and LE were linked 'possibly through the common factor of disturbed immunological response... this group of cases had been provisionally designated as "lupoid hepatitis" since "lupus" has now acquired a far broader significance than the original term suggests... we consider that immunological destruction of the host's liver cells best explains the perpetuation of the hepatitis and progression to cirrhosis. If this is so, it would be rational to use therapeutic measures (e.g., cortisone therapy) designed to modify this process, and our experience suggests that cortisone is of benefit in this autoimmune hepatitis' (Mackay et al., 1956).

At the same time, Bearn et al. (1956) at the Rockefeller Institute in New York, published a detailed report on their cases, documenting the features described in the 1951 abstract (Kunkel et al., 1951). Thus the cases were predominantly young women with a severe, progressive and often fatal chronic hepatitis, and emphasis was given to multisystem involvement and marked plasmacytosis in the liver. Additional points were that extreme hyperglobulinaemia was noted as 'an uncommon though well-recognized feature of some cases of cirrhosis unquestionably due to infectious hepatitis', whereas 'the generalized nature of the disease in certain persons, the involvement of joints, pericardium and lungs as well as liver raises the possibility that some other disorder possibly related to the collagen diseases, may play an important part in the disease process' and finally, 'striking improvement followed the use of cortisone in some cases'.

The early indications, from observations in Sweden, Melbourne and New York, and subsequent confirmation, that corticosteroids were of therapeutic benefit in this newly recognized type of chronic hepatitis are described in Section 6.

2.4. Past 1960

After 1960, CAH became generally accepted as a distinct clinical entity, and the lupoid type began to attract considerable attention and was described under a variety of different names (Mackay, 1975). However, there developed sharp controversies over the uncertain relationship between lupoid hepatitis and SLE on the one hand, and 'garden-type' CAH on the other (Mackay, 1991b). To exemplify this, the initial description from Melbourne of patients with lupoid hepatitis by Mackay et al. (1956) included several of the features later listed in the revised criteria for SLE (Tan et al., 1982), notably malar rash, non-erosive arthritis, serositis, renal disorder, haematologic disorder with cytopenias, and immunologic disorder. Case series of lupoid hepatitis published in subsequent years were to a varying degree in accord with this. Thus the 26 cases of Bearn et al. (1956) included a 'surprising number' with joint pains associated in some cases with actual arthritis, which together with serositis, pneumonia or erythema multiforme, raised the suspicion of collagen disease. Krook (1961) described 9 patients with liver cirrhosis in whom a diagnosis of a 'lupus erythematosus-like syndrome' could be made and, of these, 5 had Sjögren's syndrome. The two cases of Applebaum and Job (1961) had 'probable DLE with cirrhosis or severe hepatitis', and Robson (1959) reported on a single patient with chronic hepatitis who developed the classical syndrome of SLE with pericarditis, pleurisy and joint pains. On the other hand, Mackay et al. (1959) differentiated the hepatic expressions of lupoid hepatitis and SLE. Read et al. (1963) tabulated 81 cases of 'active juvenile cirrhosis' and, although observing rashes, arthralgia, 'lupus kidney', autoimmune thyroid disease and ulcerative colitis, concluded that 'this form of chronic liver disease cannot be equated with systemic lupus erythematosus'. Miescher et al. (1966) reported 4 cases of 'progressive hyperglobulinemic hepatitis' with coexisting extra-hepatic features, but also concluded that the syndrome appeared different from that associated with classical SLE.

It is of interest that two quite detailed case studies, 1964 and 1965, provided differing interpretations. That of Reynolds et al. (1964) was based on 15 patients, 13 with lupoid hepatitis and two considered to have SLE with a coexisting liver disease, viral hepatitis or alcoholic cirrhosis. In the former 13, the liver disease was dominant and the systemic features were unspectacular: arthralgia in 8 cases and fever in one case, and a weakly reactive Venereal Disease Research Laboratory (VDRL) test in 3 cases. The conclusion was that 'there was no convincing evidence of systemic lupus erythematosus'. On the other hand, MacLachlan et al. (1965) reported on 20 patients with CAH of whom most had a positive test for anti-nuclear antibody (ANA), and systemic features were very prominent: arthritis or arthralgia, 16 cases; pleurisy, 4 cases; pericarditis, 3 cases; nephritis of lupus type, 3 cases; rashes, 5 cases; ulcerative colitis, 3 cases; convulsions, 2 cases; and cytopenias, 11 cases. Moreover, among the families of 9 cases, there was a high incidence of stigmata of autoimmunity, including SLE in two members. The conclusion was that the disease expressions 'in some of these patients are remarkably similar to those encountered in systemic lupus erythematosus'.

The large experience of 'archetypal' CAH accumulated at the Mayo Clinic, Rochester, U.S.A., has been well reported on, from 1958 (Bartholomew et al., 1958) and subsequently, including 88 cases by Soloway et al. (1972a) and 126 cases by Czaja et al. (1983, 1986). The Mayo criteria were that patients should be seronegative for the hepatitis B surface antigen (HBsAg), have no other known aetiologies for CAH, and that corticosteroids be indicated for therapy. In the initial series, an associated autoimmune disease was recorded in 37 of 88 cases and in the latter series, in 21 of 126 cases. Notwithstanding these frequencies, and the presence of ANA in over 50% of the cases, the Mayo authors discounted any relationship of the disease to SLE. Czaja et al. (1983) questioned whether lupoid features defined a subset distinguishable from other cases of HBsAg-negative CAH, or were indicative of a particular pathogenetic process: 'the autoimmune markers associated with CAH may reflect dysglobulinemia associated with the severity of hepatocellular inflammation and necrosis or uncontrolled plasma cell proliferation triggered by unknown factors'.

This conspectus of reports in the early literature on CAH illustrates the blurred viewpoints on the 'lupus–hepatitis connection' (Mackay, 1991b). In fact, there may not have been any greater insights subsequent to those cited in an analysis from Melbourne (Mackay et al., 1965) some 25 years ago:

'(1) there is probably an initial episode of hepatocellular damage which in most instances would be due to virus infection: other damaging agents would be malnutrition, alcohol, hepatotoxins and drug allergy;
(2) in persons predisposed either genetically or for reasons as yet unkown, antigens derived from damaged liver cells provoke a continuing immune response

which is damaging; this causes self-perpetuating disease, with continuing necrosis, regeneration, nodular cirrhosis, and impairment of liver function;

(3) extension of the autoimmune response will result in systemic phenomena and various autoimmune serological reactions including L.E. cell production, thus defining the entity of lupoid hepatitis;

(4) occasional cases eventually resemble true systemic lupus erythematosus'.

As a concluding point on clinical aspects, the earlier (1950–1970) literature on CAH clearly indicates a degree of merging towards SLE, as judged by at least some cases fulfilling American Rheumatism Association (ARA) criteria for that disease. On the other hand, major case studies on patients presenting as classical SLE seldom reveal evidence of CAH, nor does this appear to evolve during periods of observation. This is not to say that the liver is spared in SLE, since there is hepatomegaly in 30–50% of cases due to fatty infiltration or congestion, and increased aminotransferase enzyme levels and functional abnormalities in 30–60% of cases (Dubois and Wallace, 1987). The most informative analysis, by Runyon et al. (1980), is that of the frequency of hepatitis features in 238 patients diagnosed as SLE and fulfilling 4 or more of the initial ARA criteria. This analysis included 124 patients with at least one abnormal liver function test result, and 43 (21%) who met the authors' criteria for 'liver disease'. Liver tissue from 33 patients showed 'cirrhosis' in 4, CAH in 4, and other histological changes in the remainder. Runyon et al. (1980) concluded that 'patients who satisfy the ARA criteria for SLE and have clinical and histologic evidence of chronic active hepatitis as well, should probably be considered as having both diseases'.

2.5. Heterogeneity of chronic active hepatitis

Writers on CAH throughout the 1950s and 1960s considered this as a single disease entity. Their descriptions mostly tallied with the features of what is now regarded as the autoimmune type. The recognition in the mid-1960s that the particle originally described as the 'Australia antigen' was related to infection with HBV led to new perceptions of CAH. The particle was identified as a derivative of the surface envelope of the virus, and hence called HBsAg, and became a marker of acute and chronic infection with HBV. It was soon recognized that a substantial proportion of cases of CAH were carriers of HBsAg and, in such cases, the core antigen of the virus (HBcAg) and HBsAg could be re-cognized in the liver immunohistochemically. These findings called for a re-examination of autoimmune aspects in CAH and it became evident from several centres that cases tended to segregate into those that were autoantibody-positive and HBsAg-negative or autoantibody-negative and HBsAb-positive (Mackay, 1975).

In 1972, a request to one of us (I.R.M.) to write on 'The Prognoses of Chronic Active Hepatitis' led to the initial specification that CAH was indeed a hetero-genous disease entity (Mackay, 1972). As well as the autoimmune and HBV-associated types of CAH, there were types associated with adverse reactions to drugs, ethanol, Wilson's disease, haemochromatosis, etc. Other subtypes included non-A, non-B virus infection and a 'cryptogenic' subtype in which no pathogenesis was evident; the recent recognition of the hepatitis C virus (HCV) has led to a merging of the non-A, non-B and 'cryptogenic' types, since most cases of what was termed cryptogenic CAH are explainable by chronic infection of the liver with HCV (Mackay, 1990). An analysis was made by Hodges et al. (1982) of the relative frequencies in the U.K. of the different aetiological types of CAH based on a defined population of 404,000, and a 5-year study period during which 61 cases were ascertained and diagnosed according to the criteria of an International Group (1977). The frequencies reported included alcohol-related 26%, autoimmune 23%, HBV 20%, non-A, non-B virus infection 15%, α_1-antitrypsin deficiency 13% and drug-related 3%. These frequencies could be regarded as regionally and temporally biased, since virus-related types of CAH would predominate at present in most parts of the world. Notwithstanding, the only published set of criteria for the diagnosis of CAH (Leevy et al., 1976) gives consideration only to the archetypal CAH of the 1960s.

Previously, the various types of CAH were specified by an alphabetical suffix, A (autoimmune), B (HBV associated) etc. (Mackay, 1987), but in view of the alphabetical classification of hepatitis viruses, autoimmune CAH is now abbreviated as AI-CAH, and viral types of CAH as CAH-B, CAH-C, etc.

This discussion on heterogeneity requires reference to heterogeneity within the AI-CAH group itself. First, there appears to be an immunogenetic heterogeneity, as discussed by Tait and Mackay (Chapter 15). There is also serological heterogeneity, according to the profile of autoantibody reactivity of serum. The classical type of AI-CAH is that marked by nuclear and/or smooth muscle (actin) antibody. An alternative autoantibody marker, to liver–kidney microsomes (LKM) was recognized by Rizzetto et al. (1973), but it was not until 1987 that a clinical syndrome was clearly attributed to the anti-LKM subtype (Homberg et al., 1987). It is now customary to refer to classical AI-CAH as type 1 and anti-LKM-positive as type 2. Further subgrouping according purely to serological criteria has been proposed, e.g., AI-CAH marked by reactivity only to a soluble cytoplasmic antigen (Manns, 1991) or to the asialoglycoprotein receptor (ASGP-R) (Johnson et al., 1991).

3. *The pathological aspects*

Liver biopsy was introduced in 1939 and was used during the 1940s to assess chronicity in acute viral hepatitis. This technique revealed that changes interpreted as Laennec's cirrhosis could occur after acute viral hepatitis, according to reports from Krarup and Roholm (1941) and Dible et al. (1943). However, the typical histological appearances of CAH were not clearly delineated until the disease itself was identified, during the 1950s.

In the paper of Bearn et al. (1956), their Fig. 5, of the macroscopic appearance of the liver, shows a macronodular cirrhosis and their Fig. 6, of the microscopic appearance, shows a chronic inflammatory process with evident fibrosis, plasma cell–lymphocytic infiltrates and disarray of hepatic parenchymal cells. This plasma cell increase was likewise noted in the case described by Zimmerman et al. (1951) and attracted much subsequent attention (Page and Good, 1960; Mackay et al., 1965), to the extent that the descriptive name of 'plasma cell hepatitis' was coined by Page and Good (1962). Bearn et al. (1956) in their cases noted correlation between the number of plasma cells in the liver and levels (markedly elevated) of serum γ-globulin.

'Bridging lesions' are characterized by confluence of zones of hepatic necrosis, inflammation and parenchymal collapse linking adjacent portal areas or portal areas and central veins. This type of lesion was first emphasized by Klatskin (1958) and later by Tisdale (1963). These authors drew upon older terms, 'subacute hepatic necrosis' and 'subacute hepatitis', to describe it. Bridging was considered by Boyer and Klatskin (1970) to be a critical transitional lesion between acute viral hepatitis and CAH with cirrhosis. However, bridging lesions appear to be a component of all forms of chronic hepatitis undergoing evolution to cirrhosis.

The most characteristic of the histological features of CAH is the inflammatory activity and liver cell necrosis that appears to erode the hepatic lobule or the cirrhotic nodule. The name given to this process of piecemeal necrosis by Popper et al. (1965) has become cemented into the histological nomenclature of hepatitis.

Piecemeal necrosis describes extensive erosive necrosis of hepatocytes which line the portal area and constitute the 'limiting plate' of the lobule, together with dense portal and periportal lymphocyte–plasma cell infiltrates. The intensity of periportal necrosis tends to correlate with transaminase levels in serum. Small groups of damaged and ballooned hepatocytes in periportal areas form pseudo-acinar structures, referred to as rosettes (Klatskin, 1958).

The numerous histological descriptions of CAH were rationalized by a consensus statement from an International Group of Pathologists (de Groote, 1968) who nominated definitions and a nomenclature which distinguished predictably progressive lesions as chronic active (aggressive) hepatitis, and predictably non-progressive lesions (as seen in some instances of chronic viral hepatitis) as chronic persistent hepatitis. The International Group (1977) later 'revisited' chronic hepatitis and allocated levels of importance for various histological criteria for the diagnosis of CAH: piecemeal necrosis and lymphocytic infiltration were seen as important pathogenetic and prognostic features.

Finally, reference can be made to the acidophilic 'Councilman' body seen by light microscopy as a shrunken eosinophilic structure representing the remains of a liver cell. Ultrastructural observations in 1971 by Kerr on these bodies in toxic liver injury led to the introduction of the term 'apoptosis' to describe a form of cell death associated with shrinkage of the cytoplasm and preservation of organelles, in contrast to the usual coagulative necrosis (Searle et al., 1987). First described in the context of liver injury, the term apoptosis has now come in wide usage to describe random or programmed fall-out of cells in various tissues. In the context of autoimmune hepatitis, apoptosis of hepatocytes could indicate cytotoxic effects of activated T-cells.

4. *The serological aspects*

Concurrent in time (1945–1946) with early descriptions of subacute or progressive hepatitis (then attributed to persisting viral hepatitis), observations were appearing on anti-liver antibodies, although these observations were made quite independently of the subsequent clinical descriptions (vide supra) of CAH with hypergammaglobulinaemia. Eaton et al. (1944) had detected by CF, in the serum of cases of acute viral hepatitis, the presence of broadly reactive 'heterogenetic' antibodies, against saline extracts of normal human liver, and also sheep erythrocytes. However, liver specificity of this reaction was shown by absorption with normal human liver. Eaton et al. (1944) made the following comment: 'An additional interesting speculation is the possibility that the liver antibody once produced combines with additional antigen in situ in the liver cells and causes further liver damage after the acute infectious process has subsided. This might be the explanation for some of the fatal cases in which the disease was greatly prolonged, with findings at autopsy resembling those of subacute yellow atrophy of the liver'. Gear (1946) observed that a liver emulsion prepared from a rhesus monkey that had died from a viral hepatitis (yellow fever) elicited antibodies to liver when injected into a normal rhesus monkey and he speculated that the presence of virus in liver cells could make such cells antigenic; similarly other infections exemplified by malaria might likewise serve to make normal tissues antigenic, so accounting for the haemolysis of blackwater fever.

The first serological indication of autoimmunity in liver disease was the LE cell response indicating the presence of ANA. This served as the laboratory marker for lupoid hepatitis until this cumbersome test was replaced by immunofluorescence for the detection of ANA in the early 1960s, particularly since it was found (Holborow et al., 1963) that ANAs were demonstrable in cases of CAH despite a negative LE cell test. Even today, immunofluorescence remains the routine laboratory procedure for detecting ANA. Whilst great advances have been made in standardization and calibration of the immunofluorescence procedure for ANA, the actual range of nuclear constituent(s) reactive with CAH sera has not been resolved at the molecular level. Anti-histone could account for much of the homogeneously-reactive ANA in CAH. Anti-dsDNA was detected in some 10% of cases by Smeenk et al. (1982), but was not demonstrable when more specific assays were used (Gurian et al., 1985). A notable substrate specificity for the ANA reaction in autoimmune CAH is the granulocyte nucleus (Smalley et al., 1968);

the restriction of the antigen to the nucleus of mature neutrophils gives it the property of a differentiation marker (Whittingham et al., 1981).

Autoantibodies to smooth muscle (SMA) were recognized by immunofluorescence in the mid-1960s (Johnson et al., 1965; Whittingham et al., 1966a) and a broader reactivity became evident when SMA-positive sera were found to react with glomerular mesangium (Whittingham et al., 1966b). Later, in 1972, the pattern of reactivity of SMA-positive sera with cells of foetal liver and lung in cultured monolayers indicated reactivity with the contractile protein actomyosin in cell membranes (Holborow, 1972). It was subsequently ascertained (Gabbiani et al., 1973; Lidman et al., 1976; Kurki et al., 1980) that SMA reactivity was directed against cytoskeletal filaments. The SMA reactivity in autoimmune hepatitis is accounted for by anti-actin (Toh, 1979; Pedersen et al., 1982; Kurki et al., 1983).

There has been a long and rather confusing history of serological reactivity with putative liver-specific antigens: the finale is still to come (Swanson et al., 1990). The research dates back to attempts to purify and characterize a liver-specific autoantigenic protein (Meyer zum Büschenfelde and Miescher, 1972), and a fractionated preparation from a liver homogenate (LP-1) appeared capable of inducing a facsimile of autoimmune hepatitis in rabbits. This preparation, later designated as liver-specific membrane lipoprotein (LSP), gave positive responses for lymphokine release in a migration inhibition assay (Meyer zum Büschenfelde et al., 1974) and hence seemed a good candidate for the organ-specific antigenic target to which an autoimmune response could be directed. Evidence was obtained in 1976 that cellular damage in autoimmune hepatitis could result from antibody-dependent K-cell activity, facilitated by the attachment of anti-LSP to the liver cell membrane (Cochrane et al., 1976). In 1978, a radioimmunoassay was described that demonstrated circulating antibody against LSP; however, raised levels of anti-LSP were present in both autoimmune and HBV-associated CAH and levels correlated with the degree of periportal necrosis rather than with a presumed pathogenesis of the disease (Jensen et al., 1978). Since LSP has a MW upwards of 4×10^6, it must be regarded more as a 'reactant' than an 'antigen'; moreover LSP itself is not to be regarded as either an organ- or species-specific preparation (Chisari, 1980; Mackay and Frazer, 1984; Meyer zum Büschenfelde and Manns, 1984).

At present, there is no absolute consensus as to whether LSP preparations do or do not contain an identifiable organ-specific and disease-specific antigen moiety, but the hepatic ASGP-R is a candidate. ASGP-R, a protein that is normally expressed on the hepatocyte surface, was recognized as an antigenic component of LSP by McFarlane et al. (1984). The development of an immunoassay for antibodies to ASGP-R (McFarlane et al., 1986) has promoted interest in this as a liver-specific autoantigen, and reactant in autoimmune hepatitis. The recent literature on ASGP-R is reviewed by Poralla et al. (1991) who make the point that patients with autoimmune hepatitis have antibodies to ASGP-R that react predominantly with human ASGP-R, whereas in other liver diseases, the antibodies react predominantly with rat/rabbit ASGP-R. Levels of anti-ASGP-R correlate with the degree of activity of disease and therefore reflect the occurrence of quiescence after immunosuppressive treatment. Although recombinant ASGP-R has been derived, assays using this preparation and investigation of immunodominant sites on ASGP-R, are not yet reported on. In view of previous uncertainties on the significance of immune responses to LSP, an even wider confirmation of the recent data including T-cell responses (Wen et al., 1990) would be desirable.

In contrast to CAH type 1, knowledge on the LKM reactant increased rapidly by application of immunoblotting and recombinant DNA technology. The antigenic molecule is a P-450 cytochrome enzyme, and usually P-450-2D6, although other P-450 cytochromes may serve as reactants (Manns, 1991). The sequence of the 2D6 molecule contains an immunodominant site within which possible crossreactive homologies with extrinsic molecules can be discerned (Gueguen et al., 1991).

5. *The immunogenetic aspects*

The immunogenetic basis for predisposition to autoimmune CAH is described in detail by Tait and Mackay (Chapter 15). The historical aspects are described briefly in this section. The major genetic influence in autoimmune hepatitis, female gender, became evident when the disease was first recognized in the 1950s. Interest in immunogenetic aspects developed after the recognition by Mackay and Morris (1972) of an association between autoimmune hepatitis and HLA-A1 (60% of cases) and HLA-B8 (68% of cases). These results were soon confirmed from other centres, with the highest level of association of HLA-B8 reported from West Germany, 82% of 108 cases versus 19% of 5046 controls, representing a relative risk of disease for HLA-B8 of 15 (Freudenberg et al., 1977). Subsequently D and DR locus associations were identified and also haplotype associations, initially HLA-A1-B8-DR3 and subsequently the 'ancestral' extended haplotype A1-B8-C4AQ0-C4B1-BfS-DR3. Evidence for immunogenetic heterogeneity according to the age of patients has come from Histocompatibility Workshop data (Mackay et al., 1991), and was reported by Donaldson et al. (1991) who found an increase HLA-DR4 in older patients with autoimmune hepatitis. Despite the LKM-positive type of autoimmune hepatitis being described in 1973, and clearly delineated by Homberg et al. in 1987, there do not appear to be any reports as yet on HLA associations with this subset of the disease.

As for other diseases associated with HLA-B8-DR3, no pathogenetic explanation for the association has emerged, but various possibilities are discussed (Mackay et al., 1991). These include polymorphisms in DRβ chains that could result in enhanced presentation of particular antigens, as postulated for the DRβ molecules of the DR4 specificity and predisposition to rheumatoid arthritis.

There are notable geographical differences in the prevalence of autoimmune hepatitis, with the highest rates among populations of Northern European origin and lower rates among Asian populations. The disease is recognized in Japan, with HLA-DR4 and -Bw54, rather than -DR3 as risk-associated alleles (Seki et al., 1990). Further investigations among Japanese cases (Seki et al., 1992), using DNA amplified by the polymerase chain reaction, followed by enzymatic digestion, have revealed disease-associated increases in frequencies in alleles specified as DRB1-0405, DQA1-0301 and DQB1-0401, with DRB1-0405 as the primary association. Disease-related polymorphisms of HLA-DR3 have not been ascertained, as yet, for autoimmune hepatitis in Caucasians. However, for thyrotoxicosis, another B8-DR3-associated disease in Caucasians, direct sequencing of the DR3 molecules of patients with this disease did not reveal differences from sequences of DR3 molecules in controls (Hu et al., 1992).

The HLA association with autoimmune hepatitis, albeit weak, creates an expectation that familial instances of the disease would be observed, but this is most infrequent (Mackay et al., 1991). Even with analysis of families on the basis of 'surrogate' phenotypes defined according to relevant autoantibodies in first-degree relatives, as described by Krawitt and Albertini (1991), there was no evident segregation to support a single autosomal dominant or recessive inheritance for the antibody-positive phenotypes. As for other autoimmune diseases, there are likely to be (as yet undisclosed) environmental determinants, and possibly multiple non-HLA 'background' genes operating through as yet poorly understood immunological pathways.

6. *The therapeutic aspects*

It was suspected by Waldenström (1950) that treatment of chronic hepatitis with corticosteroids (adrenocorticotrophic hormone (ACTH) was cited) could be successful. In the initial report on patients with CAH and a positive LE cell test, treatment with cortisone resulted in a symptomatic improvement (Mackay et al., 1956). In the New York cases (Bearn et al. 1956), a possible relationship of chronic hepatitis to the collagen diseases was noted, and cautious administration of cortisone to patients in the acute stages of the disease was considered of probable therapeutic value. Thus Bearn et al. (1956) stated that 'while on cortisone therapy the patients usually improved symptomatically, the size of the liver and spleen frequently diminished, the serum bilirubin fell and the serum proteins reverted towards normal', and that 'withdrawal of cortisone from two patients resulted in prompt clinical and biochemical relapse', but their proviso that 'there was no conclusive evidence that cortisone modified the disease process or that it will alter the eventual outcome'. The initial experience with corticosteroids in cases of CAH in Melbourne (Saint et al., 1953) was 'equivocal', but subsequently, in a limited study, was more favourable (Last, 1957).

The recognition in 1955 that serum transaminase could serve as a marker of recent tissue damage, whether of the heart or elsewhere, prompted our use of this serum assay to monitor the effectiveness of prednisolone in the treatment of lupoid hepatitis. The results were very striking in that there was a prompt fall in levels of serum transaminase within hours of dosage (O'Brien et al., 1958). Improvement in symptoms and biochemical features was found to occur with treatment with prednisolone and later, prednisolone and azathioprine in combination (Mackay et al., 1964). This led to a 3-year trial of suppressive treatment during which indices of liver function were obtained at 3-month intervals and compared with pretreatment values. There were significant differences at all time points after the zero time point, for both prednisolone alone, and prednisolone with azathioprine (Mackay, 1968). This study established that a steroid-induced decrease in levels of transaminases was accompanied by synchronous improvements in measures of actual liver function (bilirubin level, albumin level and bromsulphalein excretion), and a presumed decrease in the autoimmune response as judged by serum levels of γ-globulin.

However, placebo-controlled trials of treatment of autoimmune hepatitis, with prednisolone or prednisolone and azathioprine were called for, and a number have been reported (Copenhagen Study Group, 1969; Cook et al., 1971; Soloway et al. 1972b; Murray-Lyon et al., 1973). The decisive trial reported by Cook et al. (1971) included 49 patients: for 22 treated cases the survival was 90%; and for 27 non-treated cases the survival was 44%. Kirk et al. (1980) report on later results of this trial. Treatment policies that developed during the 1970s–1980s involve a long period (up to 3 years) of therapy with prednisolone, usually combined with azathioprine, and then gradual tapering of drugs. A proportion of patients relapse during withdrawal of prednisolone and these will require indefinite continuation of treatment. Current views on treatment policies and survival expectations are presented by Davis and Czaja (1986), Mackay (1987) and Czaja (1991).

7. Conclusions: history merging into the future

This historical analysis of autoimmune hepatitis has, here and there, become so contemporary as to resemble a review. This seems inevitable for a disease with such a recent and controversial history, and for which there remain so many unanswered questions. Thus, with history in this essay having already merged into the present, it could be allowed to merge into the future! If so, the historian of the year 2000 might be able to give answers to the following unknowns of 1992: the environmental agent(s) that initiates autoimmune hepatitis and how this (or these) may act; the identity of the putative liver-specific autoantigen and its disease-relevant epitopes; the way in which MHC molecules relate to susceptibility; the significance of the serological subtypes of CAH, specified as ANA/SMA-positive or anti-LKM-positive; the immunological effector process that damages hepatocytes; the nature of immunoregulatory defects that may operate to allow perpetuation of autoimmune hepatitis; the explanation for the difficulty in creating a reliable experimental model; and, finally, what is the reason for the decreasing incidence of the archetypic autoimmune hepatitis, as seen in young females in the 1950s–1960s? These and other questions on autoimmune hepatitis still await solution.

References

Applebaum, J.J., Job, H. and Kern, F. (1961) Hepatitis associated with disseminated lupus erythematosus. Gastroenterology 40, 766–771.

Barker, M.H., Capps, R.B. and Allen, F.W. (1945) Chronic hepatitis in the Mediterranean theater: a new clinical syndrome. J. Am. Med. Assoc. 129, 653–659.

Bartholomew, L.G., Hagedorn, A.B., Cain, J.C. and Baggenstoss, A.H. (1958) Hepatitis and cirrhosis in women with positive clot tests for lupus erythematosus. N. Engl. J. Med. 259, 947–956.

Bearn, A.G., Kunkel, H.G. and Slater, R.J. (1956) The problem of chronic liver disease in young women. Am. J. Med. 21, 3–15.

Boyer, J.L. and Klatskin, G. (1970) Pattern of necrosis in acute viral hepatitis: prognostic value of bridging (subacute hepatic necrosis). N. Engl. J. Med. 237, 1063–1071.

Capps, R.B. (1948) Clinical aspects of the sequelae of acute hepatitis. Gastroenterology 11, 680–684.

Chisari, F. (1980) Liver specific protein in perspective. Gastroenterology 78, 168–170.

Cochrane, A.M.G., Moussouros, A., Thomson, A.D., Eddleston, A.L.W.F. and Williams, R. (1976) Antibody-dependent cell-mediated (K cell) cytotoxicity against isolated hepatocytes in chronic active hepatitis. Lancet i, 441–444.

Cook, G.C., Mulligan, R. and Sherlock, S. (1971) Controlled prospective trial of corticosteroid therapy in active chronic hepatitis. Q.J. Med. 40, 159–185.

Copenhagen Study Group for liver diseases (1969) Effect of prednisolone on the survival of patients with cirrhosis of the liver. Lancet i, 119–121.

Czaja, A.J. (1986) Autoimmune chronic active hepatitis. In: A.J. Czaja, and E.R. Dickson (Eds.) Chronic Active Hepatitis. The Mayo Clinic Experience. Dekker, New York, pp. 105–126.

Czaja, A.J, (1991) Diagnosis, prognosis, and treatment of classical autoimmune chronic active hepatitis. In: E.L. Krawitt and R.H. Wiesner (Eds.) Autoimmune Liver Diseases. Raven, New York, pp. 143–166.

Czaja, A.J., Davis, G.L., Ludwig, J., Baggenstoss, A.H. and Taswell, H.F. (1983) Autoimmune features as determinants of prognosis in steroid-treated chronic active hepatitis of uncertain etiology. Gastroenterology 85, 713–717.

Davis, G.L. and Czaja, A.J. (1986) Immediate and long-term results of corticosteroid therapy for severe idiopathic chronic active hepatitis. In: A.J. Czaja and E.R. Dickson (Eds.) Chronic Active Hepatitis. The Mayo Clinic Experience. Dekker, New York, pp. 269–283.

De Groote, J., Desmet, V.J., Gedigk, P., Korb, G.H., Popper, H., Poulsen, H., Scheuer, P.J., Schmid, M., Thaler, H., Uehlinger, E. and Wepler, W. (1968) A classification of chronic hepatitis. Lancet ii, 626–628.

Dible, J.H., McMichael, J. and Sherlock, S.P.V. (1943) Pathology of acute hepatitis: aspiration biopsy studies of epidemic, arsenotherapy and serum jaundice. Lancet ii, 402–408.

Donaldson, P.T., Doherty, D.G., Hayllar, K.M., McFarlane, I.G., Johnson, P.J. and Williams, R. (1991) Susceptibility to autoimmune chronic active hepatitis: human leucocyte antigens DR4 and A1-B8-DR3 are independent risk factors. Hepatology 13, 701–706.

Dubois, E.L. and Wallace, D.J. (1987) Clinical and laboratory manifestations of systemic lupus erythematosus. In: D.J. Wallace and E.L. Dubois (Eds.) Dubois' Lupus Erythematosus, 3rd edn., Lea and Febiger, Philadelphia, PA, pp. 317–449.

Eaton, M.D., Murphy, W.D. and Hanford, V.L. (1944) Heterogenetic antibodies in acute hepatitis. J. Exp. Med. 79, 539–557.

Freudenberg, J., Baumann, H., Arnold, W., Berger, J. and Meyer-zum Büschenfelde, K.-H. (1977) HLA in different forms of chronic active hepatitis. A comparison between adult patients and children. Digestion 15, 260–270.

Gabbiani, G., Ryan, G.B., Lamelin, J.-P., Vassalli, P., Majno, G., Bouvier, C.A., Cruchaud, A. and Luscher, E.F. (1973) Human smooth muscle autoantibody – its identification as antiactin antibody and a study of its binding to 'nonmuscular' cells. Am. J. Pathol. 72, 473–488.

Gajdusek, D.C. (1958) An 'autoimmune' reaction against human tissue antigens in certain acute and chronic diseases: I. Serological investigations. Arch. Intern. Med. 101, 9–29.

Gear, J. (1946) Autoantigens and autoantibodies in the pathogenesis of disease with special reference to blackwater fever. Trans. R. Soc. Trop. Med. Hyg. 39, 301–314.

Gueguen, M., Boniface, O., Bernard, O., Clerc, F., Cartwright, T. and Alvarez, F. (1991) Identification of the main epitope on human cytochrome P450 IID6 recognized by anti-liver kidney microsomal antibody. J. Autoimmun. 4, 607–615.

Gurian, L.E., Rogoff, T.M., Ware, A.J., Jordan, R.E., Coombes, B. and Gilliam, J.N. (1985) The immunological diagnosis of chronic active autoimmune hepatitis: distinction from systemic lupus erythematosus. Hepatology 5, 397–402.

Himsworth, H.P. (1947) Lectures on the Liver and its Diseases. Blackwell, Oxford.

Hodges, J.R., Millward-Sadler, G.H. and Wright, R. (1982) Chronic active hepatitis: the spectrum of disease. Lancet i, 550–552.

Holborow, E.J. (1972) Immunological aspects of viral hepatitis. Br. Med. Bull. 28, 142–144.

Holborow, E.J., Asherson, G.L., Johnson, G.D., Barnes, R.D.S. and Carmichael, P.S. (1963) Antinuclear factor and other antibodies in blood and liver diseases. Br. Med. J. i, 656–658.

Homberg, J.C., Abuaf, N., Bernard, O. et al. (1987) Chronic active hepatitis with anti-liver/kidney microsome antibody Type 1: a second type of autoimmune hepatitis. Hepatology 7, 1333–1339.

Hu, R., Beck, C., Chang, Y.-B. and Degroot, L. (1992) HLA Class II genes in Graves' disease. Autoimmunity 12, 102–106.

International Group of Pathologists (1977) Acute and chronic hepatitis revisited. Lancet ii, 914–919.

Jensen, D.M., McFarlane, I.G., Portmann, B.S., Eddleston, A.L.W.F. and Williams, R. (1978) Detection of antibodies directed against liver-specific membrane lipoprotein in patients with acute and chronic active hepatitis. N. Engl. J. Med. 229, 1–7.

Johnson, G.D., Holborow, E.J. and Glynn, L.E. (1965) Antibody to smooth muscle in patients with liver disease. Lancet 2, 878–879.

Johnson, P.J., McFarlane, I. G. and Eddleston, A.L.W.F. (1991) The natural course and heterogeneity of autoimmune type chronic active hepatitis. Semin. Liver. Dis. 11, 187–196.

Joske, R.A. and King, W.E. (1955) The L.E. cell phenomenon in active chronic viral hepatitis. Lancet ii, 477–480.

Kerr, J.F.R. (1971) Shrinkage necrosis: a distinct mode of cellular death. J. Pathol. 105, 13–20.

Kirk, A.P., Jain, S., Pocock, S., Thomas, H.C. and Sherlock S. (1980) Late results of the Royal Free Hospital prospective controlled trial in hepatitis B surface antigen negative chronic active hepatitis. Gut 21, 78–83.

Klatskin, G. (1958) Subacute hepatic necrosis and postnecrotic cirrhosis due to anicteric infections with the hepatitis virus. Am. J. Med. 25, 333–358.

Krarup, N.B. and Roholm, K. (1941) The development of cirrhosis of the liver after acute hepatitis, elucidated by aspiration biopsy. Acta Med. Scand. 108, 306–331.

Krawitt, E.L. and Albertini, R.J. (1991) Immunogenetic studies of autoimmune liver diseases. In: E.L. Krawitt and R.H. Wiesner (Eds.) Autoimmune Liver Diseases. Raven, New York, pp. 63–73.

Krook, H. (1961) Liver cirrhosis in patients with a lupus erythematosus-like syndrome. Acta Med. Scand. 169, 713–726.

Kunkel, H.G. and Labby, D.H. (1950) Chronic liver disease following infectious hepatitis. II. Cirrhosis of the liver. Ann. Intern. Med. 32, 433–450.

Kunkel, H.G., Labby, D.H. and Hoagland, C.L. (1974) Chronic liver disease following infectious hepatitis. I. Abnormal convalescence from initial attack. Ann. Intern. Med. 27, 202–219.

Kunkel, H.G., Ahrens, J.R., Eisenmenger, W.J., Bongiovanni, A.M. and Slater, R.J. (1951) Extreme hypergammaglobulinemia in young women with liver disease of unknown etiology (abstract). J. Clin. Invest. 30, 654.

Kurki, P.L., Miettinen, A., Linder, E., Pikkarainen, P., Vuoristo, M. and Salaspuro, M.P. (1980) Different types of smooth muscle antibodies in chronic active hepatitis and primary biliary cirrhosis. Their diagnostic and prognostic significance. Gut 21, 878–884.

Kurki, P., Miettinen A., Salaspuro, M., Virtanen, I. and Stenman, S. (1983) Cytoskeleton antibodies in chronic active hepatitis, primary biliary cirrhosis, and alcoholic liver disease. Hepatology 3, 297–302.

Last, P.M. (1957) The treatment of active chronic infectious hepatitis with ACTH (corticotrophin) and cortisone. Med. J. Aust. i, 672–676.

Leevy, C.M., Popper, H. and Sherlock, S. (1976) Diseases of the liver and biliary tract. Standardization of nomenclature, diagnostic criteria and diagnostic methodology. Fogarty International Centre Proceedings No. 22, DHEW Publication No. (NIH) 76–725. U.S. Government Printing Office, Washington D. C.

Leoni, A. (1954) A proposito della specificità del fenomeno L.E. Minerva Med. 1, 1022–1027.

Lidman, K., Biberfeld, G., Fagraeus, A., Norberg, R., Torstenssen, R., Utter, G., Carlsson, L., Luca, J. and Lindberg, U. (1976) Anti-actin specificity of human smooth muscle antibodies in chronic active hepatitis. Clin. Exp. Immunol. 24, 266–272.

Liebowitz, S. (1950) Virus hepatitis. Implications of its chronic stages. J. Insur. Med. 5, 1–8.

Mackay, I.R. (1959) Macroglobulins and macroglobulinaemia. Aust. Ann. Med. 8, 158–170.

Mackay, I.R. (1968) Chronic hepatitis: effect of prolonged suppressive treatment and comparison of azathioprine with prednisolone. Q. J. Med. 37, 378–382.

Mackay, I.R. (1972) The prognoses of chronic hepatitis. Ann. Intern. Med. 77, 649–651.

Mackay, I.R. (1975) Chronic active hepatitis. In: L. Vander Reis (Ed.) Frontiers of Gastroenterological Research, Vol. 1. Karger, Basel, pp. 142–187.

Mackay, I.R. (1987) Treatment of chronic active hepatitis and other liver diseases with corticosteroid agents. Med. J. Aust. 146, 370–374.

Mackay, I.R. (1990) The new hepatitis virus: hepatitis C virus. Med. J. Aust. 153, 247–249.

Mackay, I.R. (1991a) Pathogenesis of autoimmune chronic hepatitis. In: E. L. Krawitt and R. Weisner (Eds.) Autoimmune Liver Diseases. Raven, New York, pp. 21–42.

Mackay, I.R. (1991b) The hepatitis–lupus connection. Semin. Liver Dis. 11, 234–240.

Mackay, I.R. and Frazer, I.H. (1984) Autoantibodies, autoimmunity and chronic hepatitis. In: F.V. Chisari (Ed.) Advances in Hepatitis Research. Masson, New York, pp. 179–189.

Mackay, I.R. and Gajdusek, D.C. (1958) An 'autoimmune' reaction against human tissue antigens in certain acute and chronic diseases: II. Clinical correlations. Arch. Intern. Med. 101, 30–46.

Mackay, I.R. and Larkin, L. (1958) The significance of the presence in human serum of complement-fixing antibodies to human tissue antigens. Aust. Ann. Med. 7, 251.

Mackay, I.R. and Morris, P.J. (1972) Association of autoimmune chronic hepatitis with HL-A1, 8. Lancet ii, 793–795.

Mackay, I.R., Taft, L.I. and Cowling, D.C. (1956) Lupoid hepatitis. Lancet 2, 1323–1326.

Mackay, I.R., Taft, L.I. and Cowling, D.C. (1959) Lupoid hepatitis and the hepatic lesions of systemic lupus erythematosus. Lancet i, 65–69.

Mackay, I.R., Weiden, S. and Ungar, B. (1964) The treatment of active chronic hepatitis and lupoid hepatitis with 6-mercaptopurine and azathioprine. Lancet i, 889–902.

Mackay, I.R., Weiden, S. and Hasker, J. (1965) Autoimmune hepatitis. Ann. N.Y. Acad. Sci. 124, 767–780.

Mackay, I.R., O'Brien, R.M. Whittingham, S. and Tait, B.D. (1991) Autoimmune hepatitis and other diseases of the liver: immunogenetic aspects. In: N. Farid (Ed.) The Immunogenetics of Autoimmune Disease, Vol. 2, CRC, Boca Raton, pp. 199–213.

MacLachlan, M.J., Rodnan, G.P. and Cooper, W.M. et al. (1965) Chronic active ('lupoid') hepatitis: a clinical, serological and pathological study of 20 patients. Ann. Intern. Med. 62, 425–462.

Manns, M. (1991) Cytoplasmic autoantigens in autoimmune hepatitis: molecular analysis and clinical relevance. Semin. Liver Dis. 11, 205–214.

Manns, M.P., Johnson, E.F., Griffen, K.J., Tan, E.M. and Sullivan, K.F. (1989) Major antigen of liver kidney microsomal autoantibodies in idiopathic autoimmune hepatitis is cytochrome P450db. J. Clin. Invest. 83, 1066–1072.

McFarlane, I.G., McFarlane, B.M., Major, G.N., Tolley, P. and Williams, R. (1984) Identification of the hepatic asialoglycoprotein receptor (hepatic lectin) as a component of liver specific membrane lipoprotein (LSP). Clin. Exp. Immunol. 55, 347–354.

McFarlane, B.M., McSorley, C.G., Vergani, D., McFarlane, I.G. and Williams, R. (1986) Serum autoantibodies reacting with the hepatic asialoglycoprotein receptor protein (hepatic lectin) in acute and chronic liver disorders. J. Hepatol. 3, 196–205.

Meyer zum Büschenfelde, K.-H. and Manns, M. (1984) Immune response to liver membrane antigens in acute and chronic hepatitis. In: F.V. Chisari (Ed.) Advances in Hepatitis Research. Masson, New York, pp. 152–162.

Meyer zum Büschenfelde, K.-H. and Miescher, P.A. (1972) Liver-specific antigens, purification and characterization. Clin. Exp. Immunol. 10, 89–102.

Meyer zum Büschenfelde, K.-H., Knolle, J. and Berger, J. (1974) Celluläre Immunreaktionen gegenüber homologen leberspecifischen Antigenen (HLP) bei chronischen Leberentzündungen. Klin. Wschr. 52, 246–248.

Miescher, P.A., Braverman, A. and Amorosi, E. (1966) Progressive hypergammaglobulinaemic hepatitis. Dtsch. Med. Wschr. 91, 1525–1532.

Murray-Lyon, I.M., Stern, R.B. and Williams, R. (1973) Controlled trial of prednisolone and azathioprine in active chronic hepatitis. Lancet i, 735–737.

O'Brien, E.N., Goble, A.J. and Mackay, I.R. (1958) Plasma transaminase activity as an index of the effectiveness of cortisone in chronic hepatitis. Lancet i, 1245–1249.

Page, A.R. and Good, R.A. (1960) Plasma-cell hepatitis, with special attention to steroid therapy. Am. J. Dis. Child. 99, 288–314.

Page, A.R. and Good, R.A. (1962) Plasma cell hepatitis. Lab. Invest. 11, 351–359.

Pedersen, J.S., Toh, B.H., Mackay, I.R., Tait, B.D., Gust, I.D., Kastelan, A. and Hadzic, N. (1982) Segregation of autoantibody to cytoskeletal filaments, actin and intermediate filaments, with two types of chronic active hepatitis. Clin. Exp. Immunol. 48, 527–532.

Popper, H., Paronetto, F. and Schaffner, F. (1965) Immune processes in the pathogenesis of liver disease. Ann. N.Y. Acad. Sci. 124, 781–799.

Poralla, T., Treichel, U., Löhr, H. and Fleischer, B. (1991) The asialoglycoprotein receptor as target structure in autoimmune liver diseases. Semin. Liver Dis. 11, 215–222.

Read, A.E., Sherlock, S. and Harrison, C.V. (1963) Active 'juvenile' cirrhosis as part of a systemic disease and the effect of corticosteroid therapy. Gut. 4, 378–393.

Reynolds, T.B., Edmondson, H.A., Peters, R.L. and Redeker, A. (1964) Lupoid hepatitis. Ann. Intern. Med. 61, 650–666.

Rizzeto, M., Swana, G. and Doniach, D. (1973) Microsomal antibodies in active chronic hepatitis and other disorders. Clin. Exp. Immunol. 15, 331–344.

Robson, M.D. (1959) Systemic lupus erythematosus complicating chronic liver disease. Guy's Hosp. Rep. 108, 438–443.

Runyon, B.A., LaBreque, D.R. and Anuras, S. (1980) The spectrum of liver disease in systemic lupus erythematosus. Am. J. Med. 69, 187–194.

Saint, E.G., King, W.E., Joske, R.A. and Finckh, E.S. (1953) The course of infectious hepatitis with special reference to prognosis and the chronic stage. Aust. Ann. Med. 2, 113–127.

Searle, J., Harmon, B.V., Bishop, C.J. and Kerr, J.F.R. (1987) Significance of cell death by apoptosis in hepatobiliary disease. J. Gastroenterol. Hepatol. 2, 77–96.

Seki, T., Kiyosawa, K. and Ota, M. (1990) Association of autoimmune hepatitis with HLA-Bw54 and DR4 in Japanese patients. Hepatology 12, 1300–1304.

Seki, T., Ota, M., Furuta, S., Fukushima, H., Kondo, T., Hino, K., Mizuki, N., Ando, A., Tsuji, K., Inoko, H. and Kiyosawa, K. (1992) HLA class II molecules and autoimmune hepatitis susceptibility in Japanese patients. Gastroenterology 103, 1041–1047.

Smalley, M.J., Mackay, I.R. and Whittingham, S. (1968) Antinuclear factors and human leucocytes: reaction with granulocytes and lymphocytes. Aust. Ann. Med. 17, 28–32.

Smeenk, R., Van der Lelij, G. and Swaak, T. (1982) Specificity in systemic lupus erythematosus of antibodies to double-stranded DNA measured with the polyethylene glycol precipitation assay. Arthritis Rheum. 25, 631–638.

Soloway, R.D., Summerskill, D.M., Baggenstoss, A.H. and Shoenfield, L.J. (1972a) 'Lupoid' hepatitis, a non-entity in the spectrum of chronic active liver disease. Gastroenterology 63, 458-465.

Soloway, R.D., Summerskill, W.H.J., Baggenstoss, A.H., Geall, M.G., Gitnick, G.L., Elveback. L.R. and Schonfeld, L.J. (1972b) Clinical, biochemical and histological remission of severe chronic active liver disease: a controlled study of treatments and early prognosis. Gastroenterology 63, 820–833.

Swanson, N.R., Reed, W.D., Yarred, L.J., Shilkin, K.B. and Joske, R.A. (1990) Autoantibodies to isolated plasma membranes in chronic active hepatitis II. Specificity of antibodies. Hepatology 11, 613–621.

Tan, E.M., Cohen, A.S., Fries, J.F., Masi, A.T., McShane, D.J., Rothfield, N.F., Schaller, J.G., Talal, N. and Winchester, R.J. (1982) The 1982 revised criteria for the classification of systemic lupus erythematosus. Arthritis Rheum. 25, 1271–1277.

Tisdale, W.A. (1963) Subacute hepatitis. N. Engl. J. Med. 268, 138–142.

Toh, B.H. (1979) Smooth muscle autoantibodies and autoantigens. Clin. Exp. Immunol. 38, 621–628.

Waldenström, J. (1950) Leber, Blutproteine und Nahrungseiweiss. Dtsch Ges. Verdau. Stoffwechselkr. 15, 113–119.

Waxman, D.J., Lapenson, D.P., Krishnan, M., Bernard, O., Kreibich, G. and Alvarez, F. (1988) Antibodies to liver/kidney microsomes in chronic active hepatitis recognize specific forms of hepatic cytochrome P-450. Gastroenterology 95, 1326–1331.

Weiden, S. (1953) The zinc sulphate turbidity test in the differential diagnosis of jaundice. Med. J. Aust. i, 364–366.

Wen, L., Peakman, M., Lobo-Yeo, A., McFarlane, B.M., Mowat, A.P., Mieli-Vergani, G. and Vergani, D. (1990) T-cell-directed hepatocyte damage in autoimmune chronic active hepatitis. Lancet 336, 1527–1530.

Whittingham, S., Mackay, I.R. and Irwin, J. (1966a) Autoimmune hepatitis: immunofluorescence reactions with cytoplasm of smooth muscle and renal glomerular cells. Lancet i, 1333–1336.

Whittingham, S., Irwin, J., Mackay, I.R. and Smalley, M. (1966b) Smooth muscle autoantibody in 'autoimmune' hepatitis. Gastroenterology 51, 499–505.

Whittingham, S., Morstyn, G., Wilson, J.W. and Vadas, M.A. (1981) An autoantibody reactive with nuclei of polymorphonuclear neutrophils: a cell differentiation marker, Blood 58, 786–771.

Wood, I.J., King, W.E., Parsons, P.J., Perry, J.W., Freeman, M. and Limbrick, L. (1948) Non-suppurative hepatitis: a study of acute and chronic forms with special reference to biochemical and histological changes. Med. J. Aust. 11, 249–261.

Zimmerman, H.J., Heller, P. and Hill, R.P. (1951) Extreme hyperglobulinemia in subacute hepatic necrosis. N. Engl. J. Med. 244, 245–249.

Section II

Clinical Aspects of Autoimmune Hepatitis

Autoimmune Hepatitis
Edited by M. Nishioka, G. Toda and M. Zeniya
© 1994, Elsevier Science B.V. All rights reserved

Chapter 2

Clinical aspects of autoimmune hepatitis in North America

Albert J. Czaja

Hepatobiliary Unit, Division of Gastroenterology,
Mayo Clinic and Mayo Medical School, Rochester, MN 55905 (U.S.A.)

1. Prevalence

Autoimmune hepatitis is the predominate form of chronic active hepatitis (CAH) in those geographic regions where the human leukocyte antigen (HLA)-B8 and -DR3 phenotypes are common and the carriage frequency of chronic viral infection is low (Mackay, 1984; 1985). HLA-B8 and -DR3 are found most frequently in the populations of Northern Europe and the prevalence decreases with latitude towards the equator (Ryder et al., 1978). The frequency of autoimmune hepatitis seems to coincide with these regional changes in HLA prevalence (Mackay, 1984) and it is no surprise that the disease frequency is mirrored in the populations of North America that are largely derived from this ethnic base.

The prevalence of chronic viral infection also influences the frequency of autoimmune hepatitis (Mackay, 1985). In contrast to Hong Kong where only 1% of patients with CAH have autoimmune disease and 86% have CAH-B (Lam et al., 1980), the frequency of autoimmune hepatitis among patients with CAH is 34% in Germany (vs 36% with CAH-B) (Meyer zum Buschenfelde and Hutteroth, 1979) and 62% in Australia (vs 10% with CAH-B) (Mackay, 1985). The rough inverse relationship between chronic viral infection and autoimmune hepatitis reflects the low prevalence of HLA-B8 and -DR3 phenotypes in the Far East and the ballooning of the base population with cases of chronic viral disease.

Undoubtedly, the availability of confident diagnostic tests for hepatitis C virus infection will change the demographics of autoimmune hepatitis throughout the world, probably at the expense of the autoimmune and cryptogenic categories. Nevertheless, it is unlikely that more sophisticated virologic assays will eliminate the designation of autoimmune hepatitis. Indeed, it is probable that they will simply underscore the non-specificity of the immunoserologic markers that are currently used in the diagnosis of the disease.

The incidence of autoimmune hepatitis in North America is uncertain, but it is undoubtedly similar to that in Western Europe where there are 0.69 cases per 100,000 persons per year (Hodges et al., 1982). The frequency of autoimmune hepatitis is probably decreasing in western countries as a result of improved diagnostic methods and stricter criteria for the diagnosis. Unfortunately, autoimmune hepatitis remains a diagnosis of exclusion as it lacks a disease-specific pathognomonic marker or feature (Czaja, 1984; 1990). Consequently, newer virologic assays now divert patients with autoimmune features into viral categories and novel immunoserologic markers such as antibodies to F-actin (anti-actin) and liver/kidney microsome type 1 (anti-LKM-1) enhance diagnostic specificity (Homberg et al., 1987; Maddrey, 1987; Czaja et al., 1991a) possibly at the expense of diagnostic sensitivity.

The frequency of autoimmune hepatitis among patients with chronic liver disease in North America is estimated to be between 11 and 23%. Alcoholic liver disease remains the most common chronic liver disorder (50%) while patients with chronic viral (12%), autoimmune (11–23%), and cholestatic (10%) liver diseases are recognized with less frequency. Cirrhosis remains the fifth cause of death in individuals above 40 years of age in the U.S.A. and in Minnesota alone, the per annum rate of case discovery is 16 per 100,000 new female and 50 per 100,000 new male cases of cirrhosis each year (Rakela and Czaja, 1986). If only 10% of the female cases each year were ascribed to autoimmune hepatitis, the frequency of this diagnosis in Minnesota (1.6 cases of cirrhosis per 100,000 persons per year) would match or exceed that reported in the U.K. (Hodges et al., 1982). Importantly, of patients who underwent liver transplantation at the Mayo Clinic between March 1985 and June 1987, 29% had CAH compared to 26% with primary sclerosing cholangitis and 24% with primary biliary cirrhosis (Krom et al., 1989). Of the patients with CAH undergoing liver transplantation, the vast majority had autoimmune or cryptogenic hepatitis, thereby again emphasizing the importance of the diagnosis in patients with chronic liver disease and the aggressive potential of the condition.

Prevalence data mainly reflect disease of sufficient severity to justify medical evaluation or of sufficient aggressiveness to result in death and postmortem examination. Recent studies have indicated that asymptomatic patients with chronic aminotransferase elevations of a mild to moderate degree frequently have immunoserologic and histologic features of autoimmune hepatitis, and yet these patients may never be included in analyses of prevalence. Of 47 such patients in whom liver biopsy examination was justified only by investigational protocol, 34 had histologic features of CAH (72%), including 16 who had features of cirrhosis (Hay et al., 1989). Anti-nuclear and -smooth muscle antibodies were detected in 18 of those with CAH (53%) and the diagnostic criteria for autoimmune hepatitis were fulfilled in each. The actual size of this component of autoimmune hepatitis is unknown, but it is almost certainly not represented in any estimates of disease prevalence.

2. Types

The major type of autoimmune hepatitis in North America is type 1 ('lupoid' or 'anti-actin') autoimmune hepatitis. Conventional immunoserologic markers, including the lupus erythematosus (LE) cell phenomenon, antibodies to smooth muscle antigens (SMA), and antibodies to nuclear antigens (ANA), characterize 80% of patients with CAH that is not ascribable to virus infection or drug toxicity and these patients are now classified as having type 1 disease (Czaja, 1984; 1986). Antibodies to F-actin can be determined by immunofluorescence using actin cables and SMA reactivity can be refined by eliminating non-CAH specific reactions to tubulin and intermediate filaments (Toh, 1979). The anti-actin assay, however, is not generally available and the diagnosis of type 1 autoimmune hepatitis in North America depends mainly on the presence of conventional markers such as SMA and/or ANA in compatible clinical situations.

Seropositivity for SMA is present in 70% of patients with type 1 autoimmune hepatitis (Czaja et al., 1983; Czaja, 1984; 1986). ANAs are detected in 52% and the LE cell phenomenon can be demonstrated in 29%. The LE cell test is no longer a standard diagnostic procedure in most laboratories, but in fact only 11% of patients with type 1 autoimmune hepatitis were classifiable as such by this test only (Czaja, 1986).

Importantly, 20% of patients with type 1 autoimmune hepatitis are also seropositive for anti-mitochondrial antibodies (AMA) (Kenny et al., 1986). Typically, the AMA titer is low with only 12% of patients having AMA titers that exceed 1:160. Those who are seropositive for AMA have higher serum levels of alkaline phosphatase and an increased frequency of stainable copper in liver tissue samples (19 vs 0%) than AMA-negative counterparts. They are not distinguishable, however, by other histologic features or response to cortico-steroids (Kenny et al., 1986). The AMA reactivity was initially ascribed to antibodies that were not specific for primary biliary cirrhosis (i.e., the M4 subtype) (Berg et al., 1980) but recent studies in patients with other forms of autoimmune hepatitis indicate that the AMA specificity may not differ from that seen in classic primary biliary cirrhosis (Manns, 1991). Additionally, 27% of these patients are now recognized as actually harboring antibodies to LKM-1 (anti-LKM-1) rather than AMA (Czaja et al., 1991a).

Antibodies to double-stranded DNA may be present in more than 40% of patients with type 1 autoimmune hepatitis (Davis and Read 1975), but their presence in patients with cryptogenic CAH and CAH-B underscores the non-specificity of the finding (Wood et al., 1986). Unfortunately, immunoglobulin G antibody to double-stranded DNA has not been a satisfactory means of differentiating systemic lupus erythematosus (SLE) from type 1 autoimmune hepatitis in North America since the antibody, as determined by enzyme-linked immunosorbent assay, has been found in 64% of patients with type 1 autoimmune hepatitis, 46% with cryptogenic CAH, and 43% of patients with CAH-B, albeit the majority in low titer (Wood et al., 1986).

Type 2 (anti-LKM-1-positive) autoimmune hepatitis is characterized by the presence of anti-LKM-1 in serum and the absence of SMA and ANA (Homberg et al., 1987). It was hoped that the 20% of patients with non-viral and non-drug-related CAH who did not satisfy criteria for type 1 autoimmune hepatitis would be classifiable as type 2 disease. Unfortunately, this has not been the case and in North America, autoimmune hepatitis associated with anti-LKM-1 may be less common than that reported in Europe. Indeed, in the Mayo Clinic experience, none of 30 patients with cryptogenic CAH were seropositive for anti-LKM-1 and anti-LKM-1 seropositivity was demonstrated in only 3 of 131 patients (2%) with type 1, cryptogenic, hepatitis B virus-related, and hepatitis C virus-related CAH (Czaja et al., 1991a). The 3 patients seropositive for anti-LKM-1 had been previously classified as having AMA seropositivity and their true nature was recognized only after re-testing.

The population of patients in North America who are most likely to have type 2 autoimmune hepatitis has not been defined, but preliminary surveys suggest that adult patients with cryptogenic CAH are unlikely to be seropositive for anti-LKM-1 and it is unrealistic to presume that patients with type 2 autoim-mune hepatitis are hidden among the small group of patients with CAH and AMA seropositivity (Czaja et al., 1991a). In North America, type 2 autoimmune hepatitis may be rare or concentrated in the pediatric population that is not seen at referral centers for adults.

A third type of autoimmune hepatitis ('type 3') has been proposed. This classification is based on the presence of antibodies to soluble liver antigen (anti-SLA) in serum (Manns et al., 1987). 'Type 3' autoimmune hepatitis is not as yet established as a distinct clinical entity and its prevalence in North America is uncertain. Patients in this category lack ANA and anti-LKM-1, but they may have SMA and AMA. Consequently, it is unclear if they should be classified as a distinct group based on the presence of anti-SLA or considered a variant of type 1 disease. Surveys are in progress to assess the frequency and significance of anti-SLA-positive autoimmune hepatitis in North America and it is possible that some of the 20% of adult patients with cryptogenic CAH who continue to escape classification as viral or autoimmune disease may at last find a niche after anti-SLA testing.

3. Clinical features

The clinical expression of autoimmune hepatitis may range from the asymptomatic to the severely debilitated and moribund. Only the patients with the most severe form of the disease have been studied in a systematic fashion (Cook et al., 1971; Soloway et al., 1972; Murray-Lyon et al., 1973) and yet these patients undoubtedly comprise only a minority of patients with the diagnosis. Studies from a large referral center in Los Angeles have indicated that none of the 86 patients seen between 1973 and 1978 satisfied the Mayo criteria for severe disease (Koretz et al., 1980). Indeed, the rapidly progressive, immediately life-threatening form of autoimmune hepatitis which constitutes the core population of all controlled clinical trials represents no more than 20% of the patients with the disease.

Autoimmune hepatitis is typically insidious, but an acute clinical presentation may be evident in 40% of cases (Czaja, 1981; Czaja et al., 1983). In such instances, the disease may resemble acute 'viral' hepatitis (Davis et al., 1982; Crapper et al., 1986; Amontree et al., 1989) and liver biopsy examination is warranted to confirm the diagnosis. Prompt institution of corticosteroid therapy is indicated in such patients since delay until documentation that the disease is unresolving after 6 months may result in unnecessary morbidity and mortality. In the Mayo experience, 30% of patients with severe autoimmune hepatitis have disease of less than 6 months' duration at the time of presentation and treatment (Davis et al., 1982). Indeed, 10 weeks of unresolving severe inflammation has been our criterion for disease that is unlikely to be self-limited. In the symptomatic, incapacitated, or decompensated patient, early aggressive treatment can result in rapid clinical and biochemical improvement that offsets any advantage to the disconcerting wait for an uncertain spontaneous resolution (Davis et al., 1982).

The majority of patients with type 1 autoimmune hepatitis are women (70%) and 50% are in their third decade or less at the time of onset (mean age, 40 years) (Czaja et al., 1983; Czaja, 1984; 1986). In the Mayo experience, ages range from 13 to 81 years and the average duration of illness prior to diagnosis is 15 months. Easy fatigability is the most common symptom at presentation (85%) and 79% of patients with severe disease will describe some manifestation of jaundice (i.e., dark urine, light stools, scleral icterus). Mild right upper quadrant abdominal pain (42%), arthralgias (36%), mild itching (41%), and fever (21%) are other frequently described symptoms. Fever of 'obscure origin' was part of the early clinical description of autoimmune hepatitis (Bearn et al., 1956) and it may still be encountered as high as 40 °C. Fortunately, the young, amenorrheic, hirsute girls with acne that typified original cases of the syndrome are now rare occurrences (Bongiovanni and Eisenmenger, 1951).

Features that dissuade the diagnosis of autoimmune hepatitis include weight loss, hyperpigmentation, xanthelasmas, and severe pruritus (Czaja, 1984; 1986). Severe cholestatic features are unusual in autoimmune hepatitis and when present they usually connote an incorrect or incomplete diagnosis (Cooksley et al., 1972). Primary sclerosing cholangitis ('small duct' and 'large duct' varieties) must be considered in such patients, especially in the presence of chronic ulcerative colitis, and endoscopic retrograde cholangiography may be necessary to clarify the diagnosis (Perdigoto et al., 1992). Primary biliary cirrhosis may also be difficult to differentiate from autoimmune hepatitis, since both conditions may have histologic similarities and antimitochondrial antibodies and a treatment trial with corticosteroids may be required to establish the diagnosis (Kenny et al., 1986). Patients with hepatitis C or non-A, non-B, non-C infections may have a destructive cholangitis and they may also be confused with 'cholestatic' autoimmune hepatitis. As a general rule, the diagnosis of autoimmune hepatitis in the cholestatic patient should be regarded with skepticism.

Slit lamp examination of the eyes may rarely disclose Kayser–Fleischer rings in patients with autoimmune hepatitis (Czaja, 1984). Typically, these occur in the rare patient with cholestatic features and they are never visible grossly. Their presence requires the exclusion of Wilson's disease as well as the cholestatic diseases mentioned above.

The most common physical findings in patients with severe type 1 autoimmune hepatitis at the time of presentation are spider angiomas (57%), splenomegaly (42%), ascites (17%) and hepatic encephalopathy (12%) (Czaja et al., 1980). Splenomegaly, ascites, and hepatic encephalopathy occur more commonly in patients with cirrhosis, but each may occur in its absence. Additionally, failure to identify these features does not exclude histologic cirrhosis, since the physical findings have a low sensitivity for the diagnosis.

The most specific physical finding for cirrhosis in severe type 1 autoimmune hepatitis is hepatic encephalopathy (92%), but it occurs in only 28% of patients with cirrhosis (Czaja et al., 1980). Similarly, ascites has an 82% specificity for cirrhosis, but only a 36% sensitivity. Splenomegaly and spider angiomas have only 52 and 45% specificities for cirrhosis, respectively, and their presence should not be a basis for the diagnosis of cirrhosis (Czaja et al., 1980).

The prevalence of esophageal varices in severe type 1 autoimmune hepatitis is 15% (Czaja et al., 1979). The majority of these patients (53%) have varices prior to therapy, while the others (47%) develop them after 12–102 months of corticosteroid therapy and follow-up (mean interval to varices, 38 ± 9 months). The probability of developing varices within 1 year of treatment is 2% and it increases to 8% after 5 years (Czaja et al., 1979). Of the patients with cirrhosis, 11% will develop varices during 4.8 ± 0.3 years of treatment and follow-up. Importantly, bleeding from varices is unusual in patients undergoing therapy. Indeed, it occurs in only 5% during 4.2 ± 0.6 years of observation (Czaja et al., 1979). Death from liver failure is greater in those patients with varices at presentation than in those without varices (30 vs 6%), but mortality is not increased (as yet) in those patients who develop varices during treatment. Experiences from the randomized, controlled, clinical trials have indicated that hemorrhage and mortality are more common in untreated patients with autoimmune hepatitis (Murray-Lyon et al., 1973) and it may be that corticosteroid treatment diminishes the propensity for variceal formation and hemorrhage.

Extra-hepatic immunologic disorders commonly accompany the liver disease and they may involve a wide variety of organ systems (Table 1). In the Mayo experience, 46% of patients with type 1 autoimmune hepatitis have one or more of these manifestations. Thyroid disease is the most common associated disorder (23%), including Hashimoto's thyroiditis (16%) and Graves' disease (7%). Indeed, 20% of patients with type 1 disease have thyroglobulin antibodies in serum and 37% have microsomal thyroid antibodies. Of patients with one or both thyroid antibodies, 51% will have or develop thyroid disease. Consequently, thyroid function and antibody status should be assessed regularly and individuals with thyroid antibodies should be monitored for the emergence of a thyroid disorder.

Thirteen percent of patients have chronic ulcerative colitis. The association between chronic ulcerative colitis and autoimmune hepatitis is still valid in the era of endoscopic retrograde cholangiography and hepatitis C virus testing. All such patients, however, must have cholangiography to establish their diagnosis (Perdigoto et al., 1992). Forty-two percent of patients with the diagnosis of type 1 autoimmune hepatitis and chronic ulcerative colitis have cholangiographic features of primary sclerosing cholangitis and certainly this entity can closely resemble or coexist with type 1 disease (Ludwig et al., 1984; Perdigoto et al., 1992). Since type 1 autoimmune hepatitis and primary sclerosing cholangitis have similar HLA phenotypes, the diseases may share pathogenic mechanisms, have similar clinical expressions, or cluster in the same patient (Perdigoto et al., 1992). Importantly, those patients with normal cholangiograms respond to

Table 1
Immunologic disorders associated with autoimmune hepatitis in North America

Chronic ulcerative colitis	Leukocytoclastic vasculitis
Collagen vascular diseases	Myasthenia gravis
Coomb's positive hemolytic anemia	Panniculitis
Cryoglobulinemia	Pericarditis
Eosinophilia	Peripheral neuropathy
Erythema nodosum	Pernicious anemia
Fibrosing alveolitis	Pleuritis
Gingivitis	Primary sclerosing cholangitis
Glomerulonephritis	Pyoderma gangrenosum
Graves' disease	Rheumatoid arthritis
Hashimoto's thyroiditis	Secretory diarrhea
Idiopathic thrombocytopenia	Sjogren's syndrome
Intestinal villous atrophy	Synovitis
Iritis	Urticaria

corticosteroid therapy as satisfactorily as counterparts without ulcerative colitis, while those with abnormal cholangiograms do not.

Other extra-hepatic immunologic disorders occur less frequently and they have little impact on the outcome of treatment. Rheumatoid arthritis or synovitis (4%), pernicious anemia, nephritis, asthma, erythema nodosum, iritis, systemic sclerosis, idiopathic thrombocytopenic purpura, myositis, and Coomb's positive hemolytic anemia (1% each) occur sporadically (Table 1). Eight percent of patients have two or more extra-hepatic immunologic disorders and of those with at least one immunologic disease, 18% will have or develop another.

4. *Laboratory features*

Serum aminotransferase and γ-globulin elevations are the principal laboratory manifestations of type 1 autoimmune hepatitis and the degree of sustained abnormality defines the severity of inflammatory activity and the prognosis of the disease (Czaja et al., 1981a; Czaja, 1984; 1991). Typically, the serum aspartate aminotransferase level is less than 500 IU/l (Rakela and Czaja, 1986), but in 16% of patients it may exceed 1000 IU/l (Davis et al., 1982). Such extreme aminotransferase elevations may resemble individuals with acute viral, toxic, drug-related, or ischemic liver injuries and the diagnosis of autoimmune hepatitis may depend on the clinical suspicion, history of antecedent liver disease, or the presence of ancillary findings of chronicity such as ascites, varices, thrombocytopenia, or hypoalbuminemia (Davis et al., 1982). Importantly, these patients may not satisfy the temporal criterion for chronicity and yet delay of therapy for 6 months may be associated with early mortality. Forty-six percent of these patients have cirrhosis at presentation or they develop it later and 80% die of liver failure if untreated. In contrast, prompt institution of corticosteroid therapy reduces the immediate mortality to 14% (Davis et al., 1982). In North America, an aggressive therapeutic approach toward the ill or decompensated patient with severe non-viral liver disease and immunologic manifestations is justified and the arbitrary, usually subjective, and commonly inaccurate temporal requirement of 6 months to establish chronic disease is frequently waived.

Hypergammaglobulinemia is present in 90% of patients (Czaja et al., 1983). It is an important hallmark of the disease and a useful barometer of inflammatory activity, but its absence does not preclude the diagnosis. Typically, the γ-globulin elevation reflects a polyclonal increase in serum immunoglobulin concentrations, especially immunoglobulin G, and the finding is not indicative of a disease-specific, pathogenic antibody response (Czaja, 1984; 1990). Diverse paraproteins with antibody reactivity against bacteria (*Escherichia coli*, bacteroides, and salmonella) and viruses (measles, rubella, and cytomegalovirus) may reflect the inability of the damaged liver to sequester exogenous antigens and prevent antibody production or they may represent a non-specific increase in immunologic responsiveness to foreign antigens (Triger, 1976). The same polyclonal immunoglobulin response has been shown to confound the enzyme immunoassay for antibodies to hepatitis C virus and result in false-positive reactions, possibly by cross-reacting with hepatitis C virus-encoded antigens (McFarlane et al., 1990). Importantly, the hypergammaglobulinemia probably reflects the extent and duration of the inflammatory process rather than the immunologic nature of the disease (Czaja et al., 1981a). By selecting patients on the basis of strong seropositivity for immunoserologic markers or severe inflammatory activity, the feature of hypergammaglobulinemia is accentuated and the misperception of its diagnostic specificity perpetuated. Rarely, extremely high immunoglobulin levels may provoke coagulation abnormalities, renal insufficiency, and mental disturbances consistent with the hyperviscosity syndrome (Czaja, 1984).

Hyperbilirubinemia is present in 83% of patients with severe type 1 autoimmune hepatitis, but the bilirubin level exceeds 3 mg/dl in only 46% (Rakela and Czaja, 1986). The majority of patients, therefore, are not clinically jaundiced at the time of presentation, although up to 79% of them will describe some clinical feature of hyperbilirubinemia.

The serum alkaline phosphatase level is increased in 81% of patients at the time of presentation, but it is greater than 2-fold normal in only 33% and greater than 4-fold normal in only 10% (Kenny et al., 1986; Rakela and Czaja, 1986). A predominate alkaline phosphatase elevation is unusual and it may reflect primary sclerosing cholangitis, primary biliary cirrhosis, or an infiltrative disorder. Cholangiography is justified in such patients to secure the diagnosis. Patients with type 1 autoimmune hepatitis and marked elevation of the alkaline phosphatase level may be recalcitrant to corticosteroid therapy (Kenny et al., 1986).

Urinary copper excretion may exceed normal in nearly 50% of patients with severe inflammatory activity, but the abnormality is rarely at a level to suggest Wilson's disease (i.e., greater than 100 μg/day) (LaRusso et al., 1976). The hepatic copper concentration in liver biopsy tissue may also be increased, but it rarely exceeds 100 μg/g dry tissue weight (LaRusso et al., 1976). Serum ceruloplasmin levels are typically normal or increased at presentation as are serum α_1-antitrypsin levels. The levels return to normal as inflammatory activity subsides. In those patients who have severe impairment of hepatic synthetic function, the ceruloplasmin level can be abnormal. Although the hypoceruloplasminemia is usually not in the range of homozygous Wilson's disease, slit lamp examination and liver biopsy assessment for copper content are still essential in these individuals. Determination of the α_1-antitrypsin phenotype avoids the possibility that abnormally low levels are masked by elevations associated with inflammatory activity.

5. HLA phenotypes

Autoimmune hepatitis in North America has been associated with the HLA-A1-B8-D3 phenotype (Page et al., 1975; Mackay, 1984; 1985). HLA-B8 has been found in from 34 to 82% of patients, depending on the stringency of the diagnostic criteria for autoimmune hepatitis (Czaja et al., 1990). DR 3 is in strong linkage disequilibrium with B8 and the antigens are concurrent in 94% of instances. In the Mayo experience, HLA-B8 is present in 52% of patients, DR 3 is present in 48% and A1-B8-DR 3 is present in 40% (Czaja et al., 1992a). Patients with HLA-B8 are younger at presentation (38 ± 2 vs 48 ± 2 years, $P - 0.01$) and they have features of more active disease than HLA-B8-negative counterparts (Czaja et al., 1990). Indeed, they have higher serum levels of aspartate aminotransferase (658 ± 60 vs 465 ± 48 IU/l, $P < 0.02$) and bilirubin (7 ± 1 vs 2.8 ± 0.4 mg/dl, $P = 0.003$) at accession and they more commonly have histologic features of bridging necrosis, multilobular necrosis, and cirrhosis (85 vs 56%, $P - 0.01$) (Czaja et al., 1990). The presence of HLA-B8 has been associated with greater antibody responses to viral and non-viral antigens than other phenotypes and the B8-DR3 complex has been associated with a reduction in non-antigen-specific suppressor T-cell activity which may influence susceptibility to autoimmune hepatitis (Czaja et al., 1990). The greater degree of disease severity in patients with HLA-B8 may reflect immunoreactivity to an autoantigen or extrinsic antigen that exceeds that of patients without HLA-B8 and the younger age of these patients may reflect an earlier susceptibility to the disease because of a genetically acquired predisposition for autoimmunity (Czaja et al., 1990).

The HLA phenotype is associated with prognosis. HLA-B8-negative patients with HLA-A1 relapse less frequently after drug withdrawal than HLA-B8-positive patients and HLA-B8-negative counterparts without HLA-A1 (Czaja et al., 1990). HLA-B8 may be associated with a defect in adequately terminating an immune response and this association may explain the high relapse frequency in these patients. Additionally, HLA-A1 may modulate the immune response by promoting immune tolerance and counterbalancing the effects of HLA-B8 or other determinants on the proliferative response of antigen-reactive cells. Such an interaction would be similar to that proposed between HLA-B7, which may be linked to immunodeficiency, and HLA-B12, which may be linked to immune hyperactivity (Czaja et al., 1990).

Patients who undergo orthotopic liver transplantation for decompensated autoimmune hepatitis more commonly have the A1-B8-DR3 phenotype than those who do not (Donaldson et al., 1991; Sanchez-Urdazpal et al., 1992). This finding also implies that the A1-B8-DR3 phenotype is associated with more aggressive, corticosteroid-recalcitrant disease. The identification of such patients early in their disease might warrant closer surveillance and greater reluctance to completely withdraw corticosteroids after satisfaction of conventional remission criteria.

HLA-DR4 has been shown to be a secondary, but independent risk factor for autoimmune hepatitis in white Northern European patients (Donaldson et al., 1991), but the significance of this phenotype in the patients of North America is as yet undefined.

6. Virologic markers

By definition, autoimmune hepatitis is unassociated with an active virus infection. Serologic vestiges of previous viral infections, however, may be present and 4% of patients with type 1 autoimmune hepatitis are seropositive for antibodies to the hepatitis B core antigen (Czaja et al., 1983). Analyses of liver tissue specimens for hepatitis B virus DNA have indicated that as many as 25% of patients who are seronegative for all hepatitis B virus markers may harbor the genome of the hepatitis B virus (Brechot et al., 1985) and yet the implication of this finding in the pathogenesis of type 1 autoimmune hepatitis remains uncertain. The hepatitis B virus may be one of several different triggering agents that may initiate the immunopathogenic mechanisms responsible for the disease, and certainly patients have been described in whom this evolutionary sequence has been proposed (Laskus and Slusarczyk, 1989).

Antibodies to hepatitis C virus occur less commonly in the type 1 autoimmune hepatitis of North America (Czaja et al., 1991b; Katkov et al., 1991) than that described in Spain (Esteban et al., 1989) and the majority of the seropositive reactions in the North American patients are probably false positives (Czaja et al., 1991b; Czaja et al., 1992b). In the Mayo experience, only 6% of patients with severe type 1 disease are seropositive for antibodies to hepatitis C virus by enzyme immunoassay and of these, only 40% are reactive by recombinant immunoblot assay (Czaja et al., 1991b). Similar experiences have been reported in Boston (Katkov et al., 1991). Additionally, anti-LKM-1 seropositivity is uncommon in patients with chronic hepatitis B and C, indicating that in North America hepatitis B and C viruses are not important stimuli for the production of autoantibodies (Czaja et al., 1991a). Non-organ-specific autoantibodies, such as SMA and ANA, can occur in chronic B and C virus infections, but typically they are of low titer (Czaja et al., 1992c). These observations emphasize the diagnostic non-specificity of conventional immunoserologic markers for autoimmune disease, rather than implicate a virus as an immunogenic agent.

7. Histologic features

The histologic hallmark of autoimmune hepatitis and the sine qua non of the diagnosis is periportal hepatitis, or so-called piecemeal necrosis. Extension of the inflammatory activity between portal tracts or between portal tracts and terminal hepatic venules (bridging necrosis) or involvement of adjacent lobules with inflammatory activity resulting in architectural collapse (confluent necrosis or multilobular necrosis) are patterns of necro-inflammation that indicate more severe disease and a greater propensity for progression to cirrhosis (Schalm et al., 1977). Importantly, the pattern of histologic abnormality cannot be predicted by the clinical or laboratory findings, and all patterns occur with similar frequency in patients with disease of comparable biochemical severity. In the Mayo experience, periportal hepatitis is present in 29% of patients at presentation; bridging necrosis is present in 19%; multilobular necrosis is present in 21%; and cirrhosis is already established in 31%. These patients are indistinguishable from each other without histologic assessment (Schalm et al., 1977).

Transitions between the different histologic patterns of necro-inflammation can occur spontaneously or during corticosteroid therapy and exacerbations of the disease can be associated with the appearance of any of the histologic changes (Schalm et al., 1977). Hepatic architecture can revert entirely to normal during therapy (Czaja et al., 1984) or the histologic features can improve to those of portal hepatitis ('chronic persistent hepatitis') which at Mayo is designated 'chronic active hepatitis in remission' (Czaja et al., 1981b). 'Viral features', such as lobular disarray, Kupffer cell hyperplasia, acidophilic cell necrosis, and ballooning hepatocyte degeneration, may be present in different patients or in the same patient at different times during the course of the disease (Czaja, 1986; Dienes et al., 1989). These features have not had an etiologic connotation (Dienes et al., 1989) nor have such patients been different in age, sex, duration of illness, biochemical findings (including serum immunoglobulin G levels), immunoserologic or virologic markers, or response to corticosteroid therapy than those without these histologic features (Czaja, 1986). Tissue markers for hepatitis C virus will be necessary to fully assess the implications of these lobular changes in such patients.

Ultimately, the significance of the morphologic features of autoimmune hepatitis depend on the consistency and reproducibility of the pathologic interpretation. The application of rigid definitions for each morphologic pattern is essential in this regard. At Mayo, the reproducibility of the histologic diagnosis of cirrhosis was only 50% when the same observer was shown the same slides repeatedly in the absence of a pre-established rigidly applied definition for cirrhosis. When the definition of cirrhosis required identification of fibrosis with at least one complete regenerative nodule, the reproducibility of the interpretation improved to 78% and the presence or absence of cirrhosis was consistently diagnosed in 88% of instances (Czaja et al., 1984). The sensitivity of the histologic examination for cirrhosis probably decreased, but this compromise was necessary to maintain interpretative consistency.

The histologic diagnosis of autoimmune hepatitis in most instances depends on the assessment of a core of tissue that has been obtained by random sampling. Fortunately, the type and degree of hepatocellular inflammation can be satisfactorily determined in this fashion. The consistency of a single observer in grading the inflammatory activity is 90% (Soloway et al., 1971). The reproducibility of the morphologic interpretation by the same observer is 94% and sampling error is trivial. The ability to distinguish subtle morphologic differences has not been well tested, but studies do indicate that intra-observer variation in the grading of piecemeal necrosis may be greater than 40% (Theodossi et al., 1980). Fortunately, the range of variation in the grading of individual features is small (Theodossi et al., 1980) and it is probably insufficient to alter the morphologic diagnosis. In contrast, sampling variability is large in the assessment of cirrhosis (Soloway et al., 1971), and needle biopsy of the liver provides only a minimal estimate of its occurrence. Indeed, simultaneously obtained liver specimens from different regions of the liver in the same patient disclose a sampling error that exceeds 60% (Soloway et al., 1971).

8. *Summary*

Autoimmune hepatitis in North America is a common disease that should be considered in the differential diagnosis of all patients with chronic hepatocellular inflammation, including those with an acute presentation, asymptomatic condition, or severe decompensation. Every effort should be taken to classify patients into homogeneous subgroups according to immunoserologic manifestations as only in this fashion can differences in prognosis and pathogenesis be understood. Type 1 autoimmune hepatitis is the predominate form of the disease in North America and the prevalence, target population, and significance of anti-LKM-1-positive (type 2) disease remain uncertain in this region of the world.

Type 1 autoimmune hepatitis can afflict men as well as women and all age groups are susceptible. Stereotypic subpopulations, such as obese, amenorrheic, hirsute girls with cirrhosis, are rare and in North America, type 1 autoimmune hepatitis has no 'classic' phenotype. Cholestatic disease is unusual and other conditions, such as primary sclerosing cholangitis and primary biliary cirrhosis, must be excluded in such patients.

Extra-hepatic immunologic diseases, especially thyroid disorders, are common and they may evolve at any stage of the disease. Patients who harbor thyroid antibodies should be monitored for the emergence of Graves' disease or Hashimoto's thyroiditis. Chronic ulcerative colitis can be associated with type 1 autoimmune hepatitis without evoking the diagnoses of primary sclerosing cholangitis or chronic hepatitis C virus infection, but cholangiography is required in all such patients to establish the diagnosis.

The HLA-B8 and -DR3 define a subpopulation of patients who are younger, have more severe disease at presentation, relapse more frequently after drug withdrawal, and require liver transplantation more commonly than those with other HLA phenotypes. The A1-B8-DR3 phenotype may define patients with an increased immunoreactivity to autoantigens and their liver disease may be less manageable on corticosteroid therapy. The HLA-DR4 phenotype may be a secondary independent risk factor.

Antibodies to hepatitis C virus may be present in patients with type 1 autoimmune hepatitis, but these antibodies are usually non-specific against hepatitis

C virus-encoded antigens. True positive hepatitis C virus reactions by enzyme immunoassay in type 1 autoimmune hepatitis are unusual and there is no evidence that hepatitis C virus is an important cause of the disease in North America. Chronic active hepatitis type C may be associated with non-organ-specific autoantibodies but these are usually in low titer. Additionally, in North America, patients with chronic active hepatitis B and C lack anti-LKM-1 seropositivity, suggesting that these viruses are not important stimuli for the production of autoantibodies. In North America, the diagnosis of type 1 autoimmune hepatitis connotes the absence of hepatitis C virus infection.

Acknowledgement

Linda Grande is acknowledged for her secretarial assistance in the preparation of the manuscript.

References

Amontree, J.S., Stuart, T.D. and Bredfeldt, J.E. (1989) Autoimmune chronic active hepatitis masquerading as acute hepatitis. J. Clin. Gastroenterol. 11, 303–307.

Bearn, A.G., Kunkel, H.G. and Slater, R.J. (1956) The problem of chronic liver disease in young women. Am. J. Med. 21, 3–15.

Berg, P.A., Wiedmann, K.H., Sayers, T., Kloppel, G. and Lindner, H. (1980) Serological classification of chronic cholestatic liver disease by the use of two different types of antimitochondrial antibodies. Lancet 2, 1329–1332.

Bongiovanni, A.M. and Eisenmenger, W.J. (1951) Adrenal cortical metabolism in chronic liver disease. J. Clin. Endocrinol. 11, 152–172.

Brechot, C., Degos, F., Lugassy, C., Thiers, V., Zafrani, S., Franco, D., Bismuth, H., Trepo, C., Benhamou, J.-P., Wands, J., Isselbacher, K., Tiollais, P. and Berthelot, P. (1985) Hepatitis B virus DNA in patients with chronic liver disease and negative tests for hepatitis B surface antigen. N. Engl. J. Med. 312, 270–276.

Cook, G.C., Mulligan, R. and Sherlock, S. (1971) Controlled prospective trial of corticosteroid therapy in active chronic hepatitis. Q. J. Med. 40, 159–185.

Cooksley, W.G., Powell, L.W., Kerr, J.F. and Bhathal, P.S. (1972) Cholestasis in active chronic hepatitis. Am. J. Dig. Dis. 17, 495–504.

Crapper, R.M., Bhathal, P.S., Mackay, I.R. and Frazer, I.H. (1986) 'Acute' autoimmune hepatitis. Digestion 34, 216–225.

Czaja, A.J. (1981) Current problems in the diagnosis and management of chronic active hepatitis. Mayo Clin. Proc. 56, 311–323.

Czaja, A.J. (1984) Natural history, clinical features, and treatment of autoimmune hepatitis. Semin. Liver Dis. 4, 1–12.

Czaja, A.J. (1986) Autoimmune chronic active hepatitis. In: A.J. Czaja and E.R. Dickson (Eds.), Chronic Active Hepatitis. The Mayo Clinic Experience, Marcel Dekker, New York, pp. 105–126.

Czaja, A.J. (1990) Autoimmune chronic active hepatitis – a specific entity? The negative argument. J. Gastroenterol. Hepatol. 5, 343–351.

Czaja, A.J. (1991) Diagnosis, prognosis, and treatment of classical autoimmune chronic active hepatitis. In: E.L. Krawitt and R.H. Wiesner (Eds.), Autoimmune Liver Disease, Raven, New York, pp. 143–166.

Czaja, A.J., Wolf, A.M. and Summerskill, W.H.J. (1979) Development and early prognosis of esophageal varices in severe chronic active liver disease (CALD) treated with prednisone. Gastroenterology 77, 629–633.

Czaja, A.J., Wolf, A.M. and Baggenstoss, A.H. (1980) Clinical assessment of cirrhosis in severe chronic active liver disease. Specificity and sensitivity of physical and laboratory findings. Mayo Clin. Proc. 55, 360–364.

Czaja, A.J., Wolf, A.M. and Baggenstoss, A.H. (1981a) Laboratory assessment of severe chronic active liver disease (CALD): correlation of serum transaminase and gamma globulin levels with histologic features. Gastroenterology 80, 687–692.

Czaja, A.J., Ludwig, J., Baggenstoss, A.H. and Wolf, A.M. (1981b) Corticosteroid-treated chronic active hepatitis in remission: uncertain prognosis of chronic persistent hepatitis. N. Engl. J. Med. 304, 5–9.

Czaja, A.J., Davis, G.L., Ludwig, J., Baggenstoss, A.H. and Taswell, H.F. (1983) Autoimmune features as determinants of prognosis in steroid-treated chronic active hepatitis of uncertain etiology. Gastroenterology 85, 713–717.

Czaja, A.J., Davis, G.L., Ludwig, J. and Taswell, H.F. (1984) Complete resolution of inflammatory activity following corticosteroid treatment of HBsAg-negative chronic active hepatitis. Hepatology 4, 622–627.

Czaja, A.J., Rakela, J., Hay, J.E. and Moore, S.B. (1990) Clinical and prognostic implications of human leukocyte antigen B8 in corticosteroid-treated severe autoimmune chronic active hepatitis. Gastroenterology 98, 1587–1593.

Czaja, A.J., Manns, M.P. and Homburger, H.A. (1991a) Specificity of antibodies to liver/kidney microsome type 1 for type 2 autoimmune chronic active hepatitis: evidence against overlapping syndromes and hepatitis B and C viruses as important immunogenic stimuli. Hepatology 14, 134A.

Czaja, A.J., Taswell, H.F., Rakela, J. and Schimek, C. (1991b) Frequency and significance of antibody to hepatitis C virus in severe corticosteroid-treated autoimmune chronic active hepatitis. Mayo Clin. Proc. 66, 572–582.

Czaja, A.J., Santrach, P.J., Moore, S.B. and Homburger, H.A. (1992a) Evidence against chronic viral infection as a cause of type 1 autoimmune hepatitis. Hepatology 16, 571.

Czaja, A.J., Taswell, H.F., Rakela, J. and Rabe, D. (1992b) Duration and specificity of antibodies to hepatitis C virus in corticosteroid-treated HBsAg-negative chronic active hepatitis. Gastroenterology 102, 1675–1679.

Czaja, A.J., Taswell, H.F., Rakela, J. and Schimek, C. (1992c) Frequency of antibody to hepatitis C virus in asymptomatic HBsAg-negative chronic active hepatitis. J. Hepatol. 14, 88–93.

Davis, G.L., Czaja, A.J., Baggenstoss, A.H. and Taswell, H.F. (1982) Prognostic and therapeutic implications of extreme aminotransferase elevation in chronic active hepatitis. Mayo Clin. Proc. 57, 303–309.

Davis, P. and Read, A.E. (1975) Antibodies to double-stranded (native) DNA in active chronic hepatitis. Gut 16, 413–415.

Dienes, H.P., Popper, H., Manns, M., Baumann, W., Thoenes, W. and Meyer zum Büschenfelde, K.-H. (1989) Histologic features in autoimmune hepatitis. Z. Gastroenterol. 27, 325–330.

Donaldson, P.T., Doherty, D.G., Hayllar, K.M., MacFarlane, I.G., Johnson, P.J. and Williams, R. (1991) Susceptibility to autoimmune chronic active hepatitis: human leukocyte antigens DR4 and A1-B8-DR3 are independent risk factors. Hepatology 13, 701–706.

Esteban, J.I., Esteban, R., Viladomiu, L., Lopez-Talavera, J.C., Gonzalez, A., Hernandez, J.M., Roget, M., Vargas, V., Genesca, J., Buti, M. and Guardia, J. (1989) Hepatitis C virus among risk groups in Spain. Lancet 2, 294–297.

Hay, J.E., Czaja, A.J., Rakela, J. and Ludwig, J. (1989) The nature of unexplained chronic amino-transferase elevations of a mild to moderate degree in asymptomatic patients. Hepatology 9, 193–197.

Hodges, J.R., Millward-Sadler, G.H. and Wright, R. (1982) Chronic active hepatitis: the spectrum of disease. Lancet 1, 550–552.

Homberg, J.-C., Abuaf, N., Bernard, O., Islam, S., Alvarez, F., Khalil, S.H., Poupon, R., Darnis, F., Levy, V.-G., Grippon, P., Opolon, P., Bernuau, J., Benhamou, J.-P. and Alagille, D. (1987) Chronic active hepatitis associated with antiliver/kidney microsome antibody type 1: a second type of 'autoimmune' hepatitis. Hepatology 7, 1333–1339.

Katkov, W.N., Dienstag, J.L., Cody, H., Evans, A.A., Choo, Q.-L. and Houghton, M. (1991) Role of hepatitis C virus in non-B chronic liver disease. Arch. Int. Med. 151, 1548–1552.

Kenny, R.P., Czaja, A.J., Ludwig, J. and Dickson, E.R. (1986) Frequency and significance of antimitochondrial antibodies in severe chronic active hepatitis. Dig. Dis. Sci. 31, 705–711.

Koretz, R.L., Lewin, K.J., Higgins, J., Fagen, N.D. and Gitnick, G.L. (1980) Chronic active hepatitis: who meets treatment criteria? Dig. Dis. Sci. 25, 695–699.

Krom, R.A.F., Wiesner, R.H., Rettke, S.R., Ludwig, J., Southorn, P.A., Hermans, P.E. and Taswell, H.F. (1989) The first 100 liver transplantations at the Mayo Clinic. Mayo Clin. Proc. 64, 84–94.

Lam, K.C., Lai, C.L., Wu, P.C. and Todd, D. (1980) Etiological spectrum of liver cirrhosis in the Chinese. J. Chron. Dis. 33, 375–381.

LaRusso, N.F., Summerskill, W.H.J. and McCall, J.T. (1976) Abnormalities of chemical tests for copper metabolism in chronic active liver disease: differentiation from Wilson's disease. Gastroenterology 70, 653–655.

Laskus, T. and Slusarczyk, J. (1989) Autoimmune chronic active hepatitis developing after acute type B hepatitis. Dig. Dis. Sci. 34, 1294–1297.

Ludwig, J., Czaja, A.J., Dickson, E.R., LaRusso, N.F. and Wiesner, R.H. (1984) Manifestations of nonsuppurative cholangitis in chronic hepatobiliary diseases: morphologic spectrum, clinical correlations and terminology. Liver 4, 105–116.

Mackay, I.R. (1984) Genetic aspects of immunologically mediated liver disease. Semin. Liver Dis. 4, 13–25.

Mackay, I.R. (1985) Autoimmune diseases of the liver: chronic active hepatitis and primary biliary cirrhosis. In: N.R. Rose and I.R. Mackay (Eds.), The Autoimmune Diseases, Academic, Orlando, pp. 291–337.

Maddrey, W.C. (1987) Subdivisions of idiopathic autoimmune chronic active hepatitis. Hepatology 7, 1372–1375.

Manns, M.P. (1991) Cytoplasmic autoantigens in autoimmune hepatitis: molecular analysis and clinical relevance. Semin. Liver Dis. 11, 205–214.

Manns, M., Gerken, G., Kyriatsoulis A., Staritz, M. and Meyer zum Buschenfelde, K.-H. (1987) Characterization of a new subgroup of autoimmune chronic active hepatitis by autoantibodies against a soluble liver antigen. Lancet 1, 292–294.

McFarlane, I.G., Smith, H.M., Johnson, P.J., Bray, G.P., Vergani, D. and Williams, R. (1990) Hepatitis C virus antibodies in chronic active hepatitis: pathogenetic factor or false-positive result? Lancet 335, 754–757.

Meyer zum Bushenfelde, K.-H. and Hutteroth, T.H. (1979) Autoantibodies against liver membrane antigens in chronic active liver disease. In: A.L.W.F. Eddleston, J.C.P. Weber and R. Williams (Eds.), Immune Reactions in Liver Disease, Pitman Medical, Kent, pp. 12–20.

Murray-Lyon, I.M., Stern, R.B., and Williams, R. (1973) Controlled trial of prednisone and azathioprine in active chronic hepatitis. Lancet 1, 735–737.

Page, A.R., Sharp, H.L., Greenberg, L.J. and Yunis, E.J. (1975) Genetic analysis of patients with chronic active hepatitis. J. Clin. Invest. 56, 530–535.

Perdigoto, R., Carpenter, H.A. and Czaja, A.J. (1992) Frequency and significance of chronic ulcerative colitis in severe corticosteroid-treated autoimmune hepatitis. J. Hepatol., in press.

Rakela, J. and Czaja, A.J. (1986) Clinical, biochemical, and histologic features of HBsAg-negative chronic active hepatitis. In: A.J. Czaja and E.R. Dickson (Eds.), Chronic Active Hepatitis. The Mayo Clinic Experience, Marcel Dekker, New York, pp. 69–82.

Ryder, L.P., Andersen, E. and Svejgaard, A. (1978) An HLA map of Europe. Hum. Hered. 28, 171–200.

Sanchez-Urdazpal, L., Czaja, A.J., Van Hoek, B., Krom, R.A.F. and Wiesner, R.H. (1992) Prognostic features and role of liver transplantation in severe corticosteroid-treated autoimmune chronic active hepatitis. Hepatology 15, 215–221.

Schalm, S.W., Korman, M.G., Summerskill, W.H.J., Czaja, A.J. and Baggenstoss, A.H. (1977) Severe chronic active liver disease: prognostic significance of initial morphologic patterns. Am. J. Dig. Dis. 22, 973–980.

Soloway, R.D., Baggenstoss, A.H., Schoenfield, L.J. and Summerskill, W.H.J. (1971) Observer error and sampling variability tested in evaluation of hepatitis and cirrhosis by liver biopsy. Am. J. Dig. Dis. 16, 1082–1086.

Soloway, R.D., Summerskill, W.H.J., Baggenstoss, A.H., Geall, M.G., Gitnick, G.L., Elveback, L.R. and Schoenfield, L.J. (1972) Clinical, biochemical, and histological remission of severe chronic active liver disease: a controlled study of treatments and early prognosis. Gastroenterology 63, 820–833.

Theodossi, A., Skene, A.M., Portmann, B., Knill-Jones, R.P., Patrick, R.S., Tate, R.A., Kealey, W., Jarvis, K.J., O'Brian, D.J. and Williams, R. (1980) Observer variation in assessment of liver biopsies including analysis by kappa statistics. Gastroenterology 79, 232–241.

Toh, B.H. (1979) Smooth muscle autoantibodies and autoantigens. Clin. Exp. Immunol. 38, 621–628.

Triger, D.R. (1976) Bacterial, viral and auto antibodies in acute and chronic liver disease. Ann. Clin. Res. 8, 174–181.

Wood, J.R., Czaja, A.J., Beaver, S.J., Hall, S., Ginsburg, W.W., Kaufman, D.K. and Markowitz, H. (1986) Frequency and significance of antibody to double-stranded DNA in chronic active hepatitis. Hepatology 6, 976–980.

Autoimmune Hepatitis
Edited by M. Nishioka, G. Toda and M. Zeniya
© 1994, Elsevier Science B.V. All rights reserved

Chapter 3

Clinical characteristics of autoimmune hepatitis in Japan

Yasuyuki Ohta and Morikazu Onji

Third Department of Internal Medicine, Ehime University,
School of Medicine, Shigenobu, Ehime (Japan)

1. Introduction

Until 1980, autoimmune hepatitis (AIH), was purported to be a rare disease in Japan. However, the number of patients with AIH in Japan reported in 1985 had increased when compared to the status before 1980 (Monna et al., 1985). This number is still increasing according to a nationwide investigation. The probable reason is that AIH is now better recognized and accepted by physicians.

A nationwide survey of AIH in Japan was carried out using questionnaires during a period of 2 years between January 1988 and December 1989. In this Chapter, the clinical features of patients with AIH in Japan using the data on AIH from our clinics and the nationwide survey in Japan, are summarized.

2. Patients and methods

The Autoimmune Hepatitis Study Group, a subgroup of the Intractable Hepatitis Study Group of the Ministry of Health and Welfare of Japan, performed a nationwide survey of patients with AIH by sending out questionnaires to hospitals and clinics specializing in gastroenterologic disorders throughout the country. Data from 200 cases were collected and analyzed.

The patients included in the survey all met the following diagnostic criteria for AIH.

(1)   Hypergammaglobulinemia (≥ 2.0 g/dl).
(2)   Positive anti-nuclear antibody (ANA).

(3) Histologically verified chronic active hepatitis associated with marked lymphoid infiltration (lymphocytes, plasma cells, and notably presence of lymphoid follicles).

(4) Extra-hepatic manifestations of disease.

(5) Responsive to glucocorticoid therapy.

(6) Absence of persistent hepatitis B virus (HBV) infection: negative for HBs antigen or high titer of anti-HBc antibody.

The prognosis, therapy and relationship between AIH and chronic active type C were investigated in 17 patients in our clinics. The prevalence of antibodies to HCV (anti-C100-3) by an enzyme-linked immunosorbent assay in patients with AIH, primary biliary cirrhosis, rheumatoid arthritis and multiple myeloma were examined.

Statistical analysis of data on age at disease onset and extra-hepatic autoimmune disorders of AIH was performed by the χ^2-test.

3. Results

3.1. AIH in the nationwide survey

Of the 200 patients reported in the nationwide survey, 25 were male and 175 female. The male:female ratio was 1:7, showing a significantly greater frequency in females. The age at disease onset was 56.3 ± 15.6 years (mean ± 1 S.D.). Fig. 1 demonstrates a single peak in the age at onset of disease (40–70 years). The present data were compared with a previous survey (1975–1985) with regard to

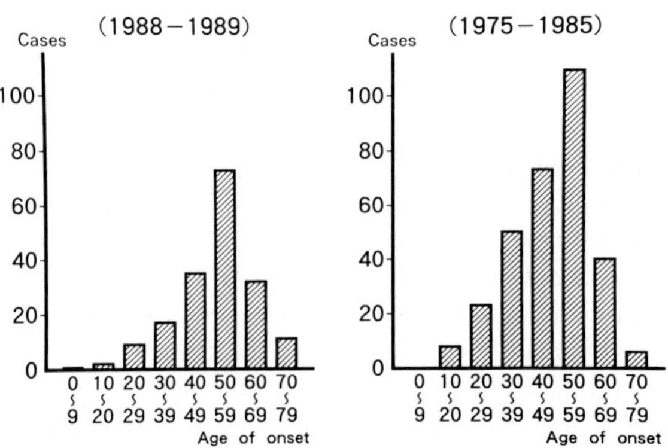

Fig. 1. Age at onset of AIH in Japanese patients. The age at onset of disease had a single peak (40–70 years). It is clear that the age at onset is shifting higher in patients in their sixties compared with the previous survey (1975–1985).

Table 1
Histology of patients with AIH

Histological diagnosis	No. of cases (out of 180)
Acute hepatitis	10 (5.6%)
Chronic active hepatitis	134 (74.4%)
Liver cirrhosis	21 (11.7%)
Others	15 (8.3%)

Table 2
Extra-hepatic autoimmune manifestations in patients with AIH

Diseases	61/187 (33%)
Rheumatoid arthritis	25 (13.4%)
Sjögren's syndrome	22 (11.8%)
Chronic thyroiditis	22 (11.8%)
Raynaud's phenomenon	7 (3.7%)
PSS-dermatomyositis	0
Primary biliary cirrhosis	0

age at onset of disease. There was an obvious increase in onset or disease in patients in their sixties.

The highest levels of total bilirubin, SGOT and SGPT were 6.7 ± 8.8 mg/dl, 432 ± 412 IU/l and 368 ± 347 IU/l, respectively. Jaundice was observed in 47.6% of patients during the observation period.

A histological examination was carried out in 180 patients: 134 (74.4%) showed chronic active hepatitis; and 21 (11.7%) showed the features of liver cirrhosis as shown in Table 1.

Extra-hepatic autoimmune disorders were present in 61 (32.6%) of 187 AIH patients. The main disorders were rheumatoid arthritis, Sjögren's syndrome and chronic thyroiditis, as illustrated in Table 2. All patients manifesting these disorders were female.

According to the nationwide survey, mortality due to AIH had decreased from 10% in 1985 to 3.1% in the present study. Liver failure was the main cause of death in 82.8% of total deaths. Only one patient died of hepatocellular carcinoma, but data on HCV markers were not available in this particular case. The incidence of hepatocellular carcinoma in AIH reported in Japan is limited. The possibility that HCV infection causes hepatocellular carcinoma in patients with AIH is currently being investigated.

Table 3
Clinical features in AIH

Data were obtained by The Third Department of Internal Medicine, Ehime University, 1976–1991. ACH, active chronic hepatitis, AIP, alkaline phosphatase; ANF, anti-nuclear factor; ASMA, anti-smooth muscle antibody; EIA, enzyme immunoassay; ESR, erythrocyte sedimentation rate; F, female; γ-glob., γ-globulin; KICG, clearance rate of ICG; LC, liver cirrhosis; LE, lupus erythematosus; LFT, liver function tests; RA, rheumatoid arthritis; RIA, radioimmunoassay; SGOT, serum glutamic-oxaloacetic transaminase; SGPT, serum glutamate pyruvate transaminase; T. bil., total bilirubin; ZTT, zinc turbidity test.

Case	Age at onset (years)	Sex	Histological diagnosis	Symptoms	Complication	LE cell	ANF (IU/l)	ASMA (IU/l)	ESR (1 h)	γ-glob. (g/dl)	T. bil. (mg/dl)	SGOT (IU/l)	SGPT (IU/l)	AIP (IU/l)	ZTT (U)	KICG	C100-3 EIA	C100-3 RIA	Blood transfusion	RA	HCV RNA
1	55	F	ACH LC	Jaundice		+	320	–	24	4.3	1.4	21	18	453	25	0.059	+	+		+	–
2	46	F	ACH LC	Jaundice, fever, arthralgia		+	80	–	78	3.8	7.7	409	418	221	28	0.137				+	–
3	50	F	ACH LC	Jaundice	Sjögren's syndrome	+	320	–	90	3.8	1.6	127	118	249	35	0.046	–	–		+	–
4	47	F	ACH LC	Jaundice, ascites		+	640	–	116	3.9	4.8	64	110	286	28	0.023	+	–	+	–	–
5	60	F	ACH	Arthralgia		+	+		8	2.0	1.5	73	34	220	16	0.080				+	–
6	60	F	ACH	Jaundice, fever	Chronic pancreatitis	+	80	160	115	3.6	3.3	207	368	1,410	32	0.070	+	–	+		
7	51	F	ACH LC	Jaundice, fever, arthralgia		+	80	160	37	4.2	4.3	82	138	165	30	0.064	+	+		+	–
8	50	F	ACH	Jaundice, eruption		–	13×10^5	–	168	4.8	24.2	91	126	145	25		+			+	–
9	45	F	ACH	Fever		–	320	320	54	3.5	1.1	175	409	406	32	0.174	+	+		–	–
10	67	F	ACH	General fatigue		–	40	–	54	2.9	9.9	126	144	258	28	0.103	–	–		–	–
11	58	F	ACH LC	Abnormal LFT		–	160	40	45	3.1	1.5	17	41	266	25	0.117					–
12	76	F	ACH	Jaundice		–	2,560	160	147	3.5	1.3	27	18	233	30	0.119	–	–		–	–
13	63	F	ACH	Jaundice		–	1,280	–	6	2.1	4.1	67	122	716	11	0.058	–	–	+	+	–
14	54	F		Jaundice general fatigue		–	2,560	160	125	3.6	3.5	48	53	223	30		–	–			
15	43	F	ACH	Myalgia arthralgia		–	320	80	21	2.4	1.1	61	137	193	18	0.183	–		–	–	–
16	58	F	ACH	Jaundice, general fatigue		–	1,280	–	25	2.0	34.4	474	309	210	15		–		+	+	–
17	29	F	ACH	Abnormal LFT		–	160	160	25	2.4	1.1	175	432	276	19		–		–	–	+

Table 4

Steroid therapy and prognosis

Data were obtained by the The Third Department of Internal Medicine, Ehime University, 1976–1991. Abbreviations and units as in Table 3 and: A, after administration of steroid; B, before administration of steroid; DA, duration of administration; GI, gastrointestinal.

Case	Age at onset (years)	Sex	Histological diagnosis	Steroid effect	DA (years)	SGPT		ANF		ESR (1 h)		γ – glob.		Prognosis	
						B	A	B	A	B	A	B	A	Survival (years)	Cause of death
1	55	F	ACH LC	Excellent	6.5	18	28	320	20	24	43	4.3	2.8	7	Hepatic failure
2	46	F	ACH LC	Excellent	7	418	25	80	–	78	12	3.8	1.1	7	GI tract hemorrhage
3	50	F	ACH LC	Excellent	13.5	118	33	320	160	90	12	3.8	1.8	13.5	
4	47	F	ACH LC	Excellent	9.3	36	40	640	160	116	13	3.9	1.2	9.3	
5	60	F	ACH	Excellent	13	110	52	+	+	8		2.0	1.8	13	Hepatic failure
6	60	F	ACH	Excellent	5	368	21	80	40	115	16	3.6	1.0	5	
7	51	F	ACH LC	Excellent	2	138	12	80	160	37		4.2	3.0	5.5	
8	50	F	ACH	Excellent	2	126	10	13×10^5	1,280	168	19	4.8	1.2	2.0	
9	45	F	ACH	Excellent	5.5	409	68	320	160	54	–	3.5	0.9	5.5	
10	67	F	ACH	Good	4.5	144	1,124	40	80	54	14	2.9	1.3	4.5	
11	58	F	ACH LC	Excellent	6.5	41	8	160	160	45	38	3.1	1.9	6.5	
12	76	F	ACH			18		2,560		147		3.5		4	Cerebral hemorrhage
13	63	F	ACH	Excellent	6 (months)	122	100	1,280	+	6	5	2.1	0.8	6 (months)	Hepatic failure
14	54	F		Excellent	4.5	67	18	2,560	320	125	33	3.6	1.4	4.5	
15	43	F	ACH	Excellent	5 (months)	137	12	320	80	21	13	2.4	1.1	5 (months)	
16	58	F	ACH	Excellent	1 (month)	389	126	1,280	1,280	25	8	2.0	1.0	2 (months)	
17	29	F	ACH	Excellent	7 (months)	432	5	160	320	25	8	2.4	1.1	1 (month)	

                              Y. Ohta and M. Onji

3.2. AIH in our clinics

We have observed 17 patients with AIH from 1976 to 1991 as shown in Table 3. The average age was 50 years, ranging from 29 to 76 years. Four patients had a history of blood transfusion. All 17 patients were female and 6 of them had progressed to liver cirrhosis. Histological examination of the patients revealed active chronic hepatitis in the last 5 years. In our cases, the symptoms were the same as those reported in the nationwide survey, and 11 of the 17 cases (65%) had obvious jaundice. In 7 cases (41%) lupus erythematosus (LE) cell test was positive. Anti-smooth muscle antibody was positive in 8 cases (47%) and this was also the same as the nationwide survey (1988–1989). In 15 cases (88%), the erythrocyte sedimentation rate was very high. The average serum γ-globulin level was 3.3 g/dl, and in only 6 cases, the γ-globulin level was between 2.0 and 3.0 g/dl.

In 3 of 16 cases, steroid therapy was very effective in normalizing serum bilirubin, γ-globulin, transaminase and the histology (Table 4). The cases who became negative for ANA after steroid therapy were very few. Three patients who stopped therapy of their own accord died due to hepatic failure.

The antibody to HCV (C100-3) was detected in 9 of 17 patients with AIH (52%), in 3 of 23 with primary biliary cirrhosis (23%), in 2 of 10 with rheumatoid arthritis (20%), and in 5 of 9 with multiple myeloma (56%). However, the optical density values for anti-C100-3 antibody in these patients were lower than those observed in non-A, non-B hepatitis (Onji et al., 1991). Anti-liver–kidney microsome antibody was negative in all 6 tested patients with AIH (Table 5). Anti-C100-3 antibody became negative immediately after the start of glucocorticoid therapy in all 4 anti-HCV-positive AIH patients treated. These results suggest that autoantibodies in AIH patients may cross-react with the HCV-related antigen. Direct association of HCV infection influencing the development of AIH is unlikely. Serum HCV RNA was positive in only one of the patients with AIH who were tested.

Therefore, care should be taken in the interpretation of anti-C100-3 positivity in patients with autoimmune diseases and multiple myeloma.

Table 5
Anti-C100-3 and -LKM antibodies in patients with AIH
LKM, liver–kidney microsome.

Anti-HCV	No.	Optical density of Anti-HCV				Anti-LKM
		<0.5	0.5–1.0	1.0–2.0	>2.0	
Positive	9	0 (0%)	7 (78%)	1 (11%)	1 (11%)	0/5
Negative	8	8 (100%)	0 (0%)	0 (0%)	0 (0%)	0/1
Total	17	8 (47%)	7 (41%)	1 (6%)	1 (6%)	0/6

4. Discussion

The geographical incidence of AIH varies considerably. As shown in Fig. 2, AIH is rather rare in Japan. The patients with AIH in the present study were characterized by a high proportion of females, especially of middle age and a high frequency of ANA positivity, as reported in previous studies (Monna et al., 1985). There are few young patients with AIH in Japan when compared with western countries. The incidence in Japan is characterized by two peaks, one in young subjects (15–25 years old) and the other around the menopause (Sherlock, 1989). Recent reports indicate that the mean age at onset of AIH has been increasing in Japan. A possible cause of the increase is considered to be related to the increase in mean life expectancy in the general population of Japan (Nishioka et al., 1988).

According to the nationwide survey, the number of patients with AIH is increasing, probably because the concept of AIH is becoming more widely accepted among physicians.

The complication rate of autoimmune disorders in patients with AIH in Japan is low, compared with cases in the U.S.A. Czaja reported that autoimmune disorders are present in up to 48% of AIH patients (Czaja, 1984). There are, however, few patients with AIH with severe complications such as hemolytic anemia in Japan.

The problem of the relationship between AIH and HCV infection is inevitable. Although a high prevalence of anti-C100-3 antibody in AIH has been reported, almost all these cases were proved to be false positive in a later study (Onji et al., 1991). There is a possibility that cases of chronic active hepatitis type C were not completely excluded in this study, because HCV infection could not be

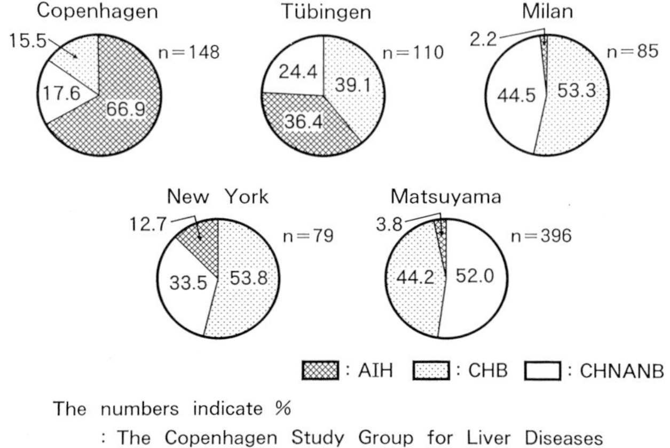

Fig. 2. The geographical incidence of AIH shows that AIH is rather rare in Japan compared with western countries.

completely excluded using the previous diagnostic criteria for AIH. Recently, we proposed a new diagnostic criteria for AIH in which HCV infection is, in principle, excluded (Ohta, 1993). However, it has been reported that HCV infection may cause AIH due to similarity of the HCV genome and the genomes of liver–kidney microsomal antigens, and antigen to GOR antibody (Mishiro et al., 1990).

In this paper, type 2 AIH patients were not reported. Some patients with type 2 AIH have been reported in Japan (Miyachi et al., 1991). Further studies are needed to reveal the characteristics of type 2 AIH cases in Japan.

In our experience, steroid therapy is highly effective for the treatment of AIH patients. We also believe that life-long steroid therapy is necessary for these patients. As the age of onset of AIH is increasing yearly, the development of osteoporosis due to steroid therapy is another problem which must be taken into consideration.

It became evident that the prognosis of patients with AIH developing liver cirrhosis was very poor and the cause of death in these patients was hepatic failure. Accordingly, it is suggested that early diagnosis and effective therapy would delay the development of liver cirrhosis and maintain a better prognosis. As the occurrence of hepatocellular carcinoma is very rare, it does not seem to be a factor affecting the prognosis of AIH.

5. *Conclusions*

In Japan, the age of onset of AIH (56.3 ± 15.6 years) has recently increased. There is no significant difference in symptoms of AIH between Japan and western countries.

The influence of HCV in the onset, disease activity and prognosis of AIH is not yet clear. Subdivisions of AIH could be established by further investigation. As it is related to therapy, early solution of this problem is warranted.

Although long-term steroid therapy has proved to be very effective in patients with AIH, the development of hepatocellular carcinoma is very limited.

References

Czaja, A.J. (1984) Natural history, clinical features, and treatment of autoimmune hepatitis. Semin. Liver Dis. 4, 1–12.

Mishiro, S., Hoshi, Y., Takeda, K. et al. (1990) Non-A, non-B hepatitis specific antibodies directed at host-derived epitope: implication for an autoimmune process. Lancet 336, 1400–1403.

Miyachi, K., Matsushima, H., Takano, S., Miyakawa, H., Matsuo, K., Nonaka, H. and Ootsuka, S. (1991) A case of chronic active hepatitis presenting with anti-liver/kidney microsome antibody. Acta Hepatol. Jap. 32, 175–179.

Monna, T., Kuroki, T. and Yamamoto, S. (1985) Autoimmune hepatitis: the present status in Japan. Gastroenterol. Jap. 20, 260–272.

Nishioka, M., Kagawa, H., Yamamoto, S. and Kuroki, T. (1988) A study of the increasing age of occurrence of autoimmune hepatitis. Acta Hepatol. Jap. 29, 1274–1275.

Ohta, Y. (1993) Report of the research subgroup of autoimmune hepatitis/primary biliary cirrhosis. Gastroenterol. Jap. 28, 128–133.

Onji, M., Kikuchi, T., Michitaka, K., Saito, I., Miyamura, T. and Ohta, Y. (1991) Detection of hepatitis C virus antibody in patients with autoimmune hepatitis and other chronic liver diseases. Gastroenterol. Jap. 26, 182–186.

Sherlock, S. (1989) Diseases of the Liver and Biliary System, 8th edn., Blackwell Scientific, London, pp. 348–349.

Chapter 4

Hepatitis C virus in type 1 autoimmune hepatitis

Gotaro Toda, Mikio Zeniya, Yoshio Aizawa and Humitoki Watanabe

First Department of Internal Medicine, The Jikei University School of Medicine, Tokyo (Japan)

1. Introduction

The etiology of autoimmune hepatitis (AIH) type 1 is unknown. Mackay et al. suggested that liver damage due to virus, malnutrition, alcohol, drugs or other hepatotoxic agents induced continuing autoimmune reactions which further damaged the liver in genetically predisposed individuals or for other unknown reasons, and that, even after the removal of these hepatotoxic agents, immunologically mediated liver injury continued (Mackay et al., 1965). When the concept of AIH was proposed, however, none of the human hepatitis viruses was isolated or identified. Discovery of the Australia antigen by Blumberg and its close association with post-transfusion hepatitis led to the isolation of the hepatitis B virus (HBV) (Blumberg et al., 1967; Okochi and Murakami, 1968). However, absence of HBsAg in the sera of AIH patients indicated that the persistence of HBV infection was not involved in the perpetuation of liver injury in AIH (Fox et al., 1969). Following the isolation of HBV, the hepatitis A virus was isolated from the feces of patients with acute hepatitis (Feinstone et al., 1973). Hepatitis A is a self-limited disease and persistent infection by the hepatitis A virus (HAV) is very rare. However, HAV infection may trigger AIH in some genetically susceptible subjects (Vento et al., 1990a).

Another hepatitis virus which persistently infected humans was provisionally named non-A, non-B (NANB) hepatitis virus. It had been impossible to evaluate the role of NANB hepatitis virus in AIH, until an assay method to detect the antibody to the C100 peptide derived from a non-structural region of the hepatitis C virus (HCV), a major etiologic agent of NANB hepatitis, was developed by the Chiron corporation (Choo and Weiner 1989; Kuo et al., 1989).

Using the Ortho-ELISA (enzyme-linked immunosorbent assay) to identify the antibody to the C100 peptide, Esteban et al. (1989) found the antibody in 44.1% of AIH patients tested. There are several lines of evidence showing that the positivity for the antibody to the C100 peptide indicates the presence of HCV infection (Kuo et al., 1989). The frequency of the HCV antibody reported by them was too high to exclude the possible involvement of HCV in the perpetuation of liver injury in AIH. Prompted by this report, several investigators in Japan tested sera from AIH type 1 patients for the antibody by the Ortho-ELISA method. As indicated in Table 1, there was a marked variation in the positivity rates among the investigators. However, Ohta et al. (1990) reported that the positivity rate was decreased when RIA (Ohtsuka) was used instead of ELISA for the detection of the antibody, suggesting that the ELISA method may produce false-positive results. McFarlane et al. (1990) also showed a close correlation between serum IgG concentration and optical density values given by sera of AIH patients, suggesting that the optical density values might not reflect the antibody activity. Although there might be several conditions where serum IgG concentration is markedly elevated, the close correlation of the optical density value with serum IgG concentration was only observed in AIH. Therefore, it seems possible that AIH serum contained IgG which bound to the epitope other than the C100 peptide, which was presented on the ELISA plate. McFarlane et al. (1990) suggested that AIH serum contained IgG which stuck to the ELISA plate. The antigen used for the detection of the antibody to the HCV-derived peptide was a fusion protein, C100-3, composed of the C100 peptide and human superoxide dismutase (SOD) (Kuo et al., 1989). Using the ELISA method, Ikeda et al. (1990) showed that all AIH sera positive for the C100 antibody by Ortho-ELISA reacted with bovine SOD fixed to the ELISA plate, suggesting that AIH serum reacted with the SOD portion of C100-3. However, the RIBA test, which differentiates

Table 1

HCV antibody in patients with autoimmune hepatitis in Japan

HCV antibody was assayed by first-generation Ortho-ELISA (enzyme-linked immunosorbent assay) or RIA (radioimmunoassay) (Ohtsuka) for the C100 peptide. The numbers and denominators in parentheses show the numbers of patients positive for HCV antibody and the total numbers of patients tested, respectively. n.t., not tested.

Authors	Positivity rate of HCV antibody (%)	
	ELISA	RIA
Akahane et al. (1990)	0.0 (0/4)	n.t.
Iino et al. (1990)	25.0 (3/12)	n.t.
Ohta et al. (1990)	61.5 (8/13)	25.0 (3/12)
Kuroki et al. (1990)	78.6 (22/28)	n.t.
Yano (1990)	58.3 (7/12)	n.t.
Ikeda et al. (1990)	71.4 (10/14)	n.t.

between serum reactivities with HCV peptides and SOD, revealed a very low frequency of SOD antibody (Nishiguchi et al., 1992). Immobilization of protein on the ELISA plate may expose an immunological epitope which is hidden in the native conformation. Taken together, these reports indicate that caution should be taken when evaluating the results obtained by Ortho-ELISA (the first generation) for HCV antibody.

Since cloning of cDNA of the HCV was accomplished, several diagnostic procedures have been developed. Using one of them, UBI (United Biomedical, Lake Success, New York, U.S.A.), which detects the antibodies to synthetic peptides from the non-structural and structural regions of the HCV genome, Lenzi et al. (1991) found the antibodies to HCV in 53 and 97% of Italian patients with type 1 and type 2 AIH, respectively. In contrast, they found the antibodies in only 13% of U.K. patients with type 1 AIH and in no U.K. patients with type 2 AIH. Furthermore, they found no close correlation between serum IgG concentration and the Ortho-ELISA value in Italian patients. This discrepancy may be due to the difference in diagnostic criteria for AIH between the two countries. Another possibility is that HCV infection may trigger autoimmunity leading to the perpetuation of liver injury at high frequency, or that persistent infection may induce an autoimmune reaction which injures hepatocytes.

2. Autoantibodies in chronic hepatitis C

An autoantibody which occurred specifically in chronic hepatitis C was reported by Mishiro et al. (Mishiro et al., 1990). This antibody, named anti-GOR, was directed to a host-derived epitope and is therefore an autoantibody. The antigen protein with which anti-GOR reacted was expressed in the nucleus of cancer cells. Manns et al. (1991) showed that the antigen of liver–kidney microsomal antibody type-1 (LKM-1), which characterizes type 2 AIH, was cytochrome P-450-IID6. Patients with type 2 AIH were shown to be frequently positive for the C100 antibody (Vento 1990b). In Italian patients with type 2 AIH, the high frequency of the HCV antibody was confirmed by a more specific assay (Lenzi, 1991). Manns et al. (1991) showed that the epitope of antigen cytochrome P-450-IID6 had partial sequence homology with HCV polyprotein, suggesting that HCV infection might induce the production of the antibody which was cross-reactive with cytochrome P-450-IID6.

Mackay et al. (1985) reported a very low frequency of autoantibodies in NANB chronic hepatitis. Using standard immunofluorescence procedures on tissue cryostat sections, they found anti-nuclear antibody (ANA) in only one of 18 patients with post-transfusion NANB chronic hepatitis. Furthermore, the titer was low. This study was carried out before the method for the detection of HCV infection had been developed. However, recent studies showed that most cases of post-transfusion hepatitis were caused by HCV (Esteban et al., 1989). Therefore, their study suggested that the occurrence of autoantibody was rare in chronic hepatitis C. However, the positivity rate of ANA was largely dependent on the assay method employed. Compatible with Mackay's report, Cassani et al. (1985) reported that none of the patients with cryptogenic non-B chronic hepatitis had ANA when their sera were tested for the antibody by immune fluorescence using tissue cryostat sections. When the same sera were tested by immunofluorescence using HEp-2 cells, however, 26% of them were found to be positive for the antibody. In AIH cases, positivity rates did not differ, whichever substrate had been employed.

Table 2 shows the positivity rates of autoantibody in patients with chronic hepatitis B and C in The Jikei University Hospital. The diagnosis of chronic hepatitis C was made by second-generation Ortho-ELISA. No patients fulfilled the diagnostic criteria of AIH proposed by a joint research group for AIH in Japan (Table 3) (Oka et al., 1988). Liver biopsy specimens showed a similar degree of histological activity of inflammation. ANA was evaluated by immunofluorescence on HEp-2 cells. Positivity rates of ANA, anti-smooth muscle antibody and anti-DNA did not differ significantly between the two groups of patients. The positivity rate for anti-LSP was lower in patients with chronic hepatitis C than in those with chronic hepatitis B. However, the difference was not statistically significant. Thus ANA was not rare in patients with chronic hepatitis C, but it occurred with almost the same frequency as in chronic hepatitis B, when assayed by immunofluorescence on HEp-2 cells.

Interferon treatment induced manifestations of AIH or exacerbation of liver cell injury in cases of AIH (Papo et al., 1992; Ruiz-Moreno et al., 1991; Ohta et al., 1991). In these cases, corticosteroid (CS) treatment was effective. In autoantibody-positive cases of chronic hepatitis C, however, CS treatment did not change

Table 2

Autoantibodies in chronic hepatitis type B and C

n = number of patients tested; ANA, anti-nuclear antibody; ASMA, anti-smooth muscle antibody.

Autoantibody	Positivity rate (%)					
	Type B			Type C		
	Male ($n = 42$)	Female ($n = 14$)	Total ($n = 56$)	Male ($n = 41$)	Female ($n = 17$)	Total ($n = 58$)
ANA	16.7	14.3	16.1	14.6	17.6	15.5
ASMA	4.8	7.1	5.4	4.9	11.8	6.9
anti-DNA	2.3	7.1	3.6	0.0	5.9	1.7
LE test	0.0	7.1	1.8	2.4	5.9	3.4
anti-LSP	26.2	35.7	28.6	14.6	29.4	19.0

Table 3

Diagnostic criteria for autoimmune hepatitis proposed by the Japanese joint research group for autoimmune hepatitis in 1988

Autoimmune hepatitis is a chronic active liver disease which is characterized by female preponderance, early progression to liver cirrhosis and beneficial effect of immunosuppressive therapy. Autoimmune mechanism is postulated as the pathogenesis and, viruses, alcohol and drugs are excluded from the causative agent. The diagnosis is made according to the criteria listed below.

Definite: I and III are fulfilled.
Highly probable: I and one of II are fulfilled.
Probable: I is fulfilled.

(I) *Major findings*
   (1) Sustained or recurrent elevation of serum transaminase activities
   (2) Serum γ-globulin or IgG over 2.0 g/dl
   (3) Seropositivity for autoantibodies, a or b
      (a) Positivity for LE cell phenomenon[a]
      (b) Seropositivity for ANA
   (4) Seronegativity for IgM class anti-HAV, HBsAg and anti-HBc, and/or low titer of anti-HBc

(II) *Accessory findings*
   (1) Presence of systemic manifestations such as arthralgia, fever and skin eruption
   (2) Complication with other autoimmune diseases or collagen diseases
   (3) Laboratory findings, a or b
      (a) Erythrocyte sedimentation rate over 30 mm/h
      (b) Positive CRP

(III) *Histology*
   Active chronic hepatitis with lobular distortion or submassive necrosis, or liver cirrhosis[b]

---

[a] When SLE is suspected, histological examination of biopsy specimen of liver should be performed and negativity for urinary protein should be confirmed.
[b] Infiltration of plasma cells is characteristic of AIH.

serum aspartate aminotransferase (AST) and alanine aminotransferase (ALT) levels, but interferon treatment normalized them (Magrin et al., 1991). As described above, HCV infection induced autoantibody reaction more frequently than previously reported. However, the occurrence of autoantibody alone does not contraindicate interferon treatment.

3. *HCV status in type 1 AIH*

As discussed above, HCV status should be carefully evaluated in type 1 AIH, especially when it was assessed by the first-generation Ortho-ELISA. According to Ikeda (1992), the positivity rate of HCV antibody in type 1 AIH was 71.4% (10/14) and 7.1% (1/14), when the antibody was assayed by the first- and second-generation Ortho-ELISA, respectively. The patient positive for HCV antibody on the second-generation ELISA was found to have HCV-RNA by polymerase chain reaction. Two other patients negative for the antibody on the second-generation ELISA were found to have HCV-RNA. Nishiguchi et al. (1992) also reported detection of HCV-RNA in AIH type 1 patients who were negative for HCV antibody by the RIBA test and second-generation Ortho-ELISA. Table 4 shows the HCV status in 20 patients with AIH type 1 who visited The Jikei University Hospital. Sera were collected at the time of the first visit, when the patients had not been treated with CS. The age of the patients of whom 16 were female ranged from 25 to 79 years. The C100 antibody was assayed by RIA (Ohtsuka) instead of ELISA. Anti-GOR was assayed according to Mishiro et al. (1990). C11 was the peptide derived from the C region of the HCV genome (Saito et al., 1992). Assay kits for the antibodies to C11 were kindly donated by Kokusai Shiyaku (Tokyo). The antibody was assayed according to the manufacturer's instructions. HCV-RNA was detected by amplification of the 5′-non-coding region of the HCV genome by reverse transcription with reverse transcriptase and the subsequent nested polymerase chain reaction. In 8 of 20

Table 4

HCV-related markers in patients with autoimmune hepatitis

Diagnosis of AIH was based on the criteria shown in Table 3. Anti-C100 was assayed by RIA (Ohtsuka).

Patient	HCV-RNA	Anti-C100	Anti-GOR	Anti-C11
S.K.	−	−	−	−
T.K.	−	−	−	−
T.Te.	−	−	−	−
K.K.	−	−	−	−
T.F.	−	−	−	−
C.E.	−	−	−	−
Y.K.	−	−	−	−
K.H.	−	−	−	−
Y.Y.	−	−	−	−
S.A.	−	−	−	−
M.Mi.	−	−	−	−
Y.N.	−	−	−	−
M.T.	−	−	−	+
T.F.	−	+	−	+
M.Ma.	−	+	+	+
K.Ts.	+	+	−	+
K.T.	+	−	+	+
T.T.	+	+	+	+
K.Ta.	+	+	+	+
M.Y.	+	+	+	+
Positivity rate (%)	25.0	30.0	25.0	40.0

patients (40%), one or more of the HCV-related markers were detected. In 5 of them, HCV-RNA was detected. Thus 8 of 20 patients diagnosed as having AIH, based on the criteria shown in Table 3, were positive for one or more of the markers.

4. Laboratory findings and frequencies of HLA phenotypes in type 1 AIH

Laboratory findings and frequencies of HLA phenotypes were compared between HCV-related marker-negative and -positive patients who were diagnosed as having AIH, based on the criteria shown in Table 3. They could not be differentiated by pathological histology (data not shown).

Serum ALT and AST activities were significantly higher in the patients negative for HCV-related marker than in those positive for it (Table 5). Serum IgG concentration did not differ significantly between the patients negative and positive for HCV-related marker (Table 5). With respect to ANA titer, all of the 12 patients negative for the HCV-related marker exhibited a titer higher than 1:40, whereas in only one of the 8 patients positive for the HCV-related marker was the antibody titer higher than 1:40 (Table 5 and Fig. 1). Thus there were significant differences between the patients negative and positive for the HCV-related marker with respect to transaminase levels and ANA titer.

The frequencies of HLA phenotypes in HCV-related marker-positive and -negative patients were compared with those in normal subjects resident in the Tokyo district and the data are shown in Table 6. All of the HCV-related marker-negative patients had HLA-DR4. The frequency of HLA-DQw4 was also significantly higher in these patients than in normal controls. In HCV-related marker-positive patients, the frequency of HLA-B35 was significantly higher than in the normal controls, and the frequency of HLA-DR4 was not significantly different from that of normal controls.

Taken together, it seems that HCV-related marker-positive and -negative patients belong to etiologically different entities, although they have several clinical and laboratory findings in common.

5. Response to corticosteroid treatment and HCV status in type 1 AIH

Response to CS was evaluated in the patients shown in Table 4. All of the patients who were negative for all of the HCV-related markers were treated with CS and followed over 6 months. In 10 of them, serum AST and ALT activities fell to within the normal range after treatment with CS and remained normalized by maintenance doses of CS throughout the observation period. Two patients in

G. *Toda et al.*

Table 5

Clinical and laboratory findings in patients with autoimmune hepatitis

Diagnosis of AIH was made according to the criteria shown in Table 3. When one or more of anti-C100, anti-GOR, anti-C11 and HCV-RNA were detected in the sera of patients, they were considered to be HCV-related marker-positive. When none of them was detected in the serum of a patient, the patient was defined to be HCV-related marker-negative. Values for age, serum ALT, AST, and IgG are means $\pm$ S.D. n = number of patients tested.

Variable	HCV-related marker	
	Negative ($n = 12$)	Positive ($n = 8$)
Sex (female/male)	10/2	6/2
Age (years)	48 ± 16	53 ± 13
ALT (mU/ml)	620 ± 342	162 ± 72
AST (mU/ml)	657 ± 528	149 ± 55
IgG (mg/100 ml)	3075 ± 719	3013 ± 377
ANA $> 1:40$	12/12	1/8
Complete response to corticosteroid[a]	10/12	3/7

[a] Serum transferase activities were normalized within 1 month after start of corticosteroid treatment and remained within normal range 6 months or longer on maintenance dose of corticosteroid (prednisolone 10 mg/day or less).

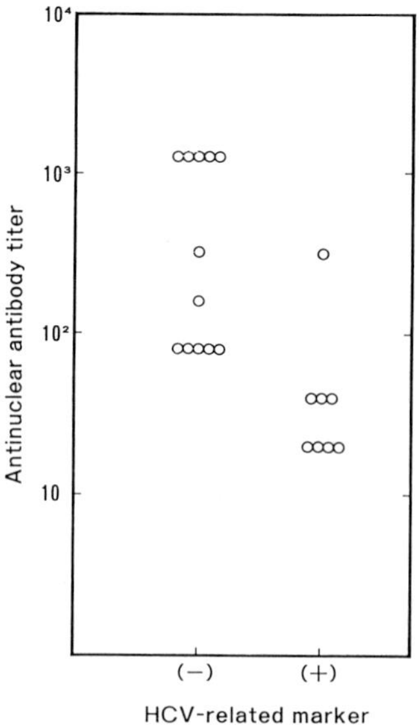

Fig. 1. Anti-nuclear antibody (ANA) titer in patients with autoimmune hepatitis. ANA was assayed by immunofluorescence on an HEp-2 cell. HCV-related markers included anti-C100 peptide, anti-GOR and anti-Cll peptide antibody, and HCV-RNA. Positivity of HCV-related marker indicates that one or more of these markers were detected. Negativity of HCV-related marker indicates that none of these markers were detected. Circles represent titers of ANA exhibited by the sera of the patients.

Table 6

Frequencies of HLA phenotypes in patients with autoimmune hepatitis

Diagnosis of AIH was made according to the diagnostic criteria shown in Table 3. When one or more of anti-C100, anti-GOR, anti-C11 and HCV-RNA were detected in the sera of patients, they were considered to be HCV-positive. When none of them was detected in the serum of a patient, the patient was considered to be HCV-negative. n = number of subjects tested.

	Frequency of HLA phenotype		
	B35 (%)	DQw4 (%)	DR4 (%)
Controls ($n = 340$)	10.6	14.4	41.5
HCV-negative patients ($n = 15$)	26.7	73.3[a]	100.0[b]
HCV-positive patients ($n = 16$)	43.8[a]	31.3	62.5

[a] $P < 0.05$ vs control.
[b] $P < 0.01$ vs control.

whom the transaminase activities were not normalized had liver cirrhosis. Out of 8 patients who had one or more of the HCV-related markers, 7 patients were treated with CS. In 3 of them, the transaminase activities were normalized by the treatment. All of those who had the transaminase activities normalized were positive for HCV-RNA. The clinical course of one of the patients is shown in Fig. 2. CS normalized the serum ALT level, whereas the HCV antibody and HCV-RNA remained positive.

Thus the response to CS treatment was observed more frequently in patients negative for HCV-related markers than in those positive for these markers. However, the difference was not statistically significant. One of the most important characteristics of AIH was the effectiveness of CS treatment. Four of 7 patients who were positive for HCV-related markers were deficient in this important characteristic of AIH. From the clinical point of view, however, it is worthy of note that, in 3 of 7 patients positive for HCV-related markers, CS treatment improved laboratory findings. HCV infection manifests itself as a chronic active liver disease characterized by a positive response to CS treatment in some subjects.

6. Outlook

AIH is characterized by female preponderance, autoantibodies, hypergamma-globulinemia, complications with autoimmune diseases and efficacy of CS therapy. The positive response to CS treatment is the most important characteristic of AIH. The causative agent of AIH is unknown. In some cases of AIH, HCV-related markers were detected. In laboratory findings, there were signifi-

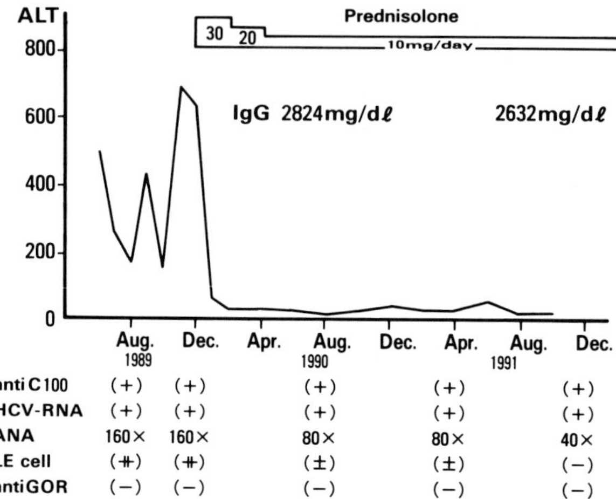

	Aug. 1989	Dec.	Apr.	Aug. 1990	Dec.	Apr. 1991	Aug.	Dec.
antiC100	(+)	(+)		(+)		(+)		(+)
HCV-RNA	(+)	(+)		(+)		(+)		(+)
ANA	160×	160×		80×		80×		40×
LE cell	(♯)	(♯)		(±)		(±)		(−)
antiGOR	(−)	(−)		(−)		(−)		(−)

Fig. 2. Clinical course of a patient with 'autoimmune hepatitis' with HCV-related markers. The patient was a 26-year-old female. Anti-C100 was assayed by first-generation Ortho-ELISA. ANA was assayed by immunofluorescence on HEp-2 cells.

cant quantitative differences between HCV-related marker-positive and -negative patients with the above characteristics of AIH. ANA titer, and serum AST and ALT levels were significantly lower in the former than in the latter. Furthermore, the high frequency of DR4 was observed in HCV-related marker-negative patients, but not in HCV-related marker-positive ones. These findings suggested that HCV-related marker-positive 'AIH' was etiologically different from HCV-related marker-negative AIH. It seems reasonable to assume that HCV infection induces an autoimmune reaction leading to chronic active liver disease (CALD) which bears a striking resemblance to AIH. Compatible with this assumption, Soga et al. (1992) reported a case of HCV-related marker-positive AIH in which the recurrence during tapering of CS was cured by the administration of interferon.

The occurrence of autoantibody to the hepatocyte surface (Hopf et al., 1976; Meliconi et al., 1983; Toda et al., 1983) and cytotoxicity of non-T-cell to autologous hepatocytes (Mieli-Vergani et al., 1979) in HBsAg-negative chronic active hepatitis were reported. These findings lead to the assumption that, in AIH, antibody-dependent cell-mediated cytotoxicity plays a role in the development of liver injury. Using isolated rabbit hepatocytes, Hopf et al. (1976) reported the occurrence of autoantibody reacting with the hepatocyte surface, liver membrane antibody (LMA), in HBsAg-negative chronic active hepatitis. However, they did not differentiate between AIH and NANB chronic active hepatitis. Meliconi et al. (1983) differentiated AIH from other CALD and showed a higher frequency of LMA in the former than in the latter. Using isolated rabbit hepatocyte plasma membrane, we (Toda et al., 1983) also reported that circulating autoantibody to the hepatocyte surface membrane occurred more frequently in the patients with AIH than in those with HBsAg-positive or NANB chronic active hepatitis. McFarlane et al. (1986) showed that autoantibody to asialoglycoprotein receptor, a normal constituent of hepatocyte plasma membrane, occurred at high frequency and titer in sera from patients with AIH. Furthermore, Treichel et al. (1990) showed that this antibody was rare in NANB chronic active hepatitis. These findings suggested that AIH and NANB chronic active hepatitis, of which a major etiologic agent was HCV, might be different with respect to mechanism of liver cell injury. In NANB chronic active hepatitis, a T-cell-mediated cytotoxic response was reported (Poralla et al., 1984). The cytopathic effect of virus to hepatocyte was also suggested. In some cases of hepatitis C, however, distinction from AIH was quite blurred and autoimmune reaction leading to hepatocyte injury may be induced. It remains for future study to ascertain whether the mechanism of liver cell injury operating in these cases of chronic hepatitis C is the same as that involved in AIH.

References

Blumberg, B.S., Gerstley, B.J.S., Hungerford, D.A., London, W.T. and Sutnick, A.I. (1967) A serum antigen (Australia antigen) in Down's syndrome leukemia and hepatitis. Ann. Intern. Med. 66, 924–931.

Cassani, F., Bianchi, F.B., Lenzi, M., Volta, U. and Pisi, E. (1985) Immunomorphological characterization of antinuclear antibodies in chronic liver disease. J. Clin. Pathol. 38, 801–805.

Choo, Q.L., Kuo, G. and Weiner, A.J. (1989) Isolation of cDNA clone derived from a blood-borne non-A, non-B viral hepatitis genome. Science 244, 359–362.

Esteban, J.I., Esteban, R., Viladomiu, I., Lopez-Talavera, J.C., Gonzallez, A., Hernandez, J.M., Roget, M., Vargas, V., Genesca, J., Buti, M. and Guardia, J. (1989) Hepatitis C virus antibodies among risk groups in Spain. Lancet ii, 294–297.

Feinstone, S.M., Kapikian, A.Z. and Purcell, R.H. (1973) Hepatitis A: detection by immune election microscopy of a virus-like particle associated with acute illness. Science 182, 1026–1028.

Fox, R.A., Niazi, S.P. and Sherlock, S. (1969) Hepatitis-associated antigen in chronic liver disease. Lancet 2, 609–612.

Hopf, U., Meyer zum Büschenfelde, K.-H. and Arnold, W. (1976) Detection of liver membrane autoantibody in HBsAg-negative chronic active hepatitis. N. Engl. J. Med. 294, 578–582.

Ikeda, Y., Toda, G., Hashimoto, N. and Kurokawa, K. (1990) Antibody to superoxide dismutase, autoimmune hepatitis, and antibody test for hepatitis C virus. Lancet 335, 1345–1346.

Kuo, G., Choo, Q.L. and Alter, H.J. (1989) An assay for circulating antibodies to a major etiologic virus of human non-A, non-B hepatitis. Science 244, 362–364.

Lenzi, M., Johnson, P.J., McFarlane, I.G., Ballandini, G., Smith, H.M., McFarlane, B.M., Bridger, C., Vergani, D., Bianch, F.M. and Williams, R. (1991) Antibodies to hepatitis C virus in autoimmune liver disease: evidence for geographical heterogeneity. Lancet 338, 227–280.

Mackay, I.R., Weiden, S. and Hasker, J. (1965) Autoimmune hepatitis. Ann. N.Y. Acad. Sci. 124, 767–780.

Mackay, I.R., Frazer, I.H., Toh, B.-H., Pederson, J.S. and Alter, H.J. (1985) Absence of autoimmune serological reactions in chronic non A, non B hepatitis. Clin. Exp. Immunol. 61, 39–43.

Magrin, S., Craxi, A., Fabiano, C., Fiorentino, G., Almasio, P., Polazzo, U. and Pinzello, G., Provenzano, G., Pagliaro, L., Choo, Q.-L., Kuo, G., Polito, A., Han, J. and Houghton, M. (1991) Hepatitis C replication in 'autoimmune' chronic hepatitis. J. Hepatol. 13, 364–367.

Manns, M.P., Griffin, K.J., Sullivan, K.F. and Johnson, E.F. (1991) LKM-1 autoantibodies recognize a short linear sequence in P45IID6, a cytochrome monooxygenase. J. Clin. Invest. 88, 1370–1378.

McFarlane, B.M., McSorley, C.G., Vergani, D., McFarlane, I.G. and Williams, R. (1986) Serum autoantibodies reacting with the hepatic asialoglycoprotein receptor protein (hepatic lectin) in acute and chronic liver diseases. J. Hepatol. 3, 196–205.

McFarlane, I.G., Smith, H.M., Johnson, P.J., Bray, G.P., Vergani, D. and Williams, R. (1990) Hepatitis C virus antibodies in chronic active hepatitis: pathogenetic factors or false-positive results? Lancet 335, 754–757.

Meliconi, R., Stanceri, M.V., Garagnani, M., Baraldini, M., Stebanini, G.F., Miglio, F. and Gabarrini, G. (1983) Occurrence and significance of IgG liver membrane autoantibodies (LMA) in chronic liver diseases of different aetiology. Clin. Exp. Immunol. 51, 567–571.

Mieli-Vergani, G., Vergani, G., Jenkins, D.J., Portmann, B., Mowat, A.P., Eddelston, A.L.W.F. and Williams, R. (1979) Lymphocyte cytotoxicity to autologous hepatocytes in HBsAg-negative chronic active hepatitis. Clin. Exp. Immunol. 38, 16–21.

Mishiro, S., Hoshi, Y., Takeda, K., Yoshikawa, K., Gotanda, T., Takahashi, K., Akahane, Y., Yoshikawa, H., Okamoto, H., Tsuda, F., Peterson, D.A. and Muchmore, E. (1990) Non-A, non-B hepatitis specific antibodies directed at host-derived epitope: implication for an autoimmune process. Lancet 336, 1400–1403.

Nishiguchi, S., Kuroki, T., Ueda, T., Fukuda, K., Takeda, T., Nakajima, S., Shiomi, S., Kobayashi, K., Otani, S., Hayashi, N. and Shikata, T. (1992) Detection of hepatitis C virus antibody in the absence of viral RNA in patients with autoimmune hepatitis. Ann. Intern. Med. 116, 21–25.

Ohta, M., Ishi, Y., Takami, S., Hayashi, K., Nishida, H., Kanaya, T., Sobajima, J., Okuda, M., Shimamoto, K., Kagawa, K., Okanoue, T. and Kashima, K. (1991) A case of autoimmune hepatitis developed by the treatment with interferon (in Japanese). Nihon Shokakibyo Gakkai Zasshi 88, 209–212.

Ohta, Y., Onji, M., Michiaki, K., Kikuchi, T., Miyamura, T., Saito, Y., Kuo, G. and Houghton, M. (1990) Assay of anti-HCV (C100-3) in autoimmune hepatitis and primary biliary cirrhosis. In: The Proceedings of the 16th Inuyama Symposium (in Japanese). pp. 183–187.

Oka, H., Toda, G., Ikeda, Y. and Hashimoto, N. (1988) A diagnostic criteria for autoimmune hepatitis. In: Annual Report of a Joint Research Group for Retractable Hepatitis 1988 (in Japanese). pp. 241–247.

Okochi, K. and Murakami, S. (1968) Observations on Australia antigen. Vox Sanguis 15, 374–385.

Papo, T., Marcellin, P., Bernau, J., Bernau, J., Durand, F., Poynard, T. and Benhamou, J.P. (1992) Autoimmune chronic hepatitis exacerbated by alpha-interferon. Ann. Intern. Med. 116, 51–53.

Poralla, T., Hutteroth, T.H. and Meyer zum Büschenfelde, K.-H. (1984) Cellular cytotoxicity against autologous hepatocytes in acute and chronic non-A, non-B hepatitis. Gut 25, 114–120.

Ruiz-Moreno, M., Rua, M.J., Carreno, V., Quiroga, J.A., Manns, M. and Meyer zum Büschenfelde, K.-H. (1991) Autoimmune chronic hepatitis type 2 manifested during interferon therapy in children. J. Hepatol. 12, 265–266.

Saito, M., Hasegawa, A., Kashiwakuma, T., Kohara, M., Sugi, M., Miki, K., Yamamoto, M., Mori, H., Ohta, Y., Tanaka, E., Kiyosawa, K., Furuta, S., Wakashima, M., Tanaka, S. and Hattori, N. (1992) Performance of ELISA system for anti-HCV using two new antigens (C11/C7). Clin. Chem., in press.

Soga, M., Yamasaki, H., Tomita, A., Iwamura, S., Iwasaki, S., Maeda, T., Miyazaki, M., Onishi, S. and Yamamoto, Y. (1992) Successful treatment with interferon for a HCV-RNA positive patient with features of 'autoimmune hepatitis' (in Japanese). Kanzo 33, 548–551.

Toda, G., Ikeda, Y., Hashimoto, N., Yamazaki, M., Torii, M. and Oka, H. (1983) Liver cell membrane antibody detected by protein A and isolated rabbit liver plasma membrane in sera of patients with chronic liver diseases. Clin. Exp. Immunol. 54, 661–670.

Treichel, U., Poralla, T., Hess, G., Manns, M. and Meyer zum Büschenfelde, K.-H. (1990) Auto-antibodies to human asialoglycoprotein receptor in autoimmune-type chronic hepatitis. Hepatology 11, 606–612.

Vento, S., Garofano, T., Di Perri, G., Dolci, L., Concia, E. and Bassetti, D. (1990a) Identification of hepatitis A virus as a trigger for autoimmune chronic hepatitis type 1 in susceptible individuals. Lancet 337, 1183–1186.

Vento, S., Perri, G., Luzzati, R., Garofano, T., Concia, E. and Bassetti, D. (1990b) Type 2 autoimmune hepatitis and hepatitis C virus infection. Lancet 335, 921–922.

Autoimmune Hepatitis
Edited by M. Nishioka, G. Toda and M. Zeniya
© 1994, Elsevier Science B.V. All rights reserved

Chapter 5

Autoimmunity in hepatitis virus infection

Kohsaku Sakaguchi, Hirofumi Kawamoto, Akinobu Takaki,
Hiroyuki Shimomura and Takao Tsuji

*First Department of Internal Medicine, Okayama University Medical School,
5-1, 2-chome, Shikata-cho Okayama 700 (Japan)*

1. Introduction

Infectious hepatitis viruses have been well described, including hepatitis A virus (HAV), hepatitis B virus (HBV) and hepatitis D virus (HDV). More recently, hepatitis C virus (HCV) has been reported to account for more than 90% of non-A, non-B (NANB) hepatitis (Kuo et al., 1989). Subsequent studies demonstrated a relatively high prevalence of anti-HCV antibodies in autoimmune hepatitis (Esteban et al., 1989, Lenzi et al., 1990), which is characterized by the clinical features of a high concentration of serum γ-globulin and the presence of autoantibodies, leading to the possibility that HCV infection might facilitate the initiation and perpetuation of autoimmune responses. From these findings, attention has been focused on autoimmune reactions in hepatitis virus infection and on hepatitis viruses as etiopathologenic agents in autoimmune hepatitis.

In this chapter we will discuss autoimmunity in viral hepatitis from the viewpoint of the production of autoantibodies and the pathological role of hepatitis virus infection as one of the candidates of etiological agents for autoimmune hepatitis.

2. Analysis of autoimmune responses in chronic hepatitis C and chronic hepatitis B: study of our cases

It is generally accepted that the frequency of autoantibodies in chronic hepatitis B seems to be low (Mackay, 1990), although occasional cases which were positive for both hepatitis B surface antigen (HBsAg) and autoimmune markers have been recognized (Soloway et al., 1972). The clinical studies of NANB hepatitis before the advent of the methods for detecting HCV infection demonstrated that the frequency of autoantibodies to nuclear, smooth muscle, cytoskeleton and liver membrane antigens was as low as chronic hepatitis B, and the few positive reactions obtained were at very low titer (Mackay et al., 1985).

The recent development of the methods for detecting hepatitis C virus-ribonucleic acid (HCV-RNA) (Okamoto et al., 1990; Weiner et al., 1990) and anti-HCV antibodies (Kuo et al., 1989) has enabled clarification of the clinical feature of chronic hepatitis C. In addition, a relatively high prevalence of anti-HCV antibodies has been reported in patients with autoimmune hepatitis (Esteban et al., 1989; Lenzi et al., 1990), although important geographical and/or genetic influences on the prevalence of anti-HCV antibodies in autoimmune hepatitis have been described (Lenzi et al., 1991). In subsequent studies on the occurrence of anti-HCV antibodies in autoimmune hepatitis, the non-specific occurrence of pseudo-positive cases accompanied by hypergammaglobulinemia was reported to be frequent (Ikeda et al., 1990; McFarlane et al., 1990). However, some cases of patients with autoimmune hepatitis, who were positive for the anti-HCV core antibodies and HCV-RNA other than the C100-3 antibodies (Tsuji and Sakaguchi, 1992), suggested the possible relationship between HCV infection and autoimmune responses.

Although possible involvement of HCV infection in the pathogenesis of autoimmune hepatitis has been suggested, as far as we know, few studies have been performed to analyze the autoimmune responses in patients with chronic hepatitis C, whose diagnosis has been confirmed by the presence of anti-HCV antibodies and/or HCV-RNA.

To investigate the relationship between hepatitis virus infection and autoimmune responses, we examined the incidence and characteristics of autoantibodies

Table 1

Incidence of anti-nuclear antibodies (ANA), anti-smooth muscle antibodies (ASMA) and anti-liver membrane antibodies (LMA)

	Cases	ANA	ASMA	LMA
Chronic hepatitis C	149	34 (22.8%)	9 (6.0%)	25 (16.8%)
Chronic hepatitis B	55	17 (30.9%)	2 (3.6%)	9 (16.4%)
Autoimmune hepatitis	11	11 (100 %)	7 (63.6%)	8 (72.7%)

and the serum γ-globulin level in 149 patients with chronic hepatitis C (positive for the anti-HCV C100-3 antibodies and/or second anti-HCV antibodies, and/or HCV-RNA), in 55 patients with chronic hepatitis B (positive for HBsAg), and in 11 patients with autoimmune hepatitis, who were confirmed to be negative for HCV infection (Kawamoto et al., 1992).

The frequency of anti-nuclear antibodies (ANA), anti-smooth muscle antibodies (ASMA) and anti-liver cell membrane antibodies (LMA) in patients with chronic hepatitis C, chronic hepatitis B and autoimmune hepatitis are listed in Table 1. The incidence of these autoantibodies was lower in patients with chronic hepatitis C and in those with chronic hepatitis B than in patients with autoimmune hepatitis. However, there was no significant difference in the incidence of these autoantibodies between chronic hepatitis B and chronic hepatitis C.

ANA were detected with an indirect immunofluorescence method using HEp-2 cells as substrates, and the titer was established by increasing double dilutions of serum diluted 1:10 until an end-point was reached. The increase in titer of ANA above 1280 was observed in 4 patients with chronic hepatitis C, whereas all the titers were below 320 in patients with chronic hepatitis B. Furthermore, we investigated serum γ-globulin levels in patients with ANA-positive chronic hepatitis (Fig. 1). It is noteworthy that some patients with chronic hepatitis C have both high levels of serum γ-globulin and high titers of ANA, as observed in those with autoimmune hepatitis.

Four patients of the 149 patients with chronic hepatitis C satisfied the immunological criteria for the diagnosis of autoimmune hepatitis (serum γ-globulin and/or IgG level of 2.5 g/dl or more, and the presence of autoantibo-

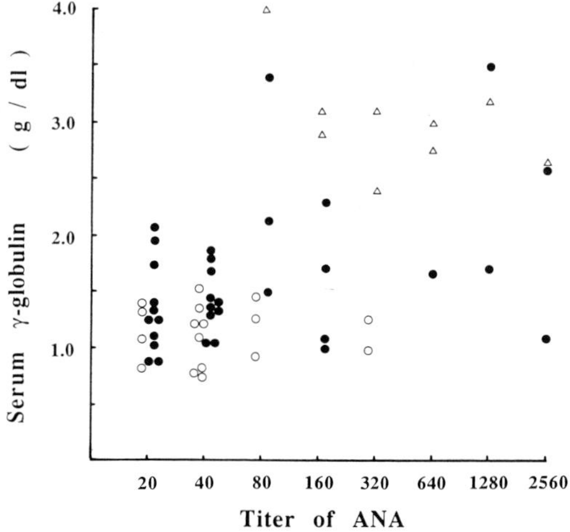

Fig. 1. Titer of anti-nuclear antibodies (ANA) and serum γ-globulin concentration in ANA-positive patients with chronic hepatitis C ($\bullet$), chronic hepatitis B ($\bigcirc$) and autoimmune hepatitis ($\triangle$).

dies including ANA), but none of the 55 patients with chronic hepatitis B did. HCV-RNA was detected in the serum of all 4 patients. The great majority of patients with chronic hepatitis C and chronic hepatitis B have negative or self-limited autoimmune responses, but a small percentage of patients with chronic hepatitis C may manifest autoimmune phenomena as observed in autoimmune hepatitis. Also, these results suggest that the autoimmune responses, as judged by the high level of serum γ-globulin and the presence of autoantibodies, might be more remarkable in chronic hepatitis C patients than in chronic hepatitis B patients.

The positive reactions for ASMA were confirmed by reacting against cytoskeletal components of the marsupial kidney cell-line, PtK2. The investigation of the specificity of anti-cytoskeleton antibodies revealed that anti-actin antibodies were found in 6 (66.7%) of the 9 ASMA-positive patients with chronic hepatitis C and in 6 (85.7%) of the 7 ASMA-positive patients with autoimmune hepatitis (Table 2).

Anti-LMA were also identified using a frozen section of rat liver by the indirect immunofluorescence method (Tsuji et al., 1979). Anti-LMA were detected in 25 (16.8%) of the 149 patients with chronic hepatitis C, in 9 (16.4%) of the 55 patients with chronic hepatitis B and in 8 (72.7%) of the 11 patients with autoimmune hepatitis. There was no significant difference between patients with chronic hepatitis C and those with chronic hepatitis B in the incidence of LMA. IgG-LMA was identified in 8 (32%) of the 25 LMA-positive patients with chronic hepatitis C, and in 4 (50%) of the 8 LMA-positive patients with autoimmune hepatitis (Table 3). The incidence of IgG-LMA in chronic hepatitis C patients was higher than that in chronic hepatitis B patients.

Table 2

Anti-actin antibodies and anti-intermediate filament (IMF) antibodies

	ASMA-positive	Anti-actin	Anti-IMF
Chronic hepatitis C	9	6 (66.7%)	6 (66.7%)
Chronic hepatitis B	2	0	2 (100%)
Autoimmune hepatitis	7	6 (85.7%)	6 (85.7%)

Table 3

Incidence of anti-liver membrane antibodies (LMA)

	LMA-positive	IgM-LMA	IgG-LMA
Chronic hepatitis C	25	17 (68.0%)	8 (32.0%)
Chronic hepatitis B	9	9 (100%)	1 (11.1%)
Autoimmune hepatitis	8	5 (62.5%)	4 (50.0%)

Table 4
Clinical data and HLA phenotype

Patient	Age (years)	Sex	HCV 2nd RNA		ALT (IU/l)	γ-Globulin (g/dl)	ANA (10×2^n)	HLA A	B	C	DR
1	49	F	+	+	55	3.5	7	2, 24	w54, w61	w1, w8	4, –
2	53	F	+	+	79	2.6	8	2, 24	35, w52	w3, –	2, 4
3	48	M	+	+	180	2.3	4	2, 24	51, w59	w1, –	4, w6
4	56	F	+	+	116	3.4	3	21, 31	w46, w54	w1, –	4, w8
5	41	F	–	–	227	3.2	7	24, 31	51, w61	w3, –	4, w8
6	42	F	–	–	258	3.1	4	2, 24	w46, w54	w1, –	4, w8
7	58	M	–	–	337	3.0	6	26, –	w61, w62	w3, –	4, 9
8	62	F	–	–	1143	2.6	8	2, w33	44, w52	–, –	2, w6

The 4 patients with chronic hepatitis C, who also satisfied the immunological criteria of autoimmune hepatitis, and 4 of the 11 patients with autoimmune hepatitis were studied for HLA association (Table 4). All 4 patients with chronic hepatitis C accompanied by autoimmune phenomena and 3 of 4 patients with autoimmune hepatitis had HLA-DR4, which is known to be strongly associated with autoimmune hepatitis in Japanese patients (Seki et al., 1990), suggesting that the autoimmune phenomena observed in chronic hepatitis C were supposed to be associated with HLA-DR4 specificity. The occurrence of autoimmune phenomena, including hypergammaglobulinemia and high titers of circulating autoantibodies in patients with chronic hepatitis C, might be in genetic control.

3. *Autoantibodies in viral hepatitis*

Several studies have shown the incidence and specificity of autoantibodies in viral hepatitis as detailed in Table 5.

ANA are the most characteristic marker for the diagnosis of autoimmune hepatitis. However, these autoantibodies are also found in a proportion of patients with viral hepatitis with lower titer reactivity than that in autoimmune hepatitis. The nuclear antigens specifically recognized by ANA in viral hepatitis have not been identified, although autoantibodies reacting with lamin C have been specifically found in some patients with hepatitis B virus and hepatitis D virus co-infection (Wesierska-Gadek et al., 1990).

ASMA have also been found to be associated with liver diseases. There is no significant difference in the incidence of ASMA among types of chronic viral hepatitis, although the incidence of ASMA in chronic viral hepatitis is lower than that in autoimmune hepatitis. Some of their reactivities can be accounted for by

Table 5
Autoantibodies observed in viral hepatitis
CAH, chronic active hepatitis; IMF, intermediate filaments; MF, microfilaments; MT, microtubules.

Viral hepatitis	Autoantibodies	Reference
Viral hepatitis A	Anti-IMF (Vimentin) Acute phase: 29/31 (93.5%)	Pedersen et al., 1981
Viral hepatitis B	ANA 8/25 (32%) Anti-cytoskeleton	Cassani et al., 1985
	CAH: anti-MF 3%, anti- IMF 32%, anti-MT 15%	Zauli et al., 1985
	Acute phase: anti-IMF 17/31 (54.8%)	Pedersen et al., 1981
	Anti-desmin	Pedersen et al., 1981, 1982
	Anti-ASGP-R 7/107 (6.5%)	Treichel et al., 1990
Viral hepatitis NANB	ANA 2/18 (11.1%) Anti-cytoskeleton	Mackay et al., 1985
	Anti-actin 1/18 (5.6%)	Mackay et al., 1985
	Anti-IMF 3/18 (16.7%)	Mackay et al., 1985
	LMA	Tsuji et al., 1985
	Anti-ASGP-R 2/83 (2.4%)	Treichel et al., 1990
Viral hepatitis D	Anti-lamin C	Wesierska-Gadek et al., 1990
and viral hepatitis B	Anti-keratin	Pisi et al., 1987
	Anti-LKM-3	Crivelli et al., 1983

antibodies to cytoskeletal components including actin (Kurki et al., 1980; Pedersen et al.,1982), vimentin (Pedersen et al., 1981), tubulin (Kurki et al., 1983) and others. Anti-actin autoantibodies are found in autoimmune hepatitis (Kurki et al., 1980; Pedersen et al., 1982), whereas anti-intermediate filaments (vimentin, cytokeratin) autoantibodies are identified in some instances of patients with viral hepatitis (Pedersen et al., 1981). There is segregation of autoimmune hepatitis and viral hepatitis according to reactivities with actin or other cytoskeletal filaments. The specificity of the reactivity of anti-cytoskeleton autoantibodies may be linked with the degree of stimulation of immune system in autoimmune hepatitis and viral hepatitis.

Autoantibodies employed in serodiagnosis of autoimmune hepatitis contain antibodies against liver cell membrane antigens (LMAg) (Meyer zum Bushenfelde et al., 1979), liver specific protein (LSP) (Meyer zum Büshenfelde and Miescher, 1972), asialoglycoprotein-receptor (ASGP-R) (McFarlane et al., 1986) and sulfatide antigens (Ikeda et al., 1990). These antibodies have been found in a large proportion of autoimmune hepatitis and in some patients with viral hepatitis. The differences in the frequency of these autoantibodies among the types of viral hepatitis were not significant.

Autoantibodies to liver–kidney microsome (anti-LKM) are mainly found in patients with idiopathic autoimmune hepatitis (Manns, 1989). The major antigen specific for anti-LKM autoantibodies in autoimmune hepatitis is reported to be cytochrome P-450 (Manns et al., 1989). Three subsets of anti-LKM autoantibodies are now recognized. Anti-LKM-1 autoantibodies characterize type 2 autoimmune hepatitis (Homberg et al., 1987), and are not associated with classical type 1 autoimmune hepatitis which is positive for ANA (Manns et al., 1987). Recently, a high prevalence of anti-HCV has been reported in patients seropositive for anti-LKM-1 autoantibodies, suggesting involvement of HCV infection in the pathogenesis of type 2 autoimmune hepatitis (Lenzi et al., 1990). Anti-LKM-3 autoantibodies have been described in some patients with chronic hepatitis B-associated hepatitis D virus infection (Crivelli et al., 1983).

Autoantibodies observed in the clinical course of viral hepatitis are generally weaker and more transiently positive than those observed in autoimmune hepatitis. These reactivities of autoantibodies are not regarded as specifying hepatitis virus infection, since they have been reported in association with various viral infections, including human immunodeficiency virus-1 (HIV-1) infection, where ANA, ASMA and anti-intermediate filaments were found in 30% of the patients (Cassani et al., 1991). Also, these autoantibodies have been described in cytomegalovirus infection (Andersen and Andersen, 1975) and Epstein–Barr virus infection (Kaplan and Tan, 1968).

These findings support a virtually clear serological segregation between 'autoimmune phenomena' observed in autoimmune hepatitis which are characterized by high titer reactions to autoantigens, particularly nuclei and smooth muscle, and 'secondary serological autoimmune reactions' in viral infection in which the titer of such reactions is relatively low. However, clinical markers which draw a clear distinction between the autoimmune phenomena observed in autoimmune hepatitis and hepatitis virus-related autoimmune reactions have not been identified.

As mentioned above, we believe that the population of patients with chronic hepatitis C includes a subset of patients associated with autoimmune phenomena, as assessed by hypergammaglobulinemia and the high titer of autoantibodies, which are similar to those observed in patients with autoimmune hepatitis. Interferon (IFN) treatment is generally accepted as beneficial in the treatment of chronic hepatitis C (Hoofnagle et al., 1986). However, at present no therapeutic methods for chronic hepatitis C associated with autoimmune phenomena have been established, since in a previous report, IFN-α therapy has been proposed to induce the development of autoantibodies and marked exacerbations in type 2 autoimmune hepatitis-associated HCV infection (Vento et al., 1989). Therefore, it is of considerable importance to identify which cases of viral hepatitis will respond to INF therapy by distinguishing between patients who have true autoimmune phenomena and those who have hepatitis-induced secondary autoimmune reactions.

4. *Hypergammaglobulinemia in viral hepatitis*

A high serum γ-globulin level with an increased level of immunoglobulin G (IgG) is recognized as a laboratory marker for the diagnosis of autoimmune hepatitis (Mackay et al., 1965). The IgG response in autoimmune hepatitis includes increased levels of antibodies to rubella and measles (Mackay, 1975). On the other hand, sera from patients with systemic lupus erythematosus (SLE) have elevated antibody titers to multiple viruses (Phillips, 1975), suggesting polyclonal B-cell stimulation rather than responses to specific viruses.

The high level of serum γ-globulin and IgG above 2.5 g/dl occurs in some cases of patients with chronic hepatitis C. Also, chronic hepatitis C has been reported to be associated with mixed cryoglobulinemia, that was successfully treated with IFN-α (Durand et al., 1992), suggesting the relation between HCV infection and the pathogenesis of mixed cryoglobulinemia. Taken together, HCV infection might be related to the mechanism of polyclonal activation of B-cells in some instances.

5. *T-cell responses involved in autoimmune responses in viral hepatitis*

Phenotypic analysis of lymphocytes infiltrating the liver tissue of patients with autoimmune hepatitis as well as of patients with viral hepatitis revealed the accumulation of CD8-positive and CD4-positive T-lymphocytes (Pape et al., 1983; Frazer et al., 1985; Hata et al., 1992), suggesting that these cells play an important role in the mechanism leading to tissue injury. Also, the functional analysis of the infiltrating T-cell clones is of great importance in understanding their involvement in the autoimmune responses associated with chronic liver diseases. Recent studies report the isolation of autoreactive T-cell clones (Franco et al., 1990) and ASGP-R specific T-cell clones from patients with autoimmune hepatitis (Löhr et al., 1992). Löhr et al. have demonstrated that the liver-infiltrating T-cell clones, which showed a proliferative response to ASGP-R, were able to induce anti-ASGP-R antibody secretion by autologous B-cells via cellular interaction in vitro, and suggested that in autoimmune hepatitis, the autoantibody production was connected to the occurrence of specific T-cell reactivity. Although T-cell responses that lead to autoimmune response in viral hepatitis are not fully understood, the helper function for autoantibody secretion by B-cells may be provided not only by autoantigen-reactive CD4-positive T-helper cells which are generated during viral hepatitis, but also by activated CD4-positive T-helper cells responding to viral proteins.

Suppressor T-cells might control liver-derived autoreactivity during viral hepatitis. Several studies have postulated a major role of defective suppressor T-cell functions in the pathogenesis of autoimmune hepatitis (Vento et al., 1984;

Vergani et al., 1989). Also, patients with chronic viral hepatitis associated with autoimmune phenomena are supposed to have increased numbers of activated T-helper cells and decreased antigen-specific and/or non-antigen-specific T-suppressor function. The uncontrolled expansion of liver-specific T-effector and B-lymphocytes found in these patients may be due to the inequality of these subpopulations of lymphocytes. However, it is unclear whether autoimmune phenomena in viral hepatitis occur in individuals who have a genetically determined defect of regulating mechanisms including suppressor T-cells or in individuals with a persisting impairment of regulating mechanisms, which is caused by hepatitis virus infections. In the patients with autoimmune hepatitis after hepatitis A virus infection, the genetically determined defect in suppressor–inducer T-lymphocytes specifically controlling immune responses to the ASPG-R has been identified (Vento et al., 1991).

6. *Mechanisms of autoimmune responses in viral hepatitis*

The complex process of the mechanisms of autoimmune responses in viral hepatitis involves two crucial steps: triggering events and perpetuating them.

Potential viral-mediated mechanisms in the initiation of autoimmune reactions in hepatitis viral infection are summarized as follows.

(1) Because intracellular antigen would not be exposed to stimulate B-lymphocytes, one possibility is that lysis of hepatitis virus-infected hepatocytes could result in the stimulation of B-lymphocytes by soluble protein.

(2) Autoantibodies may be induced against cell components which are antigenically related to hepatitis virus. A potential role for molecular mimicry in the induction of autoantibodies is suggested by amino acid homology and antibody cross-reactivity between the HCV core antigens and the cell-nuclear component (Mishiro et al., 1990), and between the HCV core antigens and LKM antigen (Manns et al., 1991).

(3) The observation that autoantibodies including ASMA develop during interferon therapy (Mayet et al., 1989) has led to the speculation that these cytokines could induce autoimmune responses by several mechanisms.

(4) Autoantibodies may be induced against virus-induced host molecules or virus-altered host molecules.

(5) Production of autoantibodies might be due to polyclonal B-cell activation mediated by T-helper cells reactive with viral protein or a T–B-bridge mediated by viral protein with superantigen properties (Friedman et al., 1991).

In general, control mechanisms must normally operate to prevent or limit autoimmune responses. Among these, the action of antigen-specific T-suppressor cells is considered to be the most likely. Therefore, in the presence of functional suppressor T-cells, autoantibodies induced by the mechanisms described above may be transient and rapidly disappear. A defect in this subpopulation may underlie the uncontrolled expansion of liver-specific T-effector and B-lymphocytes in autoimmune hepatitis. Also, impaired immunoregulation due to decreased T-cell suppressor function could play an important pathogenic role in the expansion of autoimmune responses in some cases with viral hepatitis. It may be predicted that the presence of hepatitis virus infection as a trigger and the defective suppressor T-cell mechanism could result in the persistence of autoimmune responses.

Cases of autoimmune hepatitis associated with subclinical hepatitis A virus infection are of particular use in helping to understand the effect of defective T-suppressor cells in the induction of the disease (Vento et al., 1991). Through prospective studies of healthy relatives of the patients with autoimmune hepatitis, autoimmune hepatitis type 1 has been shown to develop in individuals who have a genetically determined ASPG-R-specific defect of T-suppressor–inducer cells.

Autoimmune responses, as assessed by hypergammaglobulinemia and the presence of autoantibodies, might be more remarkable in patients with chronic hepatitis C than in those with chronic hepatitis B. This finding suggests that not only immunological factors of the host, but also viral factors might be involved in the pathogenesis of autoimmune responses in viral hepatitis. The characteristics of the hepatitis viruses that could trigger autoimmune hepatitis in the susceptible host and cause immunological abnormalities need to be defined.

7. Outlook

Although a potential role for hepatitis viruses in the pathogenesis of autoimmune hepatitis has been previously described, it was difficult to find an obvious relationship between hepatitis virus infection and autoimmune hepatitis. The recent development of methods for detecting HCV markers has enabled us to clarify the clinical features of chronic hepatitis C, and showed that the population of the patients who satisfied the immunological criteria of autoimmune hepatitis included the subset of HCV-related patients. These findings have led to the possibility that HCV infection might facilitate the initiation and perpetuation of autoimmune responses. However, many areas remain largely unknown, including the mechanism by which HCV infection may trigger and perpetuate autoimmune responses. Further detailed studies are required. In the future, they may provide further insight into the pathophysiology, not only of autoimmune hepatitis, but also of other autoimmune diseases, in which viral infection has been implicated.

References

Andersen, P. and Andersen, H.K. (1975) Smooth-muscle antibodies and other antibodies in cytomegalovirus infection. Clin. Exp. Immunol. 22, 22–27.

Cassani, F., Bianchi, F.B., Lenzi, M. et al. (1985) Immunomorphological characterization of antinuclear antibodies in chronic liver disease. J. Clin. Pathol. 38, 801–805.

Cassani, F., Baffoni L., Raise, E. et al. (1991) Serum non-organ specific autoantibodies in human immunodeficiency virus 1 infection. J. Clin. Pathol. 44, 64–68.

Crivelli, O., Lavarini, C., Chiaberge, D. et al. (1983) Microsomal auto-antibodies in chronic infection with the HBsAg associated delta (δ) agent. Clin. Exp. Immunol. 54, 232–238.

Durand, J.M., Kaplanski, G., Lefevre, P. et al. (1992) Effect of interferon-α2b on cryoglobulinemia related to hepatitis C virus infection. J. Infect. Dis. 165, 778–779.

Esteban, J.I., Esteban, R., Viladomiu, L. et al. (1989) Hepatitis C virus antibodies among risk groups in Spain. Lancet ii, 294–297.

Franco, A., Barnabara, V., Kuberti, G. et al. (1990) Liver-derived T cell clones in autoimmune chronic active hepatitis: accessory function of hepatocytes expressing class II major histocompatibility molecules. Clin. Immunol. Immunopathol. 54, 382–389.

Frazer, I.H., Mackay, I.R., Bell, J. et al. (1985) Cellular infiltrate in the liver in autoimmune chronic active hepatitis. Liver 5, 162–172.

Friedman, S.M., Posnett, D.N., Tumang, J.R. et al. (1991) A potential role for microbial superantigens in the pathogenesis of systemic autoimmune disease. Arthritis Rheum. 34, 468–480.

Hata, K., Van Thel, D.H., Herberman, R.B. et al. (1992) Phenotypic and functional characteristics of lymphocytes isolated from liver biopsy specimens from patients with active liver disease. Hepatology 15, 816–823.

Homberg, J.-C., Abuaf, N., Bernard, O. et al. (1987) Chronic active hepatitis associated with antiliver/kidney microsome antibody type 1: a second type of 'autoimmune' hepatitis. Hepatology 7, 1333–1339.

Hoofnagle, J.H., Mullen, K.D., Jones, D.B. et al. (1986) Treatment of chronic non-A, non-B hepatitis with recombinant human alpha interferon. N. Engl. J. Med. 315, 1575–1578.

Ikeda, Y., Toda, G., Hashimoto, N. et al. (1990) Antibody to superoxide dismutase, autoimmune hepatitis, and antibody tests for hepatitis C virus. Lancet 335, 1345–1346.

Kaplan, M.E. and Tan, E.M. (1968) Anti-nuclear antibodies in infectious mononucleosis. Lancet i. 561–563.

Kawamoto, H., Sakaguchi, K., Takaki, A. et al. (1993) Difference in autoimmune responses between chronic hepatitis C and chronic hepatitis B. Acta Med. Okayama 47, 305–310.

Kuo, G., Choo, Q.-L., Alter, H.I. et al. (1989) An assay for circulating antibodies to a major etiologic virus of human non-A, non-B hepatitis. Science 244, 362–364.

Kurki, P., Miettinen, A., Linder, E. et al. (1980) Different types of smooth muscle antibodies in chronic active hepatitis and primary biliary cirrhosis: their diagnosis and prognostic significance. Gut 21, 878–884.

Kurki, P., Miettinen, A., Salaspuro, M. et al. (1983) Cytoskeleton antibodies in chronic active hepatitis, primary biliary cirrhosis and alcoholic liver disease. Hepatology 3, 297–302.

Lenzi, M., Ballardini, G., Fusconi, M. et al. (1990) Type 2 autoimmune hepatitis and hepatitis C virus infection. Lancet 335, 258–259.

Lenzi, M., Johnson, P.J., McFarlane, I.G. et al. (1991) Antibodies to hepatitis C virus in autoimmune liver disease: evidence for geographical heterogeneity. Lancet 338, 277–280.

Löhr, H., Treichel, U., Poralla, T. et al. (1992) Liver-infiltrating T helper cells in autoimmune chronic active hepatitis stimulate the production of autoantibodies against human asialoglycoprotein receptor in vitro. Clin. Exp. Immunol. 88, 45–49.

Mackay, I.R. (1975) Chronic active hepatitis. In: L. Van der Reis (Ed.), Frontiers of Gastrointestinal Research, Vol. 1. Karger, Basel, pp. 142–187.

Mackay, I.R. (1990) Autoimmune (lupoid) hepatitis: an entity in the spectrum of chronic active liver disease. J. Gastroenterol. Hepatol. 5, 352–359.

Mackay, I.R., Weiden, S. and Hasker, J. (1965) Autoimmune hepatitis. Ann. N.Y. Acad. Sci. 124, 767–780.

Mackay, I.R., Frazer, I.H., Toh, B.H. et al. (1985) Absence of autoimmune serological reactions in chronic non-A, non-B viral hepatitis. Clin. Exp. Immunol. 61, 39–43.

Manns, M.P. (1989) Autoantibodies and antigens in liver diseases – updated. J. Hepatol. 9, 272–280.

Manns, M., Gerken, G., Kyriatsoulis, A. et al. (1987) Characterisation of a new subgroup of auto-immune chronic active hepatitis by autoantibodies against a soluble liver antigen. Lancet i. 292–294.

Manns, M.P., Johnson, E.F., Griffin, K.J. et al. (1989) Major antigens of liver kidney microsomal autoantibodies in idiopathic autoimmune hepatitis is cytochrome P450 db1, J. Clin. Invest. 83, 1066–1072.

Manns, M.P., Griffin, K.J., Sullivan, K.F. et al. (1991) LKM-1 autoantibodies recognize a short linear sequence in P450 IID6, a cytochrome P-450 monooxygenase. J. Clin. Invest. 88, 1370–1378.

Mayet, W.-J., Hess, G., Gerken, G. et al. (1989) Treatment of chronic type B hepatitis with recombinant α-interferon induces autoantibodies not specific for autoimmune chronic hepatitis. Hepatology 10, 24–28.

McFarlane, B.M., McSorley, C.G., Vergani, D. et al. (1986) Serum autoantibodies reacting with the hepatic asialoglycoprotein receptor protein (hepatic lectin) in acute and chronic liver disorders. J. Hepatol. 3, 196–205.

McFarlane, I.G., Smith, H.M., Johnson, P.J. et al. (1990) Hepatitis C virus antibodies in chronic hepatitis: pathogenetic factors or false positive results? Lancet 335, 754–757.

Meyer zum Bushenfelde, K.H. and Miescher, P.A. (1972) Liver-specific antigens. Purification and characterization. Clin. Exp. Immunol. 10, 89–102.

Meyer zum Büshenfelde, K.H., Manns, M., Hutteroth, M. et al. (1979) LM-Ag and LSP – two different target antigens involved in the immunopathogenesis of chronic active hepatitis. Clin. Exp. Immunol. 37. 205–212.

Mishiro, S., Hoshi, Y., Takada, K., et al. (1990) Non-A, non-B hepatitis-specific antibodies direct at host-derived epitope: implication for an autoimmune process. Lancet 336, 1400–1403.

Okamoto, H., Okada, S., Sugiyama, Y. et al. (1990) Detection of hepatitis C virus RNA by a two state polymerase chain reaction with two pairs of primer deduced from the 5′-noncoding region. Jap. J. Exp. Med. 60, 215–222.

Pape, G.R., Rieber, E.P., Eisenburg, J. et al. (1983) Involvement of the cytotoxic/suppressor T-cell subset in liver tissue injury of patients with acute and chronic liver diseases. Gastroenterology 85, 657–662.

Pedersen, J.S., Toh, B.H., Locarnini, S.A., et al. (1981) Autoantibody to intermediate filaments in viral hepatitis. Clin. Immunol. Immunopathol. 21, 154–161.

Pedersen, J.S., Toh, B.H., Mackay, I.R. et al. (1982) Segregation of autoantibody to cytoskeletal filaments, actin and intermediate filaments with two types of chronic hepatitis. Clin. Exp. Immunol. 48, 527–533.

Phillips, P.E. (1975) The virus hypothesis in systemic lupus erythematosus. Ann. Intern. Med. 83, 709–717.

Pisi, E., Zauli, D. and Crespi, C. (1987) Autoantibodies in chronic hepatitis delta virus infection. In: The Hepatitis Delta Virus and Its Infection. Liss, New York, pp. 249–256.

Seki, T., Kiyosawa, K., Inoko, H. et al. (1990) Association of autoimmune hepatitis with HLA-Bw54 and DR4 in Japanese patients. Hepatology 12, 1300–1304.

Soloway, R.D., Summerskill, W.H.J., Baggenstoss, A.H. et al. (1972) 'Lupoid' hepatitis, a nonentity in the spectrum of chronic active liver disease. Gastroenterology 63, 458–465.

Treichel, U., Poralla, T., Hess, G. et al. (1990) Autoantibodies to human asialoglycoprotein receptor in autoimmune-type chronic hepatitis. Hepatology 11, 606–612.

Tsuji, T. and Sakaguchi, K. (1992) Autoimmune reactions in chronic hepatitis C. In: T. Tsuji and G. Yamada (Eds.), Immune Responses and Interferon Treatment in Viral Hepatitis. Nankodo, Tokyo, pp. 54–57.

Tsuji, T., Araki, K., Naitou, K. et al. (1979) Detection and characterization of antibody to liver cell membrane in sera from patients with chronic active liver diseases. Acta Med. Okayama 33, 61–66.

Tsuji, T., Takahashi, K., Sawahara, M. et al. (1985) Detection and clinical significance of acetone-insoluble liver cell membrane antigen in sera of patients with chronic active liver diseases. Gastroenterol. Jap. 20, 37–47.

Vento, S., Hegarty, J.E., Bottazzo, G.F. et al. (1984) Antigen-specific suppressor cell function in autoimmune chronic active hepatitis. Lancet i, 1200–1204.

Vento, S., Di Perri, G., Garofano, T. et al. (1989) Hazards of interferon therapy for HBV-seronegative chronic hepatitis. Lancet ii, 926.

Vento, S., Garoffano, T., Di Perri, G. et al. (1991) Identification of hepatitis A virus as trigger for autoimmune chronic hepatitis type 1 in susceptible individuals. Lancet 337, 1183–1187.

Vergani, M., Lobo-Yeo, A., McFarlane, B.M. et al. (1989) Different immune mechanisms leading to autoimmunity in primary sclerosing cholangitis and autoimmune chronic active hepatitis of childhood. Hepatology 9, 198–203.

Weiner, A.J., Kuo, G., Bradley, D.W. et al. (1990) Detection of hepatitis C viral sequences in non-A, non-B hepatitis. Lancet 335, 1–3.

Wesierska-Gadek, J., Penner, E., Hitchman E. et al. (1990) Antibodies to nuclear lamin C in chronic hepatitis delta virus infection. Hepatology 12, 1129–1133.

Zauli, D., Crespi, C., Dall 'Amore, P. et al. (1985) Relationship between cytoskeleton and smooth muscle antibodies (SMA) in chronic liver disease (CLD). J. Hepatol. 1 (Suppl.), 155.

Section III

Pathology of Autoimmune Hepatitis

Autoimmune Hepatitis
Edited by M. Nishioka, G. Toda and M. Zeniya
© *1994, Elsevier Science B.V. All rights reserved*

Chapter 6

Pathology of autoimmune hepatitis and related diseases

Yasuni Nakanuma[1], Kennichi Harada[1], Akitaka Nonomura[2],
Eiki Matsushita[3] and Masashi Unoura[3]

Departments of [1]*Pathology (II),* [2]*Diagnostic Pathology and* [3]*Internal Medicine (I),*
Kanazawa University School of Medicine, Kanazawa 920 (Japan)

1. Introduction

Autoimmune phenomena have frequently been described in various hepatobiliary diseases, such as viral hepatitis, autoimmune ('lupoid') hepatitis (AIH), primary biliary cirrhosis (PBC), drug-induced hepatitis, alcoholic liver disease, and hepatic allograft rejection (Paronetto et al., 1986; Vento and Eddleston, 1990; Foster et al., 1991; Gershwin and Mackay, 1991; Meyer zum Büschenfelde, 1991; Weisner et al., 1991). In these conditions, infiltration of immunocompetent cells, such as lymphocytes and plasma cells, is found in the liver. Autoantibodies and disturbances of immunoregulation are also known to occur. Immunologic mechanisms may primarily be involved in the initiation and/or progression of autodestructive processes in some of these diseases. These immunologic disturbances may, however, be epiphenomena in other conditions.

AIH is regarded as a prototype of immune-mediated liver disease in which hepatocytes are the main target tissues (McFarlane et al., 1986; Paronetto et al., 1986; Treichel et al., 1990). This disease, which was originally reported by Mackay (Mackay et al., 1956; Mackay and Wood, 1962; Whittingham et al., 1966), is serologically characterized by hypergammaglobulinemia, predominantly IgG, and the occurrence of organ-non-specific autoantibodies, especially anti-nuclear antibodies (ANA), and lupus erythematosus (LE) cells, and predominantly affects young and postmenopausal women. Histopathologically, AIH is characterized by progressive and continuous or discontinuous (bout-like) hepatocellular necrosis with prominent mononuclear cell infiltration, irregular regeneration of the hepatocytes and fibrosis followed by rapid development of liver cirrhosis, when untreated. However, a recent study has disclosed that the prognosis of AIH is not so unfavorable, and some patients show spontaneous remission of these necroinflammatory reactions involving the liver (Johnson et al., 1991). These necroinflammatory changes of the liver are known to often respond well to steroid or immunosuppressive therapy. The term 'steroid-sensitive chronic active hepatitis' may, therefore, be preferable to AIH (Tassoni and Kaplan, 1991).

In spite of the increasing awareness of AIH and the numerous clinical, immunologic, biochemical and histologic studies, AIH is still a challenging concept at the present time. That is, it has not yet been established whether AIH is a collective clinicopathologic condition showing progressive necroinflammation of the liver with outstanding autoimmune phenomena irrespective of etiology, or an established disease entity (Soloway et al., 1972; Johnson et al., 1991; Johnson and McFarlane, 1993). The pathognomonic histopathologic and immunopathologic findings of the liver have not been reported so far (Mackay et al., 1956; Reynolds et al., 1964; Scheuer, 1980, 1988; Dienes, 1989).

Since the hepatitis viruses and their related markers have become measurable or identifiable in the liver tissue and serum (Choo et al., 1989; Kuo et al., 1989), the participation and significance of persistent and transient viral hepatitis are now being tested in AIH patients (Esteban et al., 1989; McFarlane et al., 1990; Lenzi et al., 1991; Vento et al., 1991). Furthermore, a number of specific monoclonal antibodies and immunohistochemical techniques are now becoming available in routine pathologic practice (Hsu et al., 1981). The immunopathological features of AIH have been evaluated in viral hepatitis and other hepatobiliary diseases (Paronetto et al., 1986; Lohr et al., 1990; Van den Oord et al., 1990). The experimental basis of the disease has also been challenged (Meyer zum Büschenfelde et al., 1972; Mori et al., 1985; Schaffner, 1986; Lohse, 1991).

Recent advances in the characterization of autoantibodies and their corresponding antigens have greatly contributed to the understanding of AIH. Clinical, serologic and immunologic studies have suggested that AIH could be subclassified into several groups: types 1, 2 and 3. Type 1, or classic AIH, is characterized by periportal piecemeal necrosis accompanied by high serum titers (> 40) of non-organ-specific autoantibodies (ANA of homogeneous type and antibodies to actin) and by hypergammaglobulinemia. The asialoglycoprotein receptor (ASGP-R) of the hepatocytes is now regarded as the target antigen (McFarlane et al., 1986; Treichel et al., 1990). Type 2 AIH is positive for liver–kidney microsomal (LKM) antibody and mainly affects children (Vento et al., 1988; Manns, 1991). Type 3 AIH is characterized by the presence of antibodies against a soluble liver antigen (SLA) (Johnson et al., 1991; Manns, 1991). The relevant inciting agent(s) causing marked immune responses, mechanisms of immunological sequences for hepatocellular necrosis, characterization of another or additional target antigen(s) in liver tissue, and the natural course of this disease are under active study (Cohen and Lohse, 1991; Johnson et al., 1991;

Lohse, 1991; Manns, 1991; McFarlane, 1991; Meyer zum Büschenfelde, 1991; Poralla et al., 1991). In addition, there are also a few AIH patients presenting with atypical clinicopathologic features such as peripheral and liver tissue eosinophilia (Panush et al., 1973; Croffy et al., 1988; Foong et al., 1991; Foster et al., 1991). In addition to AIH, there are a number of autoimmune hepatobiliary diseases such as PBC, overlapping syndrome of PBC and chronic active hepatitis (CAH), primary sclerosing cholangitis (PSC) (Bianchi et al., 1987; Takegoshi et al., 1989; Dienes et al., 1991) in which autoimmune hepatocellular damage as seen in AIH is also reported.

In this chapter, we will first present the spectrum of histopathologies of AIH and representative histologic patterns. The immunopathology and pathogenesis of AIH will then be briefly discussed. Finally, the histopathologies of several autoimmune hepatobiliary diseases in which hepatocellular necrosis resembling AIH occurs, will be discussed with the emphasis on hepatocellular damage.

2. Histopathology of type 1, classic AIH

In Japan, almost all AIH cases reported so far belong to type 1 (Monna et al., 1982). We have studied 20 cases of type 1 AIH, all of which fulfil the criteria of AIH proposed by the Committee of the Japanese Health and Welfare Ministry (1982). The hepatic histopathologies of these cases, including those after steroid therapy, will be described in this section.

The necroinflammatory changes and histologic progression of the liver in AIH vary from case to case, depending upon the modes of onset and progression as well as phases (or stages) (Matsushita, 1982; Lefkowitch et al., 1984; Johnson et al., 1991; Johnson and McFarlane, 1993). Actually, Dienes et al. (1989, 1991) recently reported that AIH patients present with a broad spectrum of hepatic lesions from chronic persistent hepatitis (CPH) and acute necrotizing injury to CAH and cirrhosis.

We first describe the fundamental and also non-specific histopathologies of the liver in AIH and then several representative histologic patterns in AIH before steroid or immunosuppressive therapy. The hepatic histopathologies after these therapies will also be reviewed. Finally, the immunopathology and pathogenesis of AIH will be briefly discussed.

2.1. Fundamental hepatic histopathologies

Hepatocellular hydropic swelling and necrosis, and numerous mononuclear cell infiltrations, including plasma cells in the enlarged portal tracts and in the hepatic lobules, are fundamental and important histopathologies of the liver in AIH

(Johnson and McFarlane, 1993), though similar findings are also encountered in other chronic active hepatobiliary diseases (Tanikawa and Maeyama 1982; Dienes, 1989; Dienes et al., 1991).

2.1.1. *Hepatocellular damage and necrosis*

Hepatocellular damage and necrosis are an essential and important component of AIH. That is, the ballooning or hydropic swelling of the hepatocytes, probably followed by their lytic necrosis, are usually found to a variable extent (Figs. 1–3). These ballooning changes are diffusely found in liver specimens in some cases, while these changes are more or less pronounced in perivenular areas, adjacent to lytic necrosis and also at piecemeal necrosis in other cases. Some of these hepatocytes show clumped intra-cytoplasmic material. Hepatocyte rosettes entrapped in the enlarged portal tracts and septa also show hydropic swelling (Fig. 4). Giant cell transformation is occasionally seen in AIH with acute hepatitic changes and cholestasis (Fig. 5), while considerable giant cell transformation is also reported in adults with CAH and multiple autoimmune features (Lefkowitch et al., 1984; Thijs et al., 1985; Devaney et al., 1992).

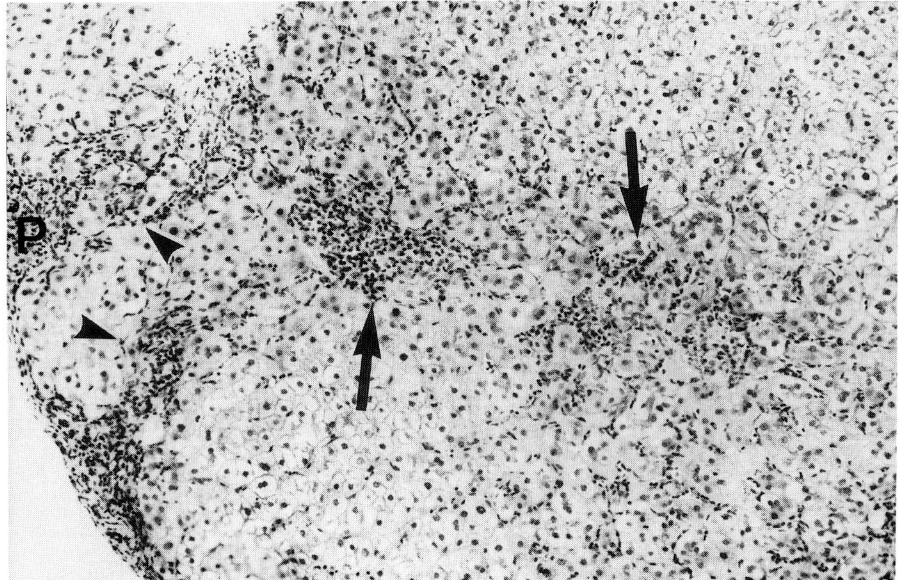

Fig. 1. Hepatocytes show diffuse hydropic changes. There are also areas of focal and spotty necrosis (arrows), piecemeal necrosis (arrowheads), and sinusoidal reaction. P, portal tract. AIH showing CAH. Hematoxylin–eosin stain.

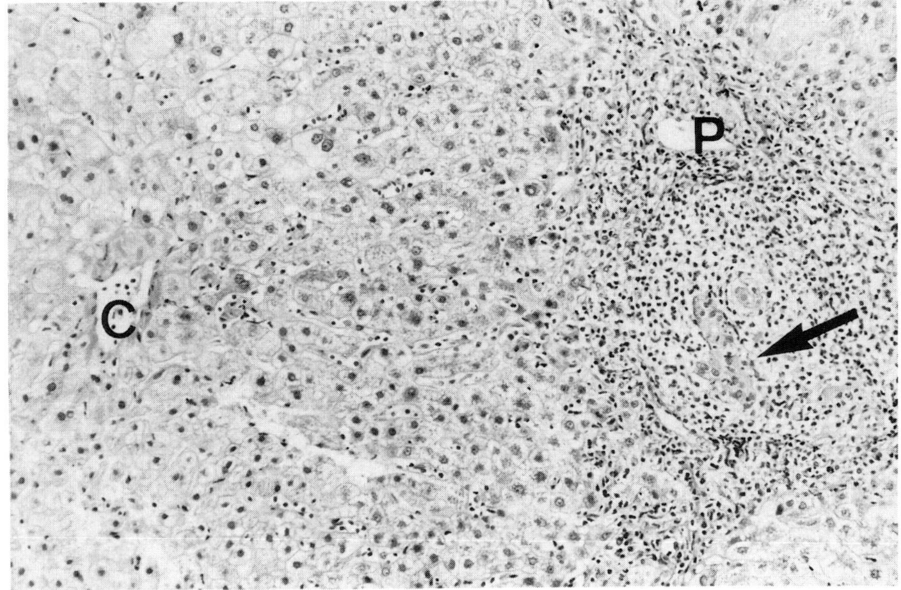

Fig. 2. A portal tract shows marked mononuclear cell infiltration and hepatitic bile duct lesion (arrow). Piecemeal necrosis and sinusoidal reaction are also found. C, central vein; P, portal tract. AIH showing CAH. Hematoxylin–eosin stain.

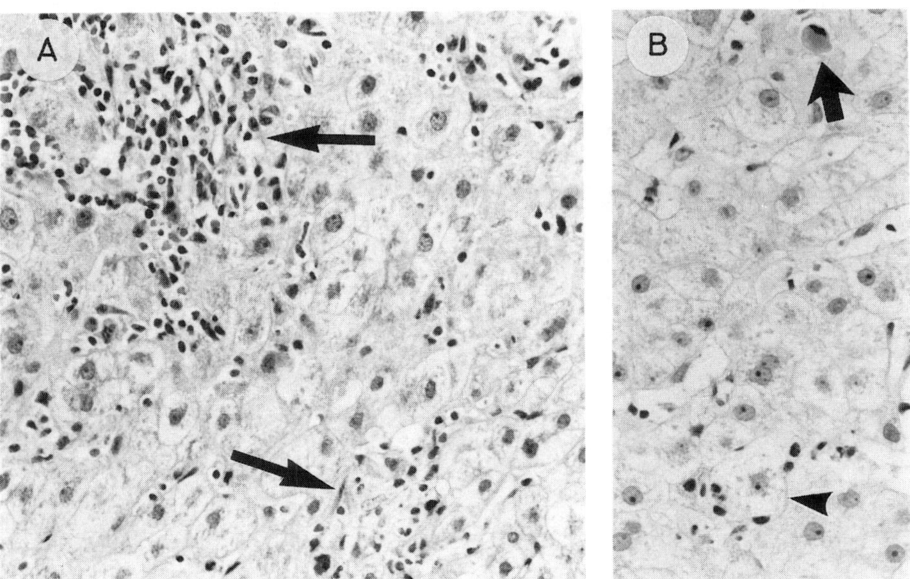

Fig. 3. A: variable-sized areas of hepatocellular necrosis (arrows) and Kupffer cell hyperplasia are seen in the hepatic parenchyma. B: acidophilic body (arrow), emperipolesis of lymphocytes and ballooning of hepatocyte (arrowhead) are seen. AIH. Hematoxylin–eosin stain.

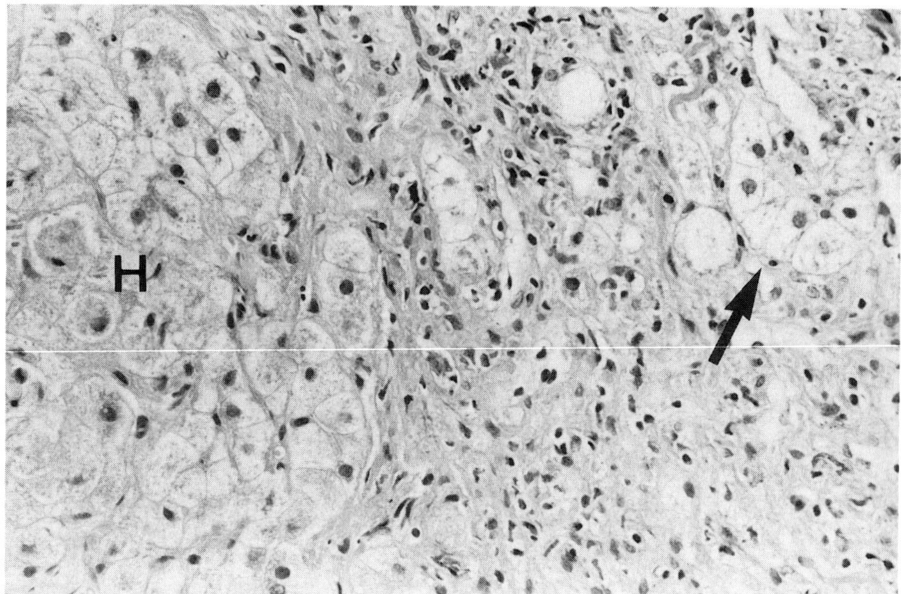

Fig. 4. Hydropic hepatocytes are entrapped in fibrous septa (rosette formation of hepatocytes) (arrows) with mild mononuclear cell infiltration. H, hepatic parenchyma. AIH. Hematoxylin–eosin stain.

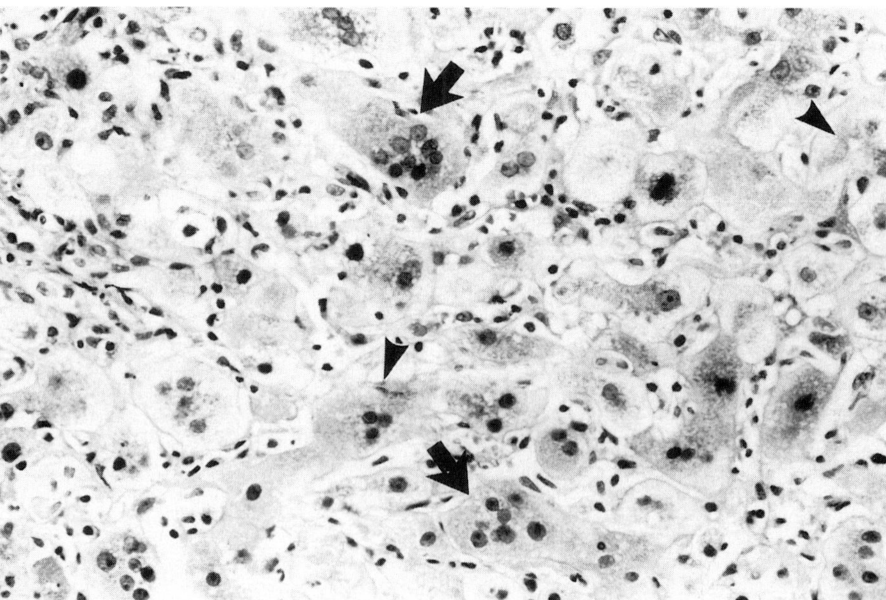

Fig. 5. Giant-cell transformation of hepatocytes (arrows), bile plugs or bile canalicular dilatation (arrowheads), and sinusoidal lymphocytic infiltration are seen. AIH with multinucleated giant cells. Hematoxylin–eosin stain.

Focal and spotty hepatocellular necroses associated with mononuclear cell infiltration and hypertrophic Kupffer cells are constantly found in the hepatic lobules (Figs. 1–3) (Dienes, 1989), although their degree is variable from lobule to lobule in the same case, or depending on the phases of disease activity. The majority of infiltrating mononuclear cells are lymphocytes, while some focal or spotty necrosis is exclusively infiltrated by plasma cells (Fig. 6). Hepatocellular necrosis associated with conspicuous emperipolesis of lymphocytes is described as one of the important findings in AIH (Fig. 3B) (Dienes, 1989; Dienes et al., 1989, 1991). Tanikawa et al. (1982) also disclosed ultrastructurally that hepatocytes adjacent to infiltrating plasma cells show severe cytopathic changes. The acidophilic bodies or apoptotic bodies (free acidophilic bodies or acidophilic cellular fragments in the sinusoid or hepatic plate framework) are also found in the majority of cases (Fig. 3B). The acidophilic cell damage appearing rhomboid or rectangle shaped, is not prominent, compared to non-A, non-B hepatitis (NANB) (Dienes et al., 1982). Confluent necrosis (zonal, bridging or submassive necrosis) is not uncommon (Figs. 7 and 8).

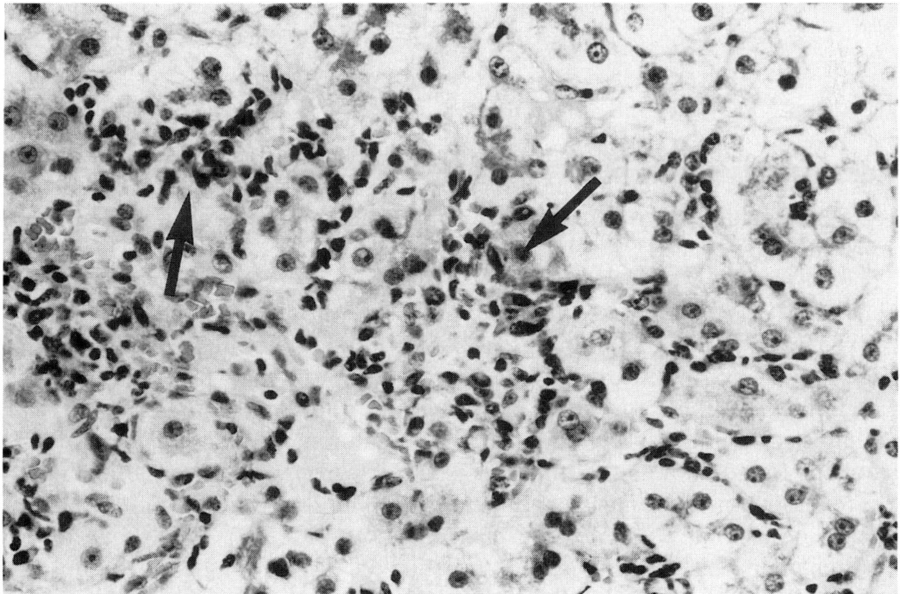

Fig. 6. Focal necroses are infiltrated by many plasma cells (arrows), and plasma cells are also predominant in sinusoids. AIH with predominant plasma cell infiltration. Hematoxylin-eosin stain.

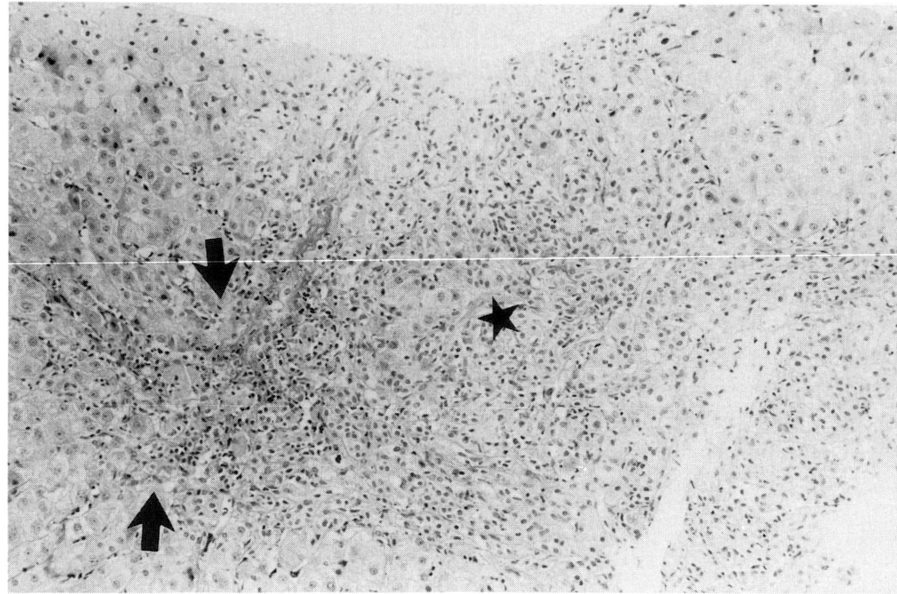

Fig. 7. Confluent necrosis or collapse with ductular proliferation and mononuclear cell infiltration is seen (★). Piecemeal necrosis (arrows) and sinusoidal reaction are also seen. AIH showing CAH with collapse and piecemeal necrosis. Hematoxylin–eosin stain.

Bile plugs and/or dilated bile canaliculi are usually seen in the perivenular areas in patients with acute hepatitic onset or CAH with bout-like exacerbations (Fig. 5). Pigmented macrophages in the portal tracts and hepatic parenchyma are also seen in these cases.

2.1.2. Marked mononuclear inflammatory cell infiltration

Marked mononuclear inflammatory cell infiltration in the enlarged portal tracts and septa and also in the surrounding parenchyma, producing piecemeal necrosis (vide infra) (Figs. 1, 2 and 10), is an important finding. The majority of these mononuclear cells are lymphocytes. Mature and immature plasma cells are also frequently found, though their number is variable from case to case or from one area to another in the same liver specimen. Lymphoid aggregates and/or follicles are also occasionally found in portal tracts (Dienes, 1989), which may reflect persistent hepatitis C virus (HCV) infection in AIH, though the pathologic significance of these lymph follicles or aggregates has not yet been ascertained (Onji et al., 1990; Lefkowitch et al., 1993). Prominent mononuclear infiltrates

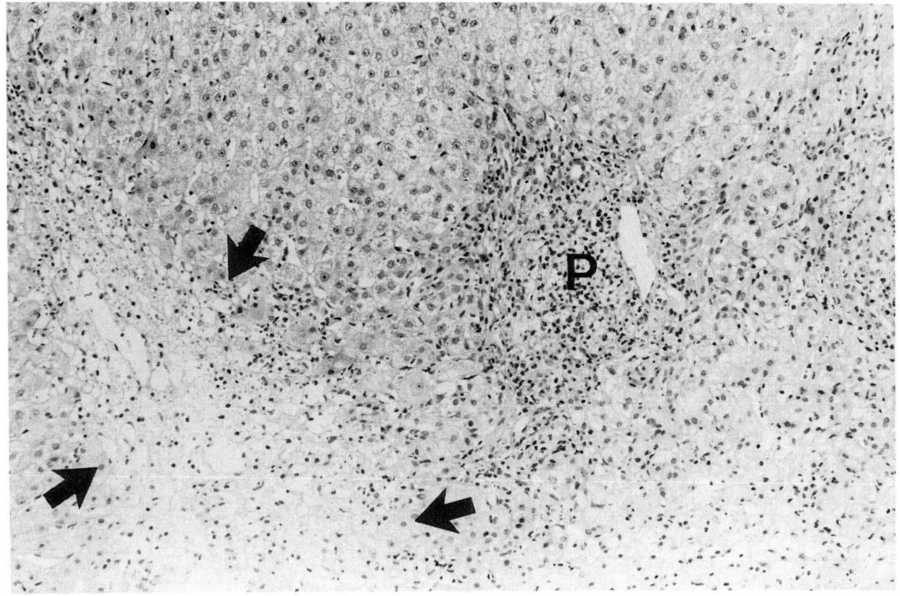

Fig. 8. Centrilobular zonal and bridging necrosis (fresh) (arrows) is seen in the liver showing CAH of the autoimmune type. Portal tract (P) shows moderate mononuclear cell infiltration and piecemeal necrosis. Hematoxylin–eosin stain.

in sinusoids with hyperplastic Kupffer cells and endothelial cells (sinusoidal reaction) are also a constant feature (Figs. 1–3, 5 and 6) (Dienes, 1989; Moteki et al., 1991).

Predominant infiltration of plasma cells, previously called plasma cell hepatitis (Good, 1956; Page and Good, 1960) was a synonym of AIH. Tanikawa and Maeyama (1982) also claimed that the identification of plasma cells is fairly easy under an electron microscope, and the degree of plasma cell infiltration in the liver is a good reflection of the serum level of γ-globulin. However, Dienes (1989) and Dienes et al. (1989, 1991) recently showed that marked plasma cell infiltration in the liver is not a prominent feature of AIH, and almost all their cases of AIH failed to show abundant plasma cell infiltration. Histologic survey of our AIH cases also disclosed that prominent plasma cell infiltration in the portal tracts (Fig. 10A), in piecemeal necrosis (Figs. 1 and 10A) or intra-lobular necrosis (Fig. 6) was found in about half the cases, while an abundance of plasma cells was not found in the rest. Furthermore, abundant plasma cell infiltration is not infrequently found in PBC and acute type A hepatitis and is, on occasion, in chronic

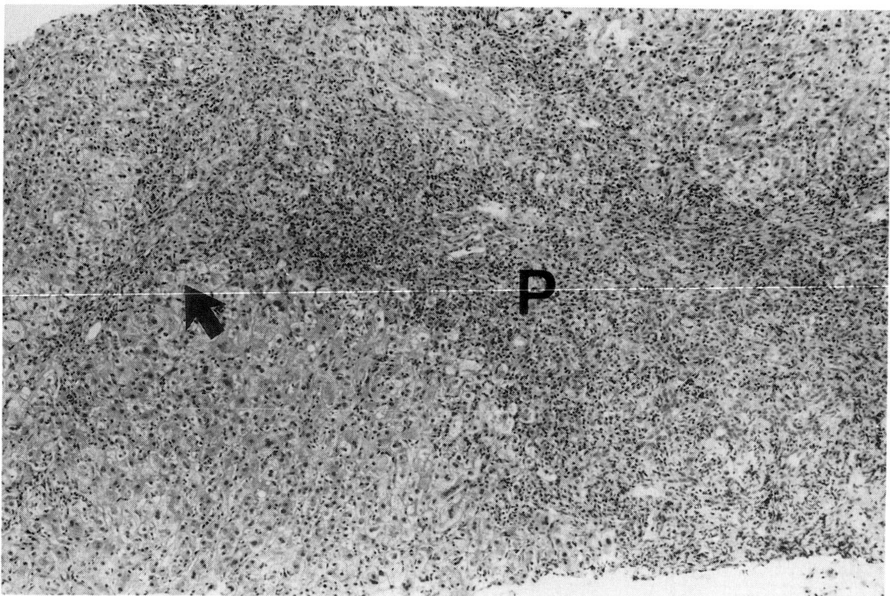

Fig. 9. Markedly enlarged portal tract (P) with mononuclear cell infiltration and bile duct proliferation. Piecemeal necrosis and fibrous bridge formation (arrow) are also seen. The parenchyma shows marked necroinflammatory cell infiltration. AIH of CAH. Hematoxylin–eosin stain.

viral hepatitis. For these reasons, Dienes et al. recommended the deletion of this name (plasma cell hepatitis) as a synonym of AIH (Dienes et al., 1989). Instead, they claimed that conspicuous emperipolesis of lymphocytes and ballooning and lytic necrosis of hepatocytes (Fig. 3B), in association with broad areas of collapse and acinar arrangement of hepatocytes, are characteristic of AIH (Dienes, 1989; Dienes et al., 1989), but these changes do not seem to be pathognomonic of AIH.

In addition to mononuclear cells, eosinophils and basophils are also reported admixed with these inflammatory cells (Fig. 10B), especially in piecemeal necrosis and around the portal venous branches, and a few AIH patients show prominent eosinophilic infiltration of the liver (Panush et al., 1973; Croffy et al., 1988; Foong et al., 1991; Foster et al., 1991). There are also variable degrees of ductular proliferation with polymorphonuclear neutrophilic infiltrates in the enlarged portal tracts and ductular cholestasis. Similar lesions are also seen in CAH of other etiologies (Wu et al., 1991) in livers with confluent necrosis. These ductular changes partially resemble large bile duct obstruction.

The peripheral zone of the hepatic parenchyma shows two remarkable alterations: piecemeal necrosis (Figs. 1, 2 and 7–9) and rosette formation (Fig. 4)

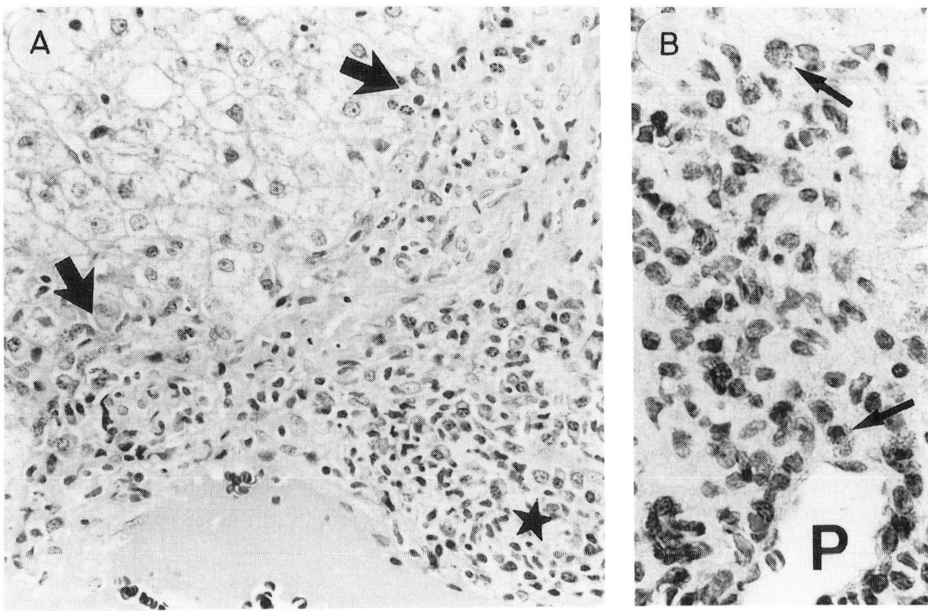

Fig. 10. A: many plasma cells are found in a portal tract (★) and also at limiting plate (arrows). B: a number of eosinophils are seen amongst the inflammatory cell infiltration in a portal tract. P, portal vein. AIH. Hematoxylin–eosin stain.

(Tanikawa and Maeyama, 1982; Hino, 1991). The former represents the destruction of limiting plates accompanied by an infiltrate of mononuclear cells. The latter is clusters of characteristic small acinar structures consisting of large, pale hepatocytes which are separated from one another and from the hepatic parenchyma by dense strands of reticulin fibers and a variable inflammatory cell infiltration. This lesion is regarded as one of the characteristic lesions in AIH and is frequently compared to CAH of other etiologies (Tanikawa and Maeyama, 1982; Hino, 1991). It may be formed by trapped hepatocytes in the fibrous septa by piecemeal or bridging necrosis. Ultrastructurally and immunohistochemically, some of the hepatocytes in rosette formation show features of bile ductules and some present findings of cell death (Tanikawa and Maeyama, 1982; Hino, 1991).

2.1.3. Regenerative process(es) of hepatocytes

Regenerative process(es) of hepatocytes are seen along with these necroinflammatory changes, as seen in other types of CAH: cluster of small and hydropic hepatocytes or cobble-stone appearance (Peters, 1978) usually around the portal tract or adjacent to the fibrous septa (Fig. 11), pleomorphic and multinucleated hepatocytes and poorly or well-developed regenerative nodules (Seki et al., 1991a, b). Acinar formation in the hepatic lobules and rosette formation (vide supra) may also reflect a process of hepatocellular regeneration (Hino, 1991). The features and degree of hepatocellular regeneration are variable, and tend to occur irregularly in the liver, and finally lead to the formation of regenerative nodules (Fig. 12) (Hino, 1991; Seki et al., 1991a, b; Lefkowitch, et al., 1993).

2.1.4. Fibrosis

Fibrosis, dense and loose, of varying degrees from enlarged portal tracts develops in the liver; incomplete septal or spur-like fibrosis and portal-to-portal (P–P) or portal-to-central (P–C) bridging fibrosis are found. The extent of fibrosis is variable within the liver specimen. Mononuclear cell infiltration in these septa is also frequently seen in AIH, suggesting an ongoing necroinflammatory process in the liver (Fig. 11). The relationship between fibrogenetic process(es) and immu-

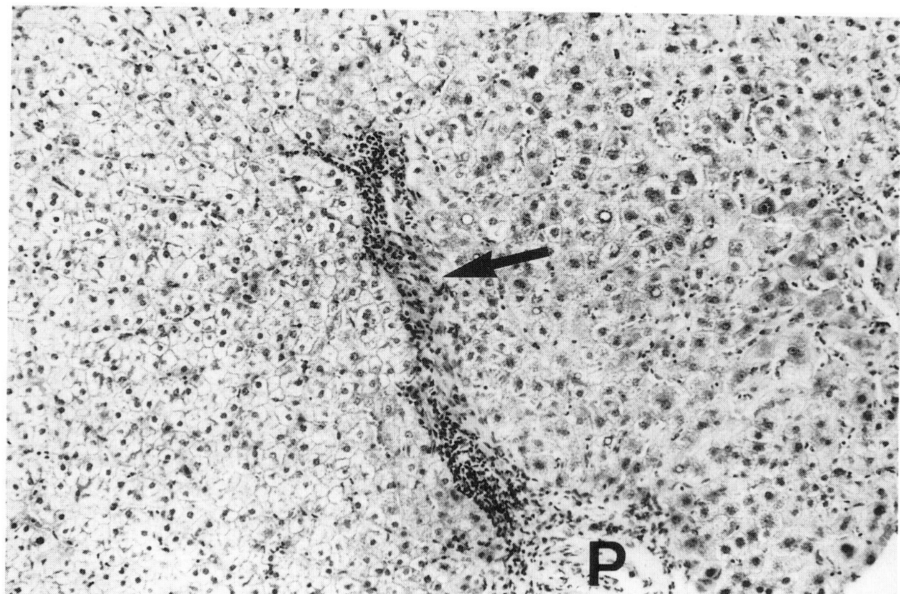

Fig. 11. Fibrous septa (arrow) extending from a portal tract (P) show mononuclear cell infiltration. The left half of the hepatic parenchyma shows cobble-stone appearance reflecting increased regenerative activity and the right half mild dysplastic change with necroinflammatory changes. AIH with CAH. Hematoxylin–eosin stain.

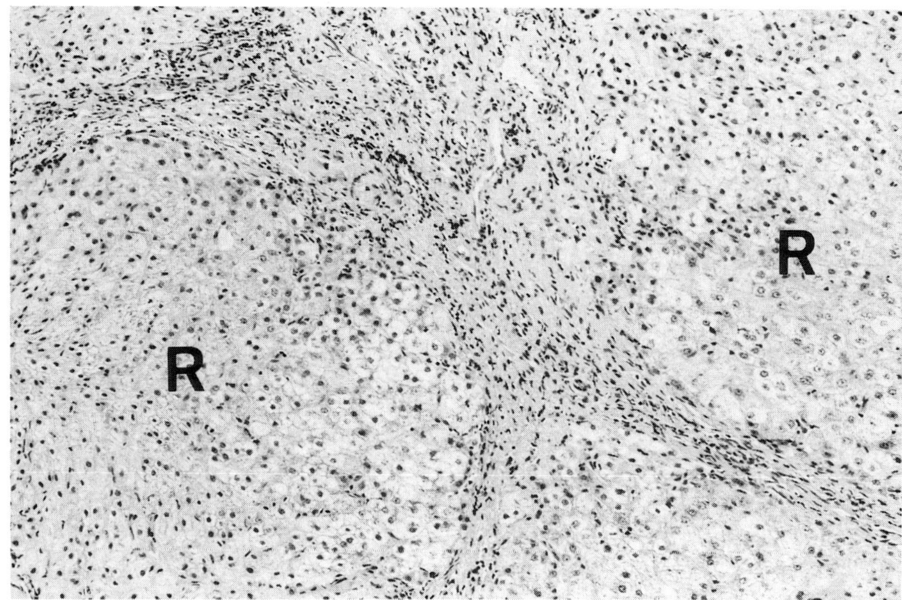

Fig. 12. Hepatocytes of regenerative nodules (R) are hydropic and piecemeal necrosis is seen here and there. Active liver cirrhosis of AIH. Hematoxylin–eosin stain.

nologic changes is only speculative in AIH. Perivenular fibrosis (Fig. 13) is more or less prominent in some cases of AIH, probably reflecting repeated and long-standing perivenular damage including zonal necrosis.

2.1.5. Hepatitic bile duct lesions

Hepatitic bile duct lesions occur infrequently in the intra-hepatic small- and, to a lesser degree, medium-sized inter-lobular bile ducts (Fig. 2) (Passwell et al., 1971; Yonekura et al., 1989), resembling those seen in chronic viral hepatitis (Poulsen–Christoffersen lesion) (Poulsen and Christoffersen, 1972; Vyberg, 1989; Lefkowitch et al., 1993). Persistent viral hepatitis infection may be related to this type of AIH. These bile ducts are surrounded by mononuclear cells or embedded in lymph follicles, and show infiltration of lymphocytes within the epithelial layer of the duct, variations in nuclear morphology and chromatinism, partial nuclear stratification, and vacuolization of biliary epithelial cells (Poulsen and Christoffersen, 1972; Scheuer 1980, 1988; Vyberg 1989; Yonekura et al., 1989). This bile duct lesion itself resembles chronic non-suppurative destructive cholangitis (CNSDC) characterizing PBC (Rubin et al., 1964), suggesting the participation of an immunologic mechanism. Several findings have been reported on the

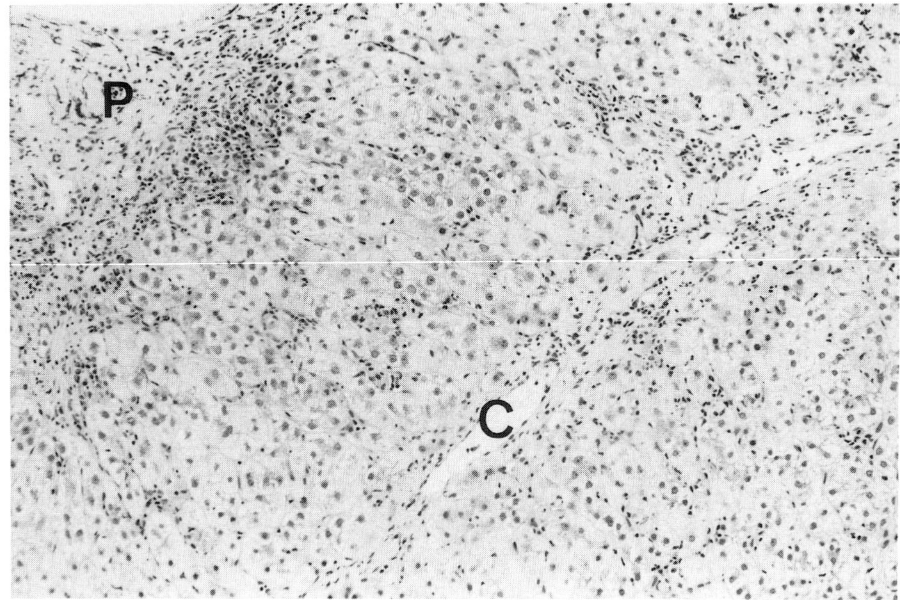

Fig. 13. A portal tract is enlarged (P) with fibrosis and mononuclear cell infiltration. Piecemeal necrosis, parenchymal necroinflammatory cell infiltration, and perivenular fibrosis (C) are seen. CAH of autoimmune type. Hematoxylin–eosin stain.

histologic differentiation from CNSDC: CNSDC is more or less widespread and frequently associated with epithelioid cell granulomas or reaction, bile epithelial rupture and acidophilic cytoplasmic alteration, while hepatitic bile duct lesions are rather focal and normal appearing bile ducts are usually found in the same portal tracts (Poulsen and Christoffersen, 1972; Scheuer, 1980, 1988; Vyberg, 1989; Carrougher et al., 1991). The former is finally followed by extensive loss of bile ducts, while the latter is not. Yonekura et al. (1989) examined the ultrastructural differences between hepatitic ductal lesions in AIH and CNSDC, and reported that in the former, there are point contacts between biliary epithelial cells and infiltrating mononuclear cells and preservation of the basal lamina, while in the latter, there are stratification of biliary epithelial cells, broad contacts between biliary epithelial cells and infiltrating mononuclear cells and also disruption of the basal lamina of the bile ducts.

2.2. Representative histologic patterns of AIH

It is generally accepted that there are several patterns of clinical presentation, including the onset and progression of AIH (Mistilis and Blackburn, 1970;

Matsushita et al., 1988). Such patterns may influence or even determine the histopathologic features of the liver. The following categories have been described in the literature: an acute onset similar to that of acute viral hepatitis, chronic hepatitis with repeated bout-like exacerbations; and an insidious and latent progressive form (Matsushita et al., 1988). Some are approaching liver cirrhosis or actually show regenerative nodules at the time of presentation. In addition, some patients fulfilling the clinical and serological criteria of AIH, especially older ones, present mild or no symptoms, and their livers show minimum to mild necroinflammatory changes.

In the great majority of AIH cases, the fundamental histologic changes mentioned above, are seen in various combinations in individual cases. The following histopathologic patterns or combinations are representative ones.

2.2.1. AIH cases presenting with acute hepatitic changes

Some cases which finally proved to be typical AIH, were initially diagnosed histologically as acute viral hepatitis (Scheuer 1980, 1988; Lefkowitch et al., 1984; Matsushita et al., 1988; Kamiyama et al., 1990; Lenzi et al., 1991). Some cases of AIH can present with clinical features of acute hepatic failure followed by death.

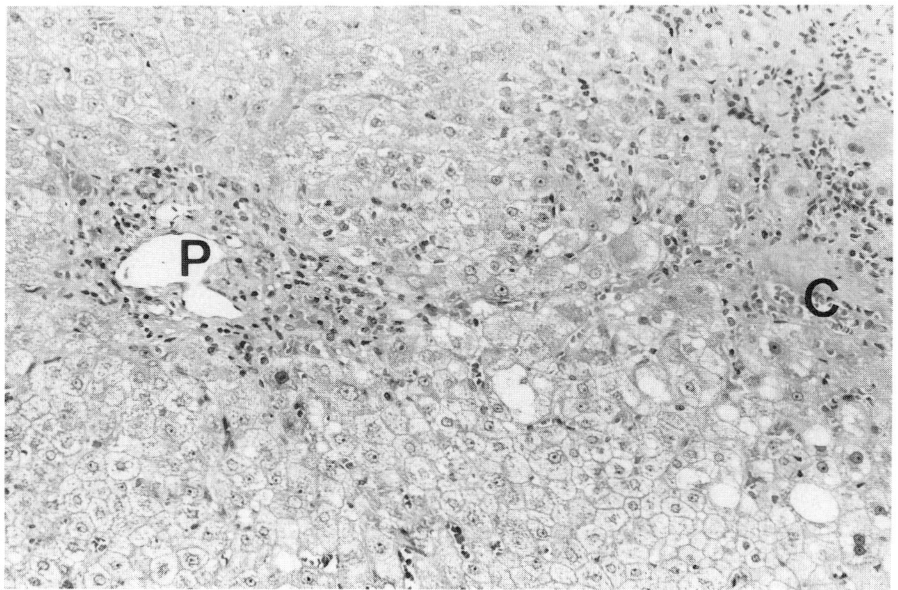

Fig. 14. Necroinflammatory changes are more or less concentrated in the perivenular area (C) (perivenular accentuation). A portal tract (P) shows mild inflammatory cell infiltration. AIH presenting with acute hepatitic changes. Hematoxylin–eosin stain.

Histologically, diffuse necroinflammatory changes with centrilobular accentuation (Fig. 14) and even perivenular zonal necrosis resembling acute viral hepatitis, particularly that of type B, are found in some cases, while such necroinflammatory changes are irregular in others. Bile plugs and/or dilated bile canaliculi are also seen. Pigmented macrophages and swollen Kupffer cells rather than mononuclear cells are prominent in these collapsed areas or confluent necrotic foci. In addition, P–P and/or P–C bridging necrosis or collapse are also frequently found. In fatal cases, submassive and massive hepatic necrosis is usually found at autopsy. The portal tracts are variably infiltrated by mononuclear cells, though the degree of infiltration is mild when compared to that of CAH (Kamiyama et al., 1990). A few portal tracts apparently lack inflammatory cell infiltration and in some cases, resemble drug-induced liver cell necrosis (Scheuer, 1980, 1988). Follow-up of these cases disclosed that some cases progressed to typical AIH after several bout-like exacerbations of hepatitic features (acute or chronic). Some survivors of confluent hepatocellular necrosis progress to CAH and active liver cirrhosis.

Some of these cases show total collapse of the left hepatic lobe or a major part of the right hepatic lobe, requiring differentiation from congenital hypoplasia of a hepatic lobe and other acquired atrophic hepatic disease.

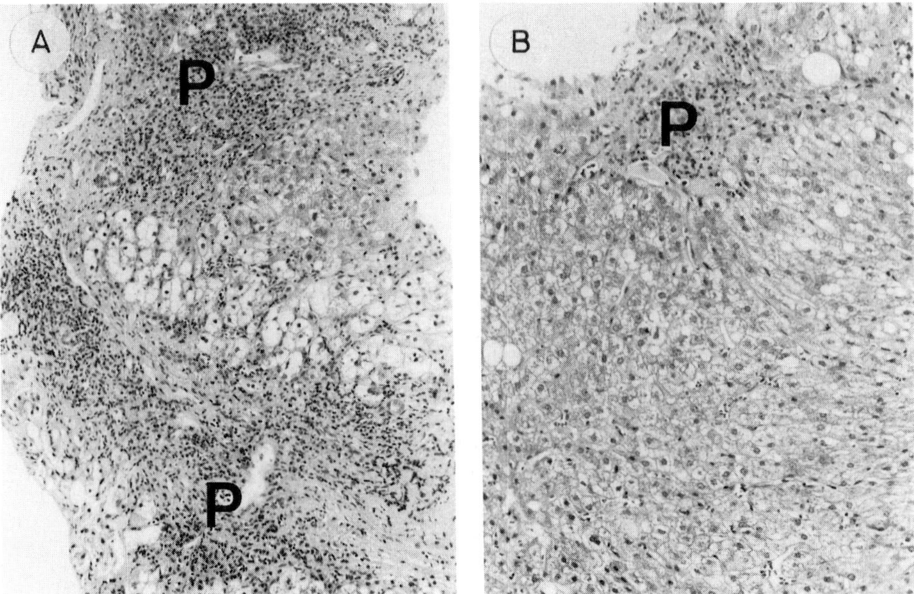

Fig. 15. Necroinflammatory changes with parenchymal loss and hepatocytic ballooning changes are seen in some parts (A) and such necroinflammatory changes are minimum in other parts (B) of the same liver specimen. P, portal tract. AIH showing CAH. Hematoxylin–eosin stain.

2.2.2. AIH cases presenting with CAH and bout-like exacerbation

The portal tracts are enlarged with marked mononuclear cell infiltration (Figs. 2 and 9), and there are areas of prominent piecemeal necrosis with mononuclear infiltration and variable fibrosis extending from the portal tracts. Considerable necroinflammatory changes are simultaneously found in the parenchyma. In addition, perivenular zonal necrosis and marked hydropic changes of the hepatocytes with occasional bile plugs are frequently found (Fig. 15). Confluent necrosis including C–C, P–C and P–P bridging necroses is not uncommon (Figs. 7 and 8). Inflammatory cell infiltration in perivenular zonal necrosis or bridging necrosis is variable, though more or less weak as seen in cases with acute hepatitic changes. Necroinflammatory changes in the hepatic parenchyma are more or less diffuse in some cases, while these changes, as well as portal tract inflammation with piecemeal necrosis, are irregularly distributed in the same liver specimen in other cases.

2.2.3. AIH cases presenting with CAH

Histologic features suggestive of viral CAH with mild to moderate portal inflammation and piecemeal necrosis are also seen in some cases of AIH. The distribution of these necroinflammatory changes is usually irregular from one hepatic lobule or portal tract to another (Peters, 1978). One or two portal tracts and hepatic lobules seem apparently normal in some parts (Fig. 15A, B), while others show moderate to marked necroinflammatory changes in the same liver specimen. Lymphoid aggregates and/or follicle formation are also variably found. It is of utmost importance that histologic differentiation is made between such types of AIH and virus-induced CAH.

2.2.4. Cirrhotic stage of AIH and complication of hepatocellular carcinoma

Liver cirrhosis in AIH tends to be of the postnecrotic type with active necroinflammatory changes (Sherlock, 1985; Motoo et al., 1988). The extent and degree of necroinflammatory changes are variable within the liver specimen; some parts are of active cirrhosis and others of inactive cirrhosis (Fig. 12). Some cases show bridging necrosis. It is generally said that about 20% of cases of AIH are already cirrhotic when they are first clinically detected (Soloway et al., 1972; Tanikawa and Maeyama, 1982). Infrequently, AIH at the cirrhotic stage, is complicated by hepatocellular carcinoma (HCC) (Arima et al., 1987; Wang and Czaja, 1988; Motoo et al., 1988). Wang and Czaja (1988) reported that AIH patients treated with corticosteroids are at risk for HCC, and this risk is greatest in patients with cirrhosis of at least 5 years' duration. However, a recent surveillance study of HCV-related protein markers and/or HCV-RNA by polymerase chain reaction (PCR) disclosed that the majority of AIH cases complicated with HCC were positive for both tests for HCV (Arima et al., 1987), and it seems likely that the majority of AIH cases associated with HCC reported so far might have been superimposed by HCV infection.

Histopathologically, this type of HCC was no different from HCC found in other types of liver cirrhosis, though some cases showed marked infiltration of lymphocytes within the HCC tissue (Imamura et al., 1991). Such infiltration is also occasionally found in HCC arising in chronic liver disease unrelated to AIH.

2.2.5. *AIH cases presenting with mild necroinflammatory changes*
Some cases fulfilling serological and clinical characteristics of AIH show mild necroinflammatory changes (mild CAH, CPH, and non-specific reactive hepatitis (NSRH), though it remains unresolved whether such patients could be regarded as having AIH or not, especially from the diagnostic, clinical and pathological standpoints. Piecemeal necrosis and inflammatory activity are mild or lower, and cellular polymorphism and anisocytosis of hepatocytes is less conspicuous or absent (Dienes et al., 1989; Dienes, 1991). However, some cases show thin fibrous septa extending from the fibrotic portal tracts. These cases represent sampling errors of liver specimens or spontaneous remission of AIH at the time of liver biopsy.

It is shown retrospectively that some of those cases of AIH with minimum to mild necroinflammatory changes finally become typical AIH with prominent necroinflammatory changes (Lefkowitch et al., 1984; Lenzi et al., 1991).

2.2.6. *AIH cases with atypical features*
A few cases of AIH show peripheral eosinophilia and also prominent eosinophilic infiltration in addition to mononuclear cells in the portal tracts and periportal regions (Panush et al., 1973; Croffy et al., 1988), suggesting that secretory products of eosinophils may also be involved in immunologic hepatocellular damage in AIH. Cytokines or chemotactic factors released from T-cells or other inflammatory cells are responsible for such liver tissue and peripheral blood eosinophilia. These patients with eosinophilia show atypical features; young men are preferentially affected, the serum gammaglobulinemia is not striking, and an association with extra-hepatic autoimmune diseases is lacking. An anti-body-dependent cell-mediated cytotoxicity (ADCC) mechanism involving eosinophils may be involved in this instance.

Thijs et al. (1985) reported that postinfantile giant-cell hepatitis presents multiple autoimmune features including positive liver membrane antibodies (LMA) and LE cells. Active necroinflammation and the occurrence of many multinucleated giant cells were found histologically. The clinical and laboratory findings responded well to immunosuppressive therapy.

It remains, however, unclarified whether or not such AIH patients with atypical features should be regarded as a subtype of AIH. More data about the characteristics of autoantibodies and target tissues are mandatory for this issue.

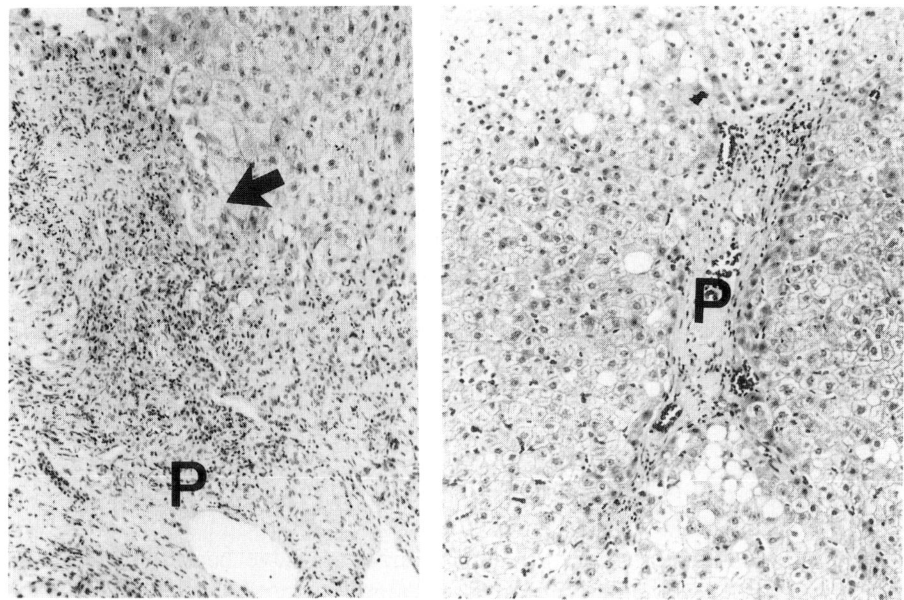

Fig. 16. Marked necroinflammatory changes with portal fibrosis and mononuclear cell infiltration and piecemeal necrosis (arrow) (left) disappear after steroid therapy (right) in the same case. Mild fatty changes may reflect an adverse effect of steroid therapy. P, portal tract. Chronic active hepatitis of the autoimmune type. Hematoxylin–eosin stain.

2.2.7. Hepatic histopathologies after steroid or immunosuppressive therapy

Almost all cases of AIH, either with a histologic pattern of acute hepatitis or CAH with or without bout-like exacerbations (Fig. 16, left), often respond well clinically, serologically and also histopathologically to specific therapies such as corticosteroids or azathioprine (Fig. 16, right) (Mackay et al., 1956; Kamiyama et al., 1990; Tassoni and Kaplan, 1991). Active cirrhosis also becomes inactive (Takahashi et al., 1977; Kuroki et al., 1984). In particular, necroinflammatory changes and hepatocellular swelling in hepatic lobules, piecemeal necrosis and portal lymphoplasmacytic infiltration regress considerably and may even disappear, and hepatocytic regenerative activities become diffuse in the liver specimen of many patients with AIH. Hepatitic bile duct lesions and liver tissue eosinophilia found in some AIH patients also regress after steroid therapy (Passwell et al., 1971; Croffy et al., 1988). Non-specific reactive changes, mild ductular proliferation in the portal tracts, CPH or mild hepatic fibrosis with acellular fibrous septa are the only histologic findings after therapy (Fig. 16, right). Some AIH cases show an almost normal liver in some parts and paren-chymal nodules surrounded by acellular and thin fibrous septa in other parts of the same liver specimen. Mild to moderate fatty changes are, on occasion, found in the hepatic parenchyma, probably reflecting an adverse effect of the steroid therapy. The prognosis of AIH patients has improved since the introduction of these immunosuppressive therapies.

While ursodeoxycholic acid (UDCA) is known to be effective against hepatic necroinflammatory changes in PBC, the overlapping syndrome of PBC and CAH, and PSC (vide infra), such therapy has not been tried in AIH to the best of our knowledge.

In relapses or acute exacerbations after the discontinuance of steroid therapy, the necroinflammatory changes flare up in the liver while these relapsed necroin-flammatory changes again regress after the resumption of steroid therapy.

3. *Immunopathology and pathogenesis of AIH*

Immunologic and immunopathologic disturbances have been found in AIH (Johnson and McFarlane, 1993). Some are causally related to AIH, while others may be the result of immunologic disturbances of the liver or an epiphenomenon of immunologic defects inherent in the AIH patients. Disturbances of the immunoregulation system, targets of autoimmune attacks and effector mechan-isms should be taken into consideration in the pathogenesis of AIH (Paronetto et al., 1986; Meyer zum Büschenfelde, 1991). In this section, the immunopatho-logic data reported so far are briefly reviewed.

The immunoregulation system, especially suppressor T-cell function, is known to be abnormal in AIH, allowing polyclonal B-cell activation and the occurrence of a kind of autoantibody and hypergammaglobulinemia (Coovadia et al., 1981; Vento et al., 1984; Paronetto et al., 1986). One hypothesis is that AIH only occurs in those individuals with a genetically determined liver cell surface antigen-specific T-cell suppressor–inducer defect, and develops T-lymphocyte reactivity to the hepatocyte-specific ASGP-R (vide infra). Some environmental factor(s) (virus, hormone or drug) may be important as a trigger of this lymphocytic reaction (Tassoni and Kaplan, 1991). However, cellular immunity to this receptor is also found in patients with PBC and viral CAH (McFarlane et al., 1986; Vento et al., 1986; Lohr et al., 1990). There have also been considerable studies on the immunological disturbances in soluble factors and also the lymphocytes in the peripheral blood in AIH patients (Vento and Eddleston, 1987).

Recent investigations have identified candidate surface membrane antigens expressed on the hepatocytes, and autoantibodies against these antigens may significantly contribute to the persistence of liver injury in AIH (Whittingham et al., 1966; Hopf et al., 1976; McFarlane, 1984; Manns et al., 1987; Lohr et al., 1990): anti-LMA; anti-LKM antibodies, and anti-liver specific protein (LSP). The anti-LSP antibodies include anti-hepatic lectin or ASGP-R antibodies (McFarlane et al., 1986; Lohr et al., 1990) which are detected in about 50% of cases of AIH (more than 80% in AIH with active phases) and are regarded as being important in the development of AIH. ASGP-R may possibly be one of numerous antigens to which autoimmune reactions are directed when unresponsiveness to 'self' antigens on the liver cells is disturbed. IgG can be detected on hepatocytes isolated from biopsy specimens from AIH patients and the pattern of immunofluorescence is generally linear, suggesting an antibody reaction against antigens diffusely distributed on the cell membranes (Hopf et al., 1976). CD4-positive T-cells and antigen-presenting cells (interdigitating and dentritic cells) are found in the mononuclear cell infiltration and at the periportal areas of the lobules in AIH (Montano et al., 1983; Bardadin and Desmet, 1984; Lohr et al., 1990). HLA-class II (HLA-DR) antigens which are cell surface glycoproteins and important in antigen presentation, are also focally positive in some of these hepatocytes where necroinflammatory changes occur (Van den Oord et al., 1990).

As to the effector system, chronic liver cell injuries in AIH are thought to be mediated by T-cells infiltrating the liver tissue by cytotoxic activity or by releasing cytokines that attract bystander T-cells or damage hepatocytes (Lohr et al., 1990). The morphologies reflecting immune-mediated hepatocellular necrosis such as emperipolesis of lymphocytes (Fig. 3B) or point or broad contacts between hepatocytes and lymphocytes are known at the foci of piecemeal necrosis and intra-lobular necrosis (Paronetto et al., 1986). Recent studies favor the concept that acidophilic bodies or apoptosis are indicative of lymphocytic immune attacks (Kerr et al., 1979). The majority of infiltrating lymphocytes at the piecemeal necrosis and in and around focal and spotty necrosis in hepatic lobules are CD8-positive cytotoxic T-cells (Lohr et al., 1990). HLA-class I or β_2-micro-globulin is strongly expressed on the hepatocytes at these necroinflammatory changes. These HLA-class I-positive hepatocytes may simultaneously present ASGP-R to the autoimmune reactive T-cells. Recent studies demonstrated the presence of a significant number of ASGP-R-specific T-cells with interleukin-2 (IL-2) receptors among the liver-infiltrating T-cells in AIH (Lohr et al., 1990). Otherwise, Hino recently disclosed that plasma cells and lymphocytes, especially natural killer cells, are in contact with the hepatocytes forming the rosettes, suggesting the participation of ADCC (Hino, 1991), and HLA-class II-restricted CD4-positive T-cells could destroy hepatocytes (Nouri-Aria et al., 1982).

There is growing evidence that the pathophysiologic manifestations of many diseases are due to the production or expression of a variety of polypeptide products known as cytokines and adhesion molecules (Van den Oord et al., 1990). Major sources of cytokines are leukocytes of the immune system, but other tissues can probably also produce them. Adhesion molecules are expressed on the target tissues and also vascular endothelial cells. The localization of these products is now being extensively studied in accordance with recent technical break-throughs in the understanding of the immune system.

Secretory products released from granules of eosinophils such as eosinophilic cationic protein and major basic proteins which are known to cause cell injuries, have recently been suspected of initiating hepatocellular damage in CAH occurring in the idiopathic hypereosinophilic syndrome (Foong et al., 1991). A similar phenomenon has also been recently reported in hepatic allograft rejection (Foster et al., 1991). Secretory products or granules were demonstrated in the extra-cellular spaces in these diseases (Foong et al., 1991; Foster et al., 1991). In the majority of AIH cases, eosinophils are found in liver tissue, especially in inflammed portal tracts (Fig. 10B). These eosinophils may play a role in liver cell necrosis by releasing secretory products. Otherwise, these eosinophils are bystander cells of inflammation or participated in down-regulation of necroinflammation rather than in the initiation and aggravation of necroinflammation.

Finally, the precise characterization and localization of target antigen(s), clarification of phenotypes and functions of infiltrating immunocompetent cells, and of immunoregulation including cytokines and adhesion molecules and also their distribution in liver tissue seem mandatory to evaluate the immunopathology and pathogenesis of AIH.

4. *Histopathology and immunopathology of immune-mediated hepatocellular damage in several other autoimmune hepatobiliary diseases, including histopathologic differentiation from AIH*

Scheuer claimed that CAH is not a disease entity, but a collective term with a histologic constellation of progressive and active necroinflammatory changes of the liver persisting more than 6 months (Scheuer, 1980). There are heterogeneous etiologies of CAH: chronic hepatitis by HBV, HCV and hepatitis D virus (HDV) infection; autoimmune processes without other evident etiologies; Wilson's disease; and adverse reactions to certain therapeutic drugs. CAH is also recognized in several hepatobiliary diseases primarily involving the biliary tree such as PBC and PSC. Piecemeal necrosis with variable parenchymal necroinflammatory changes is a hallmark of CAH and reflects an immune-mediated hepatocellular necrosis, though it remains unclear whether or not similar or identical liver histologies mean the participation of the same immunopathologic mechanism in the liver. Anyway, these necroinflammations associated with irregular hepatocellular regeneration are followed by the development of cirrhosis with CAH (Peters, 1978).

It is generally accepted that patients with CAH, especially those with marked hypergammaglobulinemia and autoimmune phenomena, tend to show similar histopathologies of the liver, irrespective of their etiologies (Soloway et al., 1972; Tassoni and Kaplan 1991). It seems impossible to make a definite diagnosis of AIH purely from the histopathological findings at present. However, several findings suggesting etiologies such as marked copper deposition and orcein-positive inclusion in the hepatocytes indicate a diagnosis of Wilson's disease and HBV infection, respectively. The exclusion of other possible etiologies is helpful in making a histologic diagnosis of AIH.

Some AIH patients presenting with an acute onset had histological features resembling acute viral hepatitis. Thus, acute viral hepatitis is also one of the diseases which needs a differential diagnosis from AIH.

The hepatobiliary diseases in which autoimmune hepatocellular necrosis may occur and histologic differentiation from AIH is necessary, are reviewed from the standpoint of hepatic histopathology.

4.1. PBC (chronic non-suppurative destructive cholangitis)

PBC and AIH are classical autoimmune diseases of the liver, though the main target antigens seem different in both diseases. In PBC, in addition to chronic cholestatic features, autoimmune phenomena, such as the occurrence of non-organ specific autoantibodies including anti-mitochondrial antibodies (AMA) (more than 90% of PBC patients), anti-actin antibody, anti-DNA antibody (about 25%), and ANA (about 50%), and also an elevation of IgM, are found (Berg and Klein, 1989; Moteki et al., 1991).

Histologically, the inter-lobular bile ducts are mainly damaged by the auto-immune mechanism, though the characterization of target antigens (probably self-antigens) of the biliary epithelial cells is challenging (Van de Water et al., 1993). This ductal lesion is characterized by mononuclear cell infiltration and epithelioid cells around the damaged bile ducts (CNSDC) (Rubin et al., 1964; Nakanuma and Ohta, 1983; Scheuer, 1980, 1988; Portmann et al., 1985; Port-mann and MacSween, 1987). Aberrant and increased expression of HLA-DR and -class I antigens on the damaged biliary epithelial cells and infiltration of CD8 + cytotoxic cells in the biliary epithelial layer are now regarded to reflect immu-nologic processes in PBC (Yamada et al., 1986; Mackay and Gershwin, 1989; Nakanuma and Kono, 1991).

In addition to the bile duct damage, there are a number of histopathologic changes in the liver in PBC. The parenchymal changes can be divided into two kinds of lesions: chronic cholestatic and hepatitic changes (Nakanuma et al., 1981; Nakanuma and Ohta, 1983; Portmann et al., 1985; Nakanuma et al., 1990). Chronic cholestatic changes which reflect biliary secretory failure due to exten-sive bile duct loss or damage, are characterized by cholate stasis, deposition of copper granules, atypical ductular proliferation, feathery degeneration, biliary fibrosis and so on (Scheuer, 1980, 1988; Nakanuma et al., 1990).

Hepatitic alterations characterized by intra-lobular hepatitic changes (focal and spotty hepatocellular necroses, acidophilic bodies, Kupffer cell hyperplasia and sinusoidal lymphocytic infiltration) (Fig. 17) and piecemeal necrosis, are

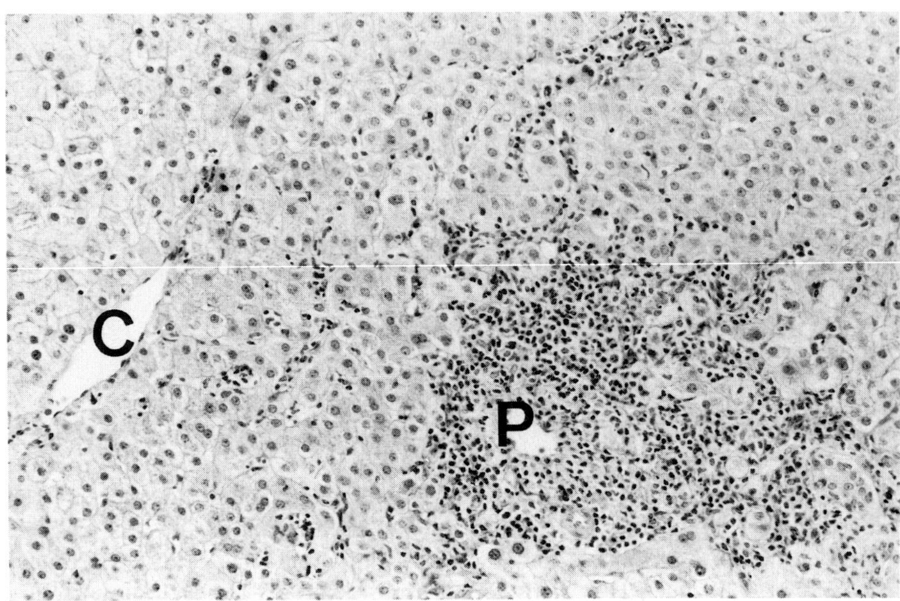

Fig. 17. Marked mononuclear cell infiltration in a portal tract (P) with marked piecemeal necrosis and parenchymal hepatitic changes. C, central vein. Stage 2 PBC.

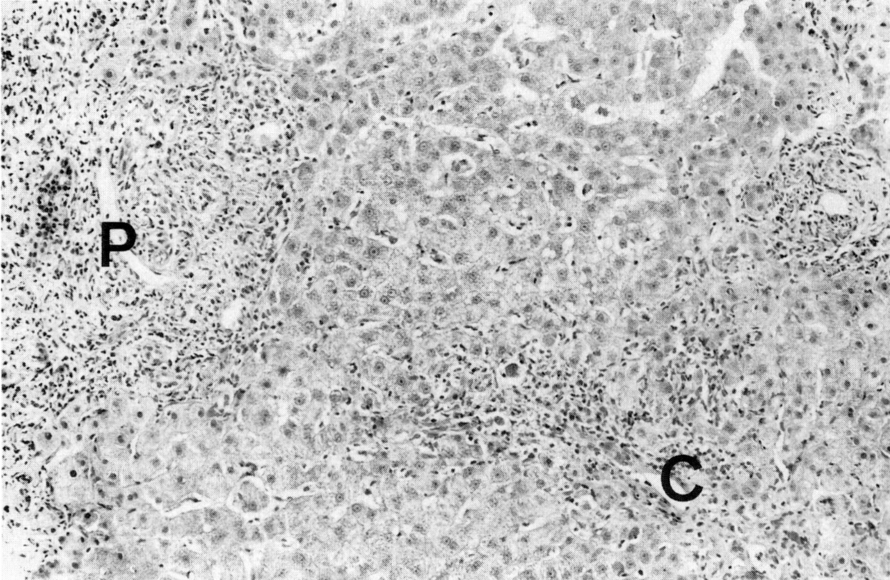

Fig. 18. A portal tract (P) is enlarged with fibrosis and mononuclear cell infiltration. In addition, there is centrilobular zonal necrosis with acidophilic bodies. C, central vein. Stage 2 PBC.

usually mild, but inherent in PBC (Hadziyannis et al., 1970; Nakanuma et al., 1990). Of great interest is that a few cases of PBC show perivenular zonal necrosis or P–P or P–C bridging necrosis (Fig. 18) (Nakanuma, 1993a). These hepatitic changes develop in the absence of measurable markers suggestive of persistent HBV and HCV infection (Nakanuma, 1993a). They tend to be found in the liver with less cholestatic changes. It is generally accepted that autoimmune process(es) are likely responsible for the development of these hepatitic changes as speculated in AIH (McFarlane et al., 1986; Vento et al., 1986; Lohr et al., 1990). Although response to steroid therapy is speculated as being valuable in the differentiation of AIH from PBC (Geubel et al., 1976), this has not yet been confirmed. Recent studies disclosed that such hepatitic changes including portal inflammation in PBC respond well to UDCA therapy (Matsuzaki et al., 1990; Terasaki et al., 1991).

Although these cholestatic and hepatitic features are found simultaneously in the same liver, semi-quantitative analysis disclosed that the great majority of PBC cases tend to belong to one of 3 types (Nakanuma et al., 1990). One type shows significant hepatitic changes (hepatitic PBC). Other cases of PBC predominantly show chronic cholestatic changes of the liver with a mild degree of necroinflammatory changes (cholestatic PBC). There are, however, no differences in the occurrence of non-organ-specific autoantibodies including AMA and ANA, serum γ-globulin, age and sex between cholestatic and hepatitic PBC (Nakanuma et al., 1990). In individual patients, both of these types tend to persist and progress to cirrhosis (Nakanuma et al., 1990).

The last type shows minimum to mild hepatitic changes as well as cholestatic changes in the hepatic parenchyma, though portal inflammation and non-suppurative cholangitis are predominant. Almost all cases of this type belong to stage 1 PBC (Scheuer, 1980, 1988; Nakanuma et al., 1981). Follow-up study of these cases shows that this type finally progresses to either the hepatitic or cholestatic type, as mentioned above.

It is generally believed that PBC progresses to true cirrhosis after extensive loss of inter-lobular bile ducts and prolonged bile secretory failure. However, some PBC patients, especially those with the hepatitic type, could progress to cirrhosis without extensive loss of inter-lobular bile ducts, that is, with less cholestatic changes (Popper, 1978; Nakanuma et al., 1990), though there has been no definite evidence of this progression.

Immunohistochemistry has disclosed that the majority of infiltrating lymphoid cells in the parenchyma and also at the limiting plates are positive for UCHL-1 and also CD8 +, suggestive of activated, cytotoxic T-cells (Van den Oord et al., 1984; Nakanuma et al., 1990), while B-cells are more or less predominant in the central parts of the portal tracts and also at the limiting plates showing ductular proliferation (Van den Oord 1984; Nakanuma et al., 1990). Infiltrating lymphocytes in hepatic lobules are also cytotoxic T-cells and similar to viral CAH or AIH. HLA-class I antigens or β_2-microglobulin are expressed on the hepatocytes at piecemeal necrosis or adjacent to intra-lobular hepatocellular necrotic foci. Some of the perivenular atrophic hepatocytes also display these antigens on their cellular membranes in PBC. HLA-DR antigens are expressed on the cell membranes of some hepatocytes at piecemeal necrosis (Terasaki et al., 1991). Recently, ASGP-R has been suspected of being a target antigen for liver-infiltrating T-cells in PBC as reported in AIH (McFarlane et al., 1986; Vento et al., 1986; Lohr et al., 1990).

In PBC, however, microgranulomatous changes or epithelioid cell reactions are frequently associated or admixed with hepatocellular necrosis, including perivenular zonal necrosis and bridging necrosis (vide supra) (Nakanuma, 1993b), appearing as a component of hepatocellular necroinflammation. Such changes are usually absent in AIH or viral CAH. Granulomatous changes are a component of CNSDC in the portal tract, suggesting that a granulomatous reaction is a basic finding of biliary as well as hepatocellular damage in PBC, probably reflecting the participation of a particular immunologic mechanism. These findings also suggest that hepatocellular necrosis could be a consistent feature of PBC.

From the standpoint of histopathologic differentiation, considerable deposition of copper granules or copper-binding proteins in periportal or periseptal hepatocytes favors a diagnosis of PBC rather than AIH (Miyamura et al., 1988).

Of great interest is that UDCA therapy restores the abnormal expression of HLA antigens on the hepatocytes in addition to the regressing necroinflammatory changes in PBC livers. We have recently shown immunohistochemically HLA-class I antigens on the hepatocytes of PBC, which disappeared after UDCA therapy (Terasaki et al., 1991). UCHL-1-positive, activated T-cells also regressed or disappeared in the hepatic parenchyma or at piecemeal necrosis. As to the expression HLA-class I antigens on hepatocellular membranes, chronic cholestasis is probably responsible in PBC (Terasaki et al., 1991). Thus, immunologic attack (probably T-cell-mediated cytotoxicity) against ASGP-R on the hepatocellular membranes which also express HLA-class I may cease after UDCA therapy. That is, UDCA restores the severely damaged liver cells caused by the toxic effects of several hydrophobic bile acids to the less damaged liver cells with less or no expression of HLA-class I antigens, and regresses, thereby, necroinflammatory changes in PBC. However, UDCA may directly alter the immunologic conditions inherent in PBC patients and then defend the hepatocytes and biliary epithelial cells from these immunologic attacks.

4.2. *Combination or overlapping syndrome of CAH and PBC (hepatitis and cholangitis)*

This combination/overlapping syndrome was originally described by Popper and Schaffner (1970). Their description was brief, but very meaningful and contributed a great deal to the progress of this field. It actually opened the new era of the immunopathological studies of PBC, CAH and cholangitis–hepatitis overlapping syndrome. Since then, several cases fulfilling the descriptions of Popper and Schaffner (1970) have been reported (Passwell et al., 1971; Kloppel et al., 1977; Brunner and Klinge, 1987; Okuno et al., 1987; Yonekura et al., 1989; Carrougher et al., 1991; Shibuya et al., 1991; Ben-Ari et al., 1993). However, this condition still remains poorly understood and incompletely characterized and defined, so that the cases and studies reported so far under the concept of an overlapping syndrome, seem heterogeneous. Several terminologies for this condition have caused some confusion in its recognition. In addition, the occurrence of AMA is also quite variable in this syndrome. AMA are negative in some cases (Carrougher et al., 1991; Shibuya et al., 1991), while some cases show positive AMA, and the occurrence of their subtypes is also variable (Kloppel et al., 1977; Moteki et al., 1991).

In this syndrome, both hepatocytes and biliary epithelial cells of the intra-hepatic small bile ducts are target tissues by autoimmune destructive attack(s). The following types or conditions are included in this syndrome.

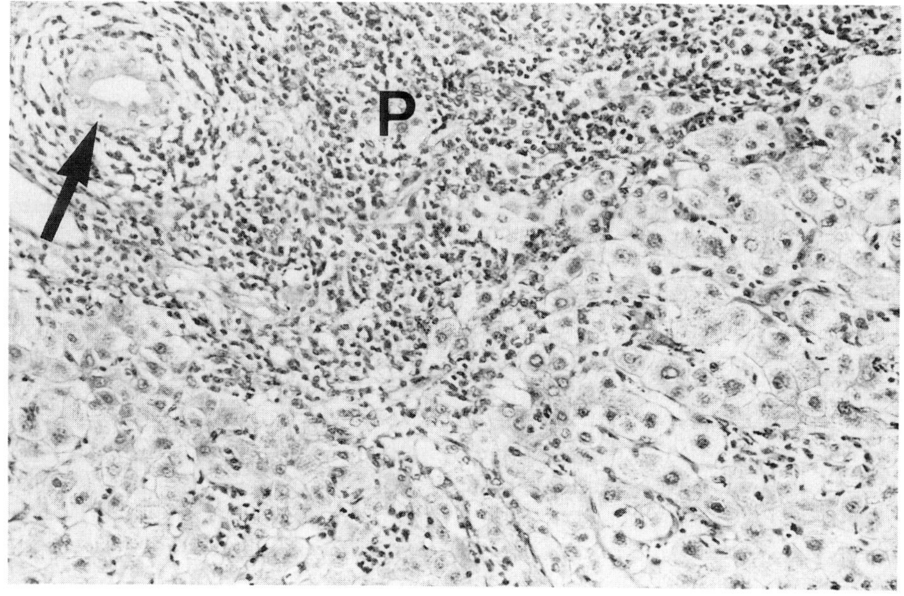

Fig. 19. Marked mononuclear cell infiltration in a portal tract (P) and piecemeal necrosis. The hepatic parenchyma also shows hepatitic changes and sinusoidal reaction. One inter-lobular bile duct (arrow) shows inflammatory change. PBC superimposed with HCV infection. Hematoxlin-eosin stain.

4.2.1. PBC associated with AIH

LE cell phenomena or high-titered ANA, antibodies to actin and hypergam-maglobulinemia are usually associated with this condition, and histologically, both of CNSDC and AIH were simultaneously found (Moteki et al., 1987). Distinction of this type of overlapping syndrome from PBC associated with systemic lupus erythematosus (SLE) is, however, necessary. Some overlapping cases begin as PBC, and AIH subsequently develops during the long course of PBC. That is, these PBC patients may present acute hepatitic changes in clinical and laboratory findings. The histopathologic findings of acute hepatitis are usually superimposed on the PBC liver, showing bile duct damage. Some cases start as AIH from the beginning and a biopsy has incidentally disclosed typical CNSDC. These cases are now regarded as a superimposition of AIH and PBC. Distinction of this syndrome from PBC with prominent hepatitic changes and with low-titered ANA is still subjective.

4.2.2. Superimposition of viral hepatitis in PBC

Persistent viral hepatitis, especially type C and type B viral infection in PBC, could explain some cases of this hepatitis–cholangitis overlapping syndrome, though the proportion of such cases is not significant. We have recently experienced a PBC patient (a 46-year-old female) who presented with repeated bout-like jaundice and elevated transaminase levels. Serial liver biopsies showed marked necroinflammatory changes including piecemeal necrosis (Fig. 19) and also the findings of PBC (CNSDC and deposition of copper-binding protein granules in periportal hepatocytes). Finally, she died of hepatic failure and several HCC nodules were found at autopsy. Her preserved serum was found to be positive for HCV-viral marker and also HCV-RNA by PCR.

Persistent HCV infection should be taken into consideration when liver histology of PBC shows marked hepatitic changes. It is generally believed that superimposition of HCV or HBV infection in PBC accelerates the histologic progress of PBC and also leads to the development of HCC in some cases, though confirmative data are not yet available.

4.2.3. PBC–CAH mixed type

Berg et al. (1980, 1985) and Kloppel et al. (1977) classified AMA into several subtypes according to their corresponding antigens (M1–8) and described several clinicopathologic features and different prognoses according to the occurrence of subtypes of AMA (Berg et al., 1980, 1985; Homberg et al., 1982; Klein et al., 1984). Among them, anti-M2 (PBC antigen, AMA directed against inner membranes of mitochondria) positive cases were typical of PBC: CNSDC and bile duct loss; chronic cholestasis leading to biliary cirrhosis; and less necroinflammatory changes of the hepatic parenchyma.

In addition, anti-M2 as well as anti-M4 AMA-positive cases with or without anti-M8 (AMA directed against outer membranes of mitochondria) showed prominent necroinflammatory changes of hepatic parenchyma and also piece-meal necrosis and positive ANA, and these cases were regarded as having the PBC–CAH mixed type. CAH patients with positive AMA so far reported may be included in this type. This type is a more severe disease with a more rapidly progressive course compared to typical PBC (Berg et al., 1986; Berg and Klein, 1989). Furthermore, Moteki et al. reported a variant of this type, that is, anti-M2- and -M4-positive in an ANA-positive patient who showed hypergammag-lobulinemia and typical histologic findings of PBC. The titer of ANA and transaminase levels responded well to steroid therapy in this case. Okuno et al. also reported a similar case (Okuno et al., 1985, 1987). On the contrary, Miyazaki et al. (1987) reported a case of asymptomatic anti-M2- and -M4-positive PBC with typical ductal lesions and minimum hepatitic activities, who also showed LE cell phenomena, ANA and hypergammaglobulinemia.

There seem to be other variations or types showing peculiar clinicolaboratory, serological, histologic and/or immunohistochemical findings in this so-called PBC–CAH mixed type. Although M2 antigens have been successfully charac-

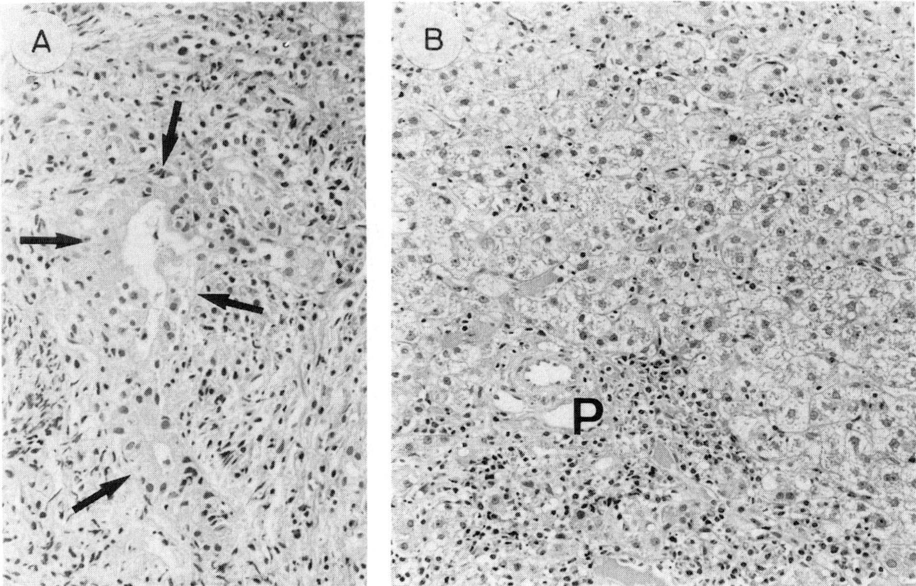

Fig. 20. An inter-lobular bile duct (arrows) shows tortuosity, disruption of the basement membrane and periductal and intra-epithelial lymphoid cell infiltration (A). A portal tract (P) shows loss of an inter-lobular bile duct and moderate mononculear cell infiltration, and the hepatic parenchyma also shows mild hepatitic changes. Overlapping syndrome of cholangitis and hepatitis (immunocholangitis). Hematoxylin–eosin stain.

terized, the identification and characterization of M4 and M8 antigens is still challenging. Thus, distinction of this PBC–CAH mixed type from PBC with prominent necroinflammatory changes of the hepatic parenchyma is still controversial.

4.2.4. Immunocholangitis

Some of the overlapping cases present additional or other features. That is, Brunner and Klinge (1987) and Ben-Ari et al. (1993) reported 3 and 4 cases, respectively, which fulfil clinically, histologically and serologically the criteria of CNSDC, though AMA was negative. Instead, their patients showed ANA at high titer and a beneficial response to steroid or immunosuppressive therapy. They called this condition 'immunocholangitis' or autoimmune cholangiopathy. Shibuya et al. (1991) reported a similar case of overlapping syndrome, although their case responded well to UDCA and the LE cell phenomena disappeared. Carrougher's case, who was negative for AMA, also seems to belong to this group, and clinicolaboratory data and histopathologic findings, including parenchymal necroinflammatory changes and ductal damage, responded well to repeated steroid or immunosuppressive therapy (Carrougher et al., 1991). We also experienced two similar cases who presented high-titer ANA, hypergammaglobulinemia and elevated biliary enzymes, but negative AMA. Serial liver biopsies disclosed CNSDC, focal bile duct loss and active necroinflammatory changes including many plasma cells (Fig. 20A, B). These two patients responded well to steroid therapy. It seems possible that these cases may be PBC, because AMA are not always positive in PBC patients. However, Ben-Ari et al. (1993) regarded these cases as a subtype of AIH.

For the time being, the above-mentioned, 4 types of overlapping hepatitis and cholangitis (CAH and PBC) are tentatively recognizable, in which target tissues attacked by autoimmune mechanism(s) may be present in the biliary epithelial cells as well as hepatocytes. More detailed studies on their clinicopathological features and biochemical analysis and characterization of AMA and their antigens are mandatory. Furthermore, criteria for the histopathologic differentiation of AIH with hepatitic duct lesions or PBC with prominent necroinflammatory changes and low-titer or negative ANA from this overlapping syndrome is necessary. Histologically, epithelioid granulomas which are usually seen in PBC, are also present in some cases and absent in other cases of this overlapping syndrome (Carrougher et al., 1991; Shibuya et al., 1991). Therefore, granulomatous reaction is not absolutely helpful in the histopathologic diagnosis.

4.3. PSC (chronic fibrous-obliterative cholangitis)

PSC is characterized by non-specific inflammation and fibrosis of the intra- and/or extra-hepatic biliary tree followed by the biliary destruction (LaRusso et al., 1984; Chapman, 1985). Several immunological abnormalities are speculated with respect to the bile duct destruction. Of interest is that a considerable number of the PSC patients disclose the occurrence of ANA in their serum and disturbed immunoregulation, especially suppressor T-cell function (LaRusso et al., 1984; Chapman, 1985). Histologically, in addition to cholestatic changes in the parenchyma, some patients show piecemeal necrosis and intra-lobular hepatocellular necrosis with Kupffer cell hyperplasia, resembling CAH. Some of these hepatitic activities may be caused by autoimmune processes as speculated in AIH, though target antigen(s) in this condition are only speculative.

Cholangiographic findings and histologic demonstration of mantle-like periductal fibrosis and fibrous obliteration of bile ducts are necessary to confirm the diagnosis of PSC. Pericholangitis associated with ulcerative colitis shows features of CAH and findings of PSC, and this condition is now called the microscopic type of PSC (Ludwig et al., 1981). The majority of cases of CAH, which have been reported as a complication of ulcerative colitis, belong to pericholangitis.

4.4. Viral hepatitis

Because the tests for hepatitis viruses (HAV, HBV, HCV, HDV, and HEV) or their markers have become or are becoming available, the differences or similarities of viral hepatitis from AIH have become evident. Recent investigations have disclosed the participation of these viruses in the initiation and progression of some AIH patients (Esteban et al., 1989; Lenzi et al., 1990, 1991; McFarlane et al., 1990). It is also well known that viral hepatitis with prominent necroinflammatory changes presents a variable autoimmune phenomenon. The relationship of viral hepatitis to AIH is now an important and debatable issue. Histopathologies of viral hepatitis are briefly reviewed relevant to AIH.

In acute *type A viral hepatitis*, abundant plasma cells are frequently and characteristically found at the periportal necrosis of hepatocytes (Dienes et al., 1989). In this sense, histologies of type A hepatitis apparently resemble AIH with acute hepatitic onset. Some susceptible cases, however, develop AIH after transient HAV infection (Vento and Eddleston, 1990).

In *type B viral hepatitis*, necroinflammatory changes and regenerative activities are rather prominent. In addition, during acute exacerbation, there frequently is zonal or confluent necrosis, partially resembling AIH. Plasma cell infiltration is prominent in some of these cases.

Serum markers for *type C viral hepatitis* and also detection of HCV-RNA by PCR have recently become available (Choo et al., 1989; Kuo et al., 1989). It was subsequently found that the majority of cases of type C hepatitis show more or less mild necroinflammatory changes in the hepatic lobules and borderline periportal destruction with lymphoid aggregates and/or follicles with germinal center in the portal tracts (Scheuer 1980, 1988; Lefkowitch et al., 1993). Steatosis is a common finding. Lymph follicles or lymphoid aggregates tend to be formed near bile ducts, some of which are variably damaged (Poulsen–Christoffersen lesion) (Poulsen and Christoffersen, 1972; Lefkowitch et al., 1993). Although the necroinflammatory changes of the liver are more or less mild, a considerable number of HCV-infected patients progress to liver cirrhosis after the long course. From the histopathological standpoint, differentiation of typical chronic hepatitis of type C from typical AIH is not difficult, though there is no reliable way or generally accepted criteria to distinguish AIH from severe CAH with autoantibodies. Response to corticosteroids may give a clue in this differentiation (Tassoni and Kaplan, 1991). Type C CAH does not respond to such immunosuppressive therapy (Tassoni and Kaplan 1991).

Recently, Cole et al. (1991) reported direct evidence of cytotoxicity associated with the expression of *hepatitis δ virus* antigen. However, hepatocellular damage mediated by an immune process may also be operative.

4.5. AIH and viral hepatitis

Most authorities agree that AIH should be diagnosed in those cases in which all known etiologic factors have been excluded. However, recent virological progress disclosed that some patients showed both the viral markers and criteria of AIH.

4.5.1. Pathogenetic relations
The relationship between AIH and viral hepatitis has been under investigation for a long time, since some AIH patients disclose transient or persistent viral markers of hepatitis virus(es) in their sera. There are several possibilities or hypotheses to date. One hypothesis is that AIH occurs in susceptible individuals who have a genetically determined ASGP-R-specific defect of suppressor–inducer T-cells and is triggered by unknown factors (possibly viruses or drugs) which induce a helper T-cell response against this liver cell surface antigen (Vento and Eddleston, 1990). That is, viral hepatitis may trigger or initiate the development of AIH in susceptible subjects. Recently, Vento et al. reported studying 58 healthy relatives of 13 patients with AIH for 4 years. Type 1 AIH developed after a subclinical HAV infection in 2 of 3 susceptible patients (relatives of AIH patients) in whom there was a defect in the suppressor–inducer T-lymphocytes controlling immune responses to the ASGP-R before HAV infection (Vento et al., 1991). During HAV infection, specific helper T-cells and antibodies to the ASGP-R persisted and increased and type 1 AIH developed 5 months after the recovery from HAV infection.

Several reports appeared, especially in Japan and Southern European countries, showing that a considerable number of AIH patients were serologically positive for HCV (Esteban et al., 1989; Lenzi et al., 1990). It was also pointed out that a considerable number of the patients with HCV infection disclosed low-titer autoantibodies such as ANA.

It was, however, soon found that the majority of these cases in Japan and England were pseudo-positive for HCV infection (Kuroki et al., 1984; Ikeda et al., 1990; McFarlane et al., 1990; Vento et al., 1991; Lefkowitch et al., 1993). However, important geographical differences and/or genetic influences have been pointed out among the different populations, and in Southern European countries, a considerable number of AIH, type 1 or type 2, cases were strongly positive for HCV-related serum markers, and these AIH patients were persistently infected with HCV (Lenzi et al., 1991). We have also experienced such cases (vide infra). The meaning(s) of these geographical differences remains unclear (Vento et al., 1991). HCV infection can also have similar pathologic processes as speculated in HAV infection (vide supra). Another possibility is that persistent HCV infection leads to the development and progression of AIH. Manns (1991) recently reported that there is molecular mimicry between HCV and autoantigens in AIH, that is, P-450 protein. He speculated that AIH, at least type 2 AIH, could be causally related to HCV infection.

4.5.2. AIH related to persistent HCV infection

Some cases of AIH are serologically positive for HCV-related antibodies as well as HCV-RNA as demonstrated by PCR and also show prominent necroinflammatory changes in the liver and high-titer ANA and LE cell phenomena. Some of these patients respond well to steroid therapy, while others respond to α-interferon therapy. It remains unclear whether these cases represent a coincidental superimposition of HCV infection on AIH or present unusual clinicopathologic manifestations of, or one phase of chronic type C hepatitis. Otherwise, HCV can induce AIH in susceptible subjects (Lenzi et al., 1991; Tassoni and Kaplan, 1991; Vento et al., 1991).

We have recently observed two cases of CAH in which HCV-RNA demonstrated by PCR as well as autoimmune features including hypergammaglobulinemia, LE cell phenomena and high-titer ANA. These cases will be presented here.

One case was a 56-year-old Japanese woman with the clinical features of acute hepatitis. This was her first form of hepatic injury. Serum transaminase and γ-globulin were elevated, and needle liver biopsy disclosed hepatocellular swelling and spotty or focal necrosis, Kupffer cell hyperplasia and acidophilic bodies which were accentuated in the perivenular areas (Fig. 21A). The histologic diagnosis was acute viral hepatitis of non-A, non-B etiology. After steroid therapy, she showed great improvement of liver functions.

After discontinuance of steroids, she again developed liver dysfunction with jaundice. Liver biopsy showed moderate portal fibrosis with heavy infiltration of lymphocytes and plasma cells, and irregularity of the limiting plates with hepatocellular hydropic changes and lymphoplasmacytic infiltration (piecemeal necrosis). In addition, there were necroinflammatory changes in the parenchyma

 Y. Nakanuma et al.

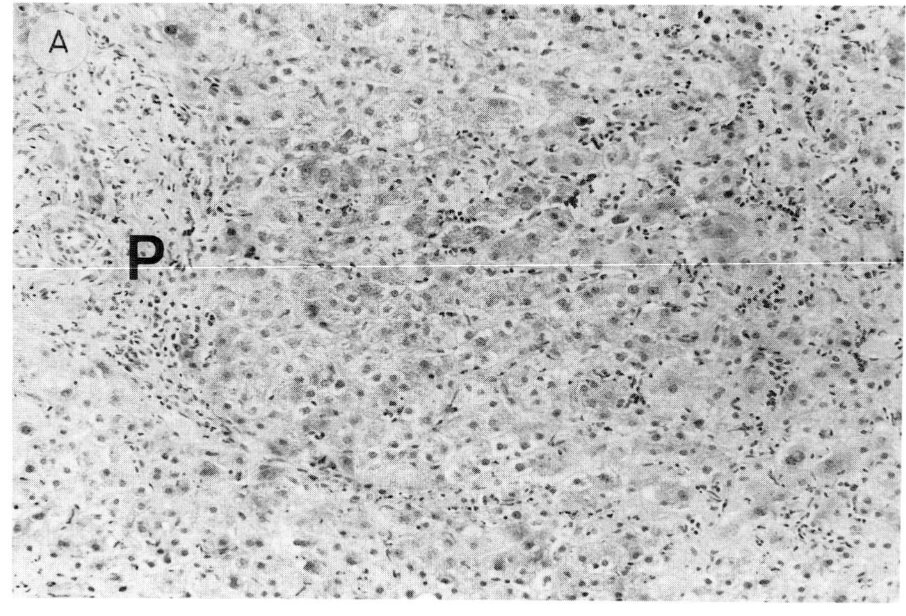

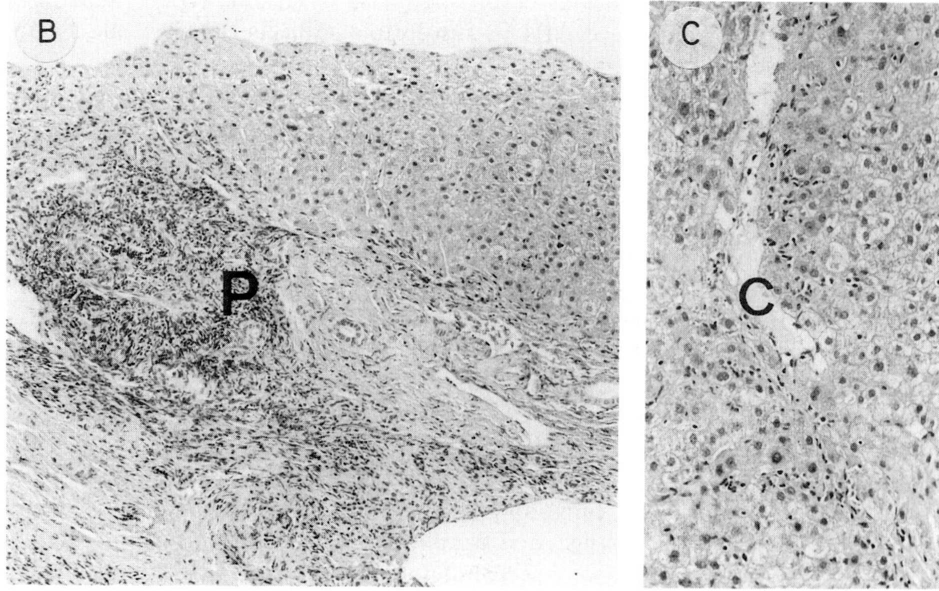

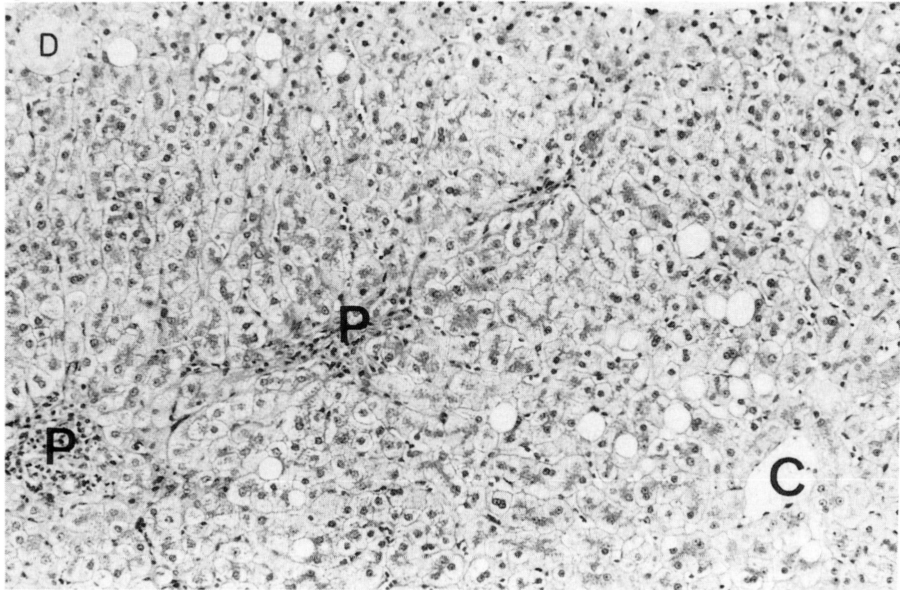

Fig. 21. A series of liver biopsies from HCV-RNA-positive autoimmune hepatitis. A: first liver biopsy shows acute hepatitic changes with parenchymal necroinflammatory changes with centrilobular accentuation. A portal tract (P) shows mild mononuclear cell infiltration. B and C: second liver biopsy shows CAH. That is, a portal tract (P) is enlarged with lymph follicle formation, fibrosis and piecemeal necrosis. The parenchyma also shows necroinflammatory changes accentuated around the central vein (C). D: third liver biopsy after steroid therapy shows marked regression of necroinflammatory changes in the portal tract (P) and also in the hepatic parenchyma. Mild fatty change reflects an adverse reaction to steroid therapy. C, central vein. Hematoxylin–eosin stain.

and perivenular zonal necrosis and C–C bridging necrosis (Fig. 21B, C). The clinical and laboratory findings greatly improved after steroid therapy, and biopsy of the liver showed mild portal fibrosis with mild ductular proliferation and no evidence of piecemeal necrosis (Fig. 21D).

Another case, a 61-year-old Japanese woman, also complained of acute features of hepatitis. Liver biopsy showed acute viral hepatitis with perivenular accentuation of necroinflammatory changes. After steroid therapy, liver histologies greatly improved. Five years later, acute exacerbation developed, and liver histology showed CAH with marked necroinflammatory changes including many plasma cells in the liver. There was centrilobular zonal necrosis, and also C–C or P–C bridging necrosis. After steroid therapy, these active necroinflammatory changes again markedly regressed.

4.6. SLE and other collagen vascular disease

While SLE and AIH present LE cell phenomena, strongly positive ANA, and hypergammaglobulinemia, the latter constantly and severely involve the liver, especially the hepatocytes, and the former preferentially affect the kidney, skin and other organs. It is generally believed that the liver is usually spared in SLE, or otherwise shows only non-specific reactive changes and mild hepatitic changes: a mild degree of hepatocellular damage with Kupffer cell hyperplasia; and mild portal inflammation (Mackay et al., 1956; Soloway et al., 1972; Takegoshi et al., 1989; Mackay, 1991). Sinusoidal lymphocytic infiltration is also reported in several cases of SLE (Takegoshi et al., 1989). These lesions are called 'hepatic lupus'.

Nevertheless, some cases of definite SLE show progressive liver disease, such as CAH and cirrhosis, and other autoimmune hepatobiliary diseases, such as PBC. Participation of hepatitis virus, especially HCV, should be considered in some of these instances. Some patients with collagen vascular and autoimmune diseases other than SLE also show hepatic dysfunction and CAH. The hepatic pathology and mechanism in the latter cases have not yet been well established.

In addition, some AIH patients present systemic changes reported in collagen vascular diseases such as vasculitis and even renal damage resembling lupus nephritis (Matsumura et al., 1987; Tsurui et al., 1988). It remains unclear whether or not these overlapping cases could be regarded as AIH.

4.7. Drug-induced hepatitis

Some cases of drug-induced hepatitis histologically show CAH and also clinically and immunologically AIH-like features, such as the occurrence of autoimmune phenomena and also organ non-specific autoantibodies including ANA (Vento and Eddleston, 1987). The following drugs are known to be capable of inducing AIH-like features: oxyphenisatin, α-methyldopa, and nitrofurantoin. In particular, oxyphenisatin present ANA and LE cell phenomena, and also, histologically, CAH with a large number of lymphoplasmacytes (Doniach and Walker, 1972). The mechanisms of drug-induced liver injury resembling AIH, especially participation of autoimmune mechanisms in the liver, remain controversial. After the withdrawal of the drug, immunological disturbances and liver injuries usually disappear, while some cases show a long persistence of autoantibodies (Vento and Eddleston, 1987).

5. Conclusions and overview

The histopathologic and immunopathologic characteristics of classic, type 1 AIH and of several other autoimmune hepatobiliary diseases in which hepatocellular necrosis is similar or identical to that of AIH, are reviewed. AIH is still a challenging concept from the clinicopathologic viewpoint and its relationship with viral hepatitis (transient or persistent) and susceptibility to this disease (genetic or environmental) is important in the understanding of the pathogenesis as well as the development and progression of AIH. HLA studies have linked AIH to HLA-B8-D3 (Manns et al., 1987; Vento and Eddleston, 1987). Immunologic and immunopathologic evaluation, especially the clarification of autoantibodies and their target tissues in the hepatocytes and immunohistochemical studies on phenotyping of infiltrating lymphocytes and identifying expressed antigens including HLA-antigens, contribute a great deal to the understanding of the evolution of this disease. The morphologic findings for an inciting agent and also for the sequences of events maintaining liver cell damage should be examined, though there have been no confirmative data or findings to date.

The lack of authorized criteria for AIH is also a frustrating issue. Characterization and clarification of hepatitis virus(es) and increasing awareness and clarification of PBC and PSC with autoimmune phenomena have led to the exclusion of cases with these diseases from ill-defined AIH. The autoimmune hepatocellular necrosis in other autoimmune hepatobiliary diseases, especially CAH of non-viral etiologies and also PBC, may provide a clue to the etiopathogenesis and pathologic progression of AIH.

References

Arima, S., Yoshida, K., Hashiguchi, O. et al. (1987) A case of lupoid hepatitis associated with hepatocelluar carcinoma. Acta Hepatol. Jap. 28, 772–777 (in Japanese).

Bardadin, K.A. and Desmet, V.J. (1984) Interdigitating and dentritic reticulum cells in chronic active hepatitis. Histopathology 8, 657–662.

Ben-Ari, Z., Dhillon, A.P. and Sherlock S. (1993) Autoimmune cholangiography: part of the spectrum of autoimmune chronic active hepatitis. Hepatology 18, 10–15.

Berg, P.A. and Klein, R. (1989) Heterogeneity of antimitochondrial antibodies. Semin. Liver Dis. 9, 103–116.

Berg, P.A., Wiedmann, K.H., Sayer, T. et al. (1980) Serological classification of chronic cholestatic liver disease by the use of two different types of antimitochondrial antibodies. Lancet 2, 1329–1332.

Berg, P.A., Weber, P., Oehring, J. et al. (1985) Significance of different types of mitochondrial antibodies in primary biliary cirrhosis. In: H. Brunner and H. Thaler (Eds.) Hepatology. A Festschrift for Hans Popper, Raven, New York, pp. 231–242.

Berg, P.A., Klein, R. and Lindenborn-Fotinos, J. (1986) Antimitochondrial antibodies in primary biliary cirrhosis. J. Hepatol. 2, 123–131.

Bianchi, L., Spichtin, H.P. and Gudat, F. (1987) Chronic hepatitis. In: R.N.M. MacSween, P.P. Anthony and P.J. Scheuer (Eds.) Pathology of the Liver. Churchill Livingstone, Edinburgh, pp. 310–341.

Brunner, G. and Klinge, G. (1987) A cholangitis with antinuclear antibodies (immunologic cholangitis) resembling chronic nonsuppurative destructive cholangitis. Dtsch Med. Woche 112, 1454–1458.

Carrougher, J.G., Shaffer, R.T., Canales, L.I. et al. (1991) A 33-year-old woman with an autoimmune syndrome. Semin. Liver Dis. 11, 256–262.

Chapman, R.W. (1985) Primary sclerosing cholangitis. J. Hepatol. 1, 179–186.

Choo, Q.L., Kuo, G., Weiner, A.J. et al. (1989) Isolation of cDNA clone derived from a blood-borne non-A, non-B viral hepatitis genome. Science 244, 359–362.

Cohen, I.R. and Lohse, A.W. (1991) Physiology and pathophysiology of autoimmunity. Semin. Liver Dis. 11, 183–186.

Cole, S., Gowans, E.J., Macnaughton, T.B. et al. (1991) Direct evidence for cytotoxicity associated with expression of hepatitis delta virus antigen. Hepatology 13, 845–851.

Coovadia, H.M., Mackay, J.R. and D'Apiece, A.J.F. (1981) Suppressor cells assayed by three different methods in patient with chronic active hepatitis and systemic lupus erythematosus. Clin. Immunol. Immunopathol. 18, 268–275.

Croffy, H., Kopelman, R. and Kaplan, M. (1988) Hypereosinophilic syndrome: association with chronic active hepatitis. Dig. Dis. Sci. 33, 233–239.

Devaney, K., Goodman, Z.D. and Ishak, K.G. (1992) Postinfantile giant-cell transformation in hepatitis. Hepatology 16, 327–333.

Dienes, H.P. (1989) Viral and autoimmune hepatitis. Gustav Fischer, Stuttgart, New York.

Dienes, H.P., Popper, H., Arnold, W. et al. (1982) Histologic observations in human hepatitis non-A, non-B. Hepatology 2, 562–571.

Dienes, H.P., Popper, H., Manns, M. et al. (1989) Histologic features in autoimmune hepatitis. Z. Gastroenterol. 27, 325–330.

Dienes, H.P., Autschbach, F. and Gerber, M. (1991) Ultrastructural lesion in autoimmune hepatitis and steps of the immune response in liver tissue. Semin. Liver Dis. 11, 197–204.

Doniach, D. and Walker, G. (1972) Immunopathology of liver disease. Prog. Liver Dis. 4, 381–402.

Esteban, J.I., Esteban, R., Viladomiu, L. et al. (1989) Hepatitic C virus antibodies among risk groups in Spain. Lancet ii, 294–297.

Foong, A., Schoks, J.V., Gleich, G.J. et al. (1991) Eosinophil-induced chronic active heptitis in the idiopathic hypereosinophilic syndrome. Hepatology 13, 1090–1094.

Foster, P.F., Bhattacharyya, A., Sankary, H.N. et al. (1991) Eosinophilic cationic protein's role in human hepatic allograft rejection. Hepatology 13, 1117–1125.

Gershwin, M.E. and Mackay, I.R. (1991) Primary biliary cirrhosis: paradigm or paradox for autoimmunity. Gastroenterology 100, 822–833.

Geubel, A.P., Baggenstoss, A.H. and Summerskill, W.H.J. (1976) Responses to treatment can differentiate chronic active hepatitis with cholangitic features from the primary biliary cirrhosis syndrome. Gastroenterology 71, 444–449.

Good, R.A. (1956) Plasma cell hepatitis and extreme hyperglobulinemia in adolescent females. Am. J. Dis. Child. 92, 508–509.

Hadziyannis, S., Scheuer, P.J., Feizi, T. et al. (1970) Immunological and histological studies in primary biliary cirrhosis. J. Clin. Pathol. 23, 95–98.

Hino, T. (1991) Studies on rosette formation in the liver of patients with autoimmune hepatitis. Acta Hepatol. Jap. 32, 997–1007 (in Japanese).

Homberg, J.C., Stelly, N., Andreis, I. et al. (1982) A new anti-mitochondria antibody (anti-M6) in iproniazid-induced hepatitis. Clin. Exp. Immunol. 47, 93–102.

Hopf, U., Meyer zum Büschenfelde, K.H., Arnold, M. et al. (1976) Detection of a livermembrane autoantibody in HBsAg negative chronic active hepatitis. N. Engl. J. Med. 294, 578–582.

Hsu, M., Raine, L. and Fanger, H. (1981) Use of avidin–biotin–peroxidase complex (ABC) in immunoperoxidase techniques: a comparison between ABC and unlabelled antibody (PAP) procedure. J. Histochem. Cytochem. 29, 557–580.

Ikeda, Y., Toda, G., Hashimoto, N. et al. (1990) Antibody to superoxide dismutase, autoimmune hepatitis, and antibody tests for hepatitis C virus. Lancet 335, 1345–1346.

Imamura, M., Seki, T., Shiro, T. et al. (1991) HCV-positive hepatocellular carcinoma with features of autoimmune hepatitis (abstract). Acta Hepatol. Jap. 32, (Suppl.) 146 (in Japanese).

Johnson, P.J. and McFarlane, I.G. (1993) Meeting report: International autoimmune hepatitis group. Hepatology 18, 998–1005.

Johnson, P.J., McFarlane, I.G. and Eddleston, A.L. (1991) The natural course and heterogeneity of autoimmune hepatitis-type chronic active hepatitis. Semin. Liver Dis. 11, 187–196.

Kamiyama, T., Izumi, N., Kojima, S. et al. (1990) A case of early autoimmune chronic active hepatitis with clinically acute onset and histological features of acute hepatitis. Acta Hepatol. Jap. 31, 565–569 (in Japanese).

Kerr, J.F.R., Searle, J., Halliday, W.J. et al. (1979) The nature of piecemeal necrosis in chronic active hepatitis. Lancet ii, 827–828.

Klein, R., Maisch, B., Berg, P.A. et al. (1984) Demonstration of organ specific antibodies against heart mitochondrial (anti-M7) in sera from patients with some forms of heart diseases. Clin. Exp. Immunol. 58, 283.

Kloppel, G., Seifert, G., Lindner, H. et al. (1977) Histologic features in mixed types of chronic aggressive hepatitis and primary biliary cirrhosis. Virchow Arch. A 373, 143–160.

Kuo, G., Choo, Q.L., Alter, H.J. et al. (1989) An assay for circulating antibodies to a major etiologic virus of human non-A, non-B hepatitis. Science 244, 362–364.

Kuroki, T., Yamamoto, S. and Monna, T. (1984) Autoimmune hepatitis. Clin. Adult Dis. 14, 781–786 (in Japanese).

LaRusso, N.F., Wiesner, R.H., Ludwig, J. et al. (1984) Primary sclerosing cholangitis. N. Engl. J. Med. 310, 899–903.

Lefkowitch, J.H., Apfelbaum, T.F., Weinberg, L. et al. (1984) Acute liver biopsy lesions in early autoimmune ('lupoid') chronic active hepatitis. Liver 4, 379–386.

Lefkowitch, H., Schiff, E.R., Davis, G.L. et al. (1993) Pathological diagnosis of chronic hepatitis C: a multicenter comparative study with chronic hepatitis B. Gastroenterology 104, 595–603.

Lenzi, M., Ballardini, G., Fusconi, M. et al. (1990) Type 2 autoimmune hepatitis and hepatitic C virus infection. Lancet 335, 258–259.

Lenzi, M., Johnson, P.J., McFarlane, I.G. et al. (1991) Antibodies to hepatitis C virus in autoimmune liver disease: evidence for geographical heterogeneity. Lancet 338, 277–280.

Lohr, H., Treichel, U., Poralla, T. et al. (1990) The human hepatic asialoglycoprotein receptor is a target antigen for liver-infiltrating T cells in autoimmune chronic active hepatitis and primary biliary cirrhosis. Hepatology 12, 1314–1320.

Lohse, A.W. (1991) Experimental models of autoimmune hepatitis. Semin. Liver Dis. 11, 241–247.

Ludwig, J., Barham, S.S., LaRusso, N.F. et al. (1981) Morphologic features of chronic hepatitis associated with primary sclerosing cholangitis and chronic ulcerative colitis. Hepatology 1, 632–640.

Mackay, I.R. (1991) The hepatitis–lupus connection. Semin. Liver Dis. 11, 234–240.

Mackay, I.R. and Gershwin, M.E. (1989) Primary biliary cirrhosis: current knowledge, perspectives, and future directions. Semin. Liver Dis. 9, 149–157.

Mackay, I.R. and Wood, I. (1962) Lupoid hepatitis: A comparison of 22 cases with other types of chronic liver diseases. Q. J. Med. 124, 485–507.

Mackay, I.R., Taft, L.I. and Cowling, D.C. (1956) Lupoid hepatitis. Lancet ii, 1323–1326.

Manns, M.P. (1991) Cytoplasmic autoantigens in autoimmune hepatitis: molecular analysis and clinical relevance. Semin. Liver Dis. 11, 205–214.

Manns, M., Gerken, G., Kyriatosoulis, A. et al. (1987) Characterization of a new subgroup of auto-immune chronic active hepatitis by autoantibodies against a soluble liver antigen. Lancet 1, 292–294.

Matsumura, K., Kajiwara, E, Tsuji, H. et al. (1987) A case of autoimmune hepatitis with high IgM class smooth muscle antibody and systemic vascular disease. Jap. J. Gastroenterol. 84, 297–301 (in Japanese).

Matsushita, E., Unoura, M., Furusawa, A. et al. (1988) Studies on the mechanisms of development of autoimmune hepatitis. Acta Hepatol Jap. 29, 1357–1361 (in Japanese).

Matsuzaki, Y., Tanaka, N., Osuga, T. et al. (1990) Improvement of biliary enzyme levels and itching as a result of long-term administration of ursodeoxycholic acid in primary biliary cirrhosis. Am. J. Gastroenterol. 85, 15–23.

Mayet, W.J., Hess, G., Gerken, G. et al. (1989) Treatment of chronic type B hepatitis with recombinant alpha-interferon induces autoantibodies not specific for autoimmune chronic active hepatitis. Hepatology 10, 24–28.

McFarlane, I.G. (1984) Autoimmunity in liver disease. Clin. Sci. 67, 569–577.

McFarlane, I.G. (1991) Autoimmunity and hepatotrophic viruses. Semin. Liver Dis. 11, 223–233.

McFarlane, I.G., McSorley, C.G, Vergani, D. et al. (1986) Serum autoantibodies reacting with the hepatic asialoglycoprotein receptor protein (hepatic lectin) in acute and chronic liver disease. J. Hepatol. 3, 196–205.

McFarlane, I.G., Smith, H.M., Johnson, P.J. et al. (1990) Hepatitis C virus antibodies in chronic active hepatitis: pathogenetic factor of false-positive result? Lancet 335, 754–757.

Meyer zum Büschenfelde, K.H.M. (1991) Autoimmunity and liver disease. Semin. Liver Dis., 11, iii–iv.

Meyer zum Büschenfelde, K.H., Kossling, F.K. et al. (1972) Experimental chronic active hepatitis in rabbits following immunization with human liver proteins. Clin. Exp. Immunol. 10, 99–108.

Mistilis, S.P. and Blackburn, C.R.B. (1970) Active chronic hepatitis. Am. J. Med. 48, 484–495.

Miyamura, H., Nakanuma, Y. and Kono, N. (1988) Survey of copper granules in liver biopsy specimens from various liver abnormalities other than Wilson's disease and biliary diseases. Gastroenterol. Jap. 23, 633–638.

Miyazaki, H., Tsubouchi, H., Kiyama, I. et al. (1987) A case of asymptomatic primary biliary cirrhosis with positive LE cell phenomenon. Acta Hepatol. Jap. 28, 1515–1520 (in Japanese).

Monna, T., Kuroki, T. and Yamamoto, S. (1982) National survey of lupoid hepatitis and related disease. Kan Tan Sui 4, 163–170 (in Japanese).

Mori, T., Mori, Y., Yoshida, H. et al. (1985) Cell mediated cytotoxity sensitized spleen cells against target liver cells – in vivo and in vitro study with a mouse model of experimental autoimmune hepatitis. Hepatology 5, 770–777.

Moteki, S., Saito, K., Saito, N. et al. (1987) A male case of primary biliary cirrhosis (PBC) complicated with lupoid hepatitis. Acta Hepatol. Jap. 28, 766–771 (in Japanese).

Motoo, Y., Wakatsuki, T., Tanaka, K. et al. (1988) Resected case of hepatocellular carcinoma associated with lupoid hepatitis. J. Gastroenterol. Hepatol. 4, 295–298.

Nakamoto, Y., Inagaki, Y., Kitano, Y. et al. (1991) A case of chronic active hepatitis type C associated with hyperthyroidism following a long-term interferon therapy. Acta Hepatol. Jap. 32, 863–867 (in Japanese).

Nakanuma, Y. (1993a) Pathology of septum formation in primary biliary cirrhosis: a histological study in the non-cirrhotic stage. Virchows Arch. A Pathol. Anat. 422, 17–23.

Nakanuma, Y. (1993b) Necroinflammatory changes in hepatic lobules in primary biliary cirrhosis with less well-defined cholestatic changes. Hum. Pathol. 24, 373–383.

Nakanuma, Y. and Kono, N. (1991) Expression of HLA-DR antigens on interlobular bile ducts in primary biliary cirrhosis and other hepatobiliary diseases: An immunohistochemical study. Hum. Pathol. 22, 431–436.

Nakanuma, Y. and Ohta, G. (1983) Quantitation of hepatic granulomas and epithelioid cells in primary biliary cirrhosis. Hepatology 3, 423–427.

Nakanuma, Y., Miyamura, H. and Ohta, G. (1981) Correlation between disappearance of the intrahepatic bile ducts and histologic changes in the liver in primary biliary cirrhosis. Am. J. Gastroenterol. 76, 506–510.

Nakanuma, Y., Saito, K. and Unoura, M. (1990) Semiquantitative assessment of cholestasis and lymphocytic piecemeal necrosis in primary biliary cirrhosis: A histologic and immuhohistochemical study. J. Clin. Pathol. 12, 357–362.

Nouri-Aria, K.T., Hegarty, J.E., Alexander, J.M. et al. (1982) Effect of corticosteroids on suppressor-cell activity in 'autoimmune' and viral chronic active hepatitis. N. Engl. J. Med. 307, 1301–1304.

Okuno, T., Seto, R., Abe, Y. et al. (1985) Overlapping syndrome of primary biliary cirrhosis and lupoid hepatitis. Acta Hepatol. Jap. 26, 88–94 (in Japanese).

Okuno, T., Seto, Y., Okanoue, T. et al. (1987) Chronic active hepatitis with histologic features of primary biliary cirrhosis. Dig. Dis. Sci. 32, 775–779.

Onji, M., Kumon, I., Nadano, N. et al. (1990) Clinicopathological significance of lymph follicle formation in primary biliary cirrhosis. Okayama Med. J. 102, 245–247 (in Japanese).

Page, A.R. and Good, R.A. (1960) Plasma-cell hepatitis with special attention to steroid therapy. Am. J. Dis. Child. 9, 288–314.

Panush, R.S., Wilkinson, L.S. and Fagin, R.R. (1973) Chronic active hepatitis associated with eosinophilia and Coombs-positive hemolytic anemia. Gastroenterology 64, 1015–1019.

Paronetto, F., Colucci, G. and Colombo, M. (1986) Lymphocytes in liver diseases. Prog. Liver Dis. 8, 191–208.

Passwell, J., Theodor, E. and Cohen, B.E. (1971). Chronic active hepatitis with unusual histologic features. Report of a case. J. Pediatr. 79, 36–41.

Peters, R.L. (1978) Acute and chronic varieties of viral hepatitis. In: T. Oda (Ed.) Hepatitis Viruses. Univ. Tokyo Press, Tokyo, pp. 197–223.

Popper, H. (1978) The problem of histologic evaluation of primary biliary cirrhosis. Virchows Arch. A 379, 99–102.

Popper, H. and Schaffner, F. (1970) Nonsuppurative destructive chronic cholangitis and chronic hepatitis. Prog. Liver Dis. 8, 336–354.

Poralla, T., Treichel, U., Lohr, H. et al. (1991) The asialoglycoprotein receptor as target structure in autoimmune liver diseases. Semin. Liver Dis. 11, 215–222.

Portmann, B. and MacSween, R.N.M. (1987) Diseases of the intrahepatic bile ducts. In: R.N.M. MacSween, P.P. Anthony and P.J. Scheuer (Eds.) Pathology of the Liver, 2nd edn. Churchill Livingstone, Edinburgh, pp. 424–453.

Portmann, B., Popper, H., Neuberger, J. et al. (1985) Sequential and diagnostic features of primary biliary cirrhosis based on serial histologic study in 209 cases. Gastroenterology 88, 1777–1790.

Poulsen, H. and Christoffersen, P. (1972) Abnormal bile duct epithelium in chronic aggressive hepatitis and cirrhosis. A review of morphology and clinical, biochemical, and immunological features. Hum. Pathol. 3, 217–225.

Reynolds, T.B., Edmondson, H.A., Peters, R.L. et al. (1964) Lupoid hepatitis. Ann Intern. Med. 61, 650–664.

Rubin, E., Schaffner, F. and Popper, H. (1964) Primary biliary cirrhosis. Chronic nonsuppurative destructive cholangitis. Am. J. Pathol. 46, 387–407.

Schaffner, F. (1986) Autoimmune chronic active hepatitis: three decades of progress. Prog. Liver Dis. 8, 485–503.

Scheuer, P.J. (1980) Liver Biopsy Interpretation, 3rd edn. Baillière-Tindall, London.

Scheuer, P.J., (1988) Liver Biopsy Interpretation, 4th edn. Baillière-Tindall, London.

Seki, S., Sakaguchi, H., Kawakita, N. et al. (1991a) Detection of proliferating hepatocytes in patients with acute hepatic failure by mitotic figures and a monoclonal antibody against DNA polymerase alpha. Liver 11, 118–126.

Seki, S., Sakaguchi, H., Kawakita, N. et al. (1991b) Identification and fine structure of proliferating hepatocytes in malignant and nonmalignant liver diseases by use of a mononclonal antibody against DNA polymerase alpha. Hum. Pathol. 21, 1020–1030.

Sherlock, S. (1985) Chronic active 'lupoid' hepatitis. In: S. Sherlock (Ed.) Diseases of the Liver and Biliary System, 7th edn. Blackwell, Oxford, pp. 287–294.

Shibuya, A., Shiratori, K., Kokubu, S. et al. (1991) A case of AMA negative primary biliary cirrhosis, overlapping with lupoid hepatitis. Acta Hepatol. Jap. 32, 926–931 (in Japanese).

Soloway, R.D., Summerfield, W.H.J., Baggenstoss, A.H. et al. (1972) Lupoid hepatitis, a nonentity in the spectrum of chronic active liver disease. Gastroenterology 63, 458–465.

Takahashi, Y., Shimizu, M., Fukuda, N. et al. (1977) Autopsy case of lupoid hepatitis: comparison of active chronic hepatitis. In: Non-B Hepatitis and Chronic Active Liver Disease. Inuyama Symposium Proceeding, Chugai, Tokyo, pp. 155–159 (in Japanese).

Takegoshi, K., Tohyama, T., Okuda, K. et al. (1989) Drug-induced mononucleosis-like hepatic injury in a patient with systemic lupus erythematosus. Gastroenterol. Jap. 24, 65–69.

Tanikawa, K. and Maeyama, T. (1982) Clinics and Pathology of lupoid hepatitis. Kan Tan Sui 4, 179–188 (in Japanese).

Tassoni, J.P. and Kaplan, M.M. (1991) Rapidly progressive liver failure in a 65-year-old woman. Gastroenterology 100, 1462–1468.

Terasaki, S., Nakanuma, Y., Ogino, H. et al. (1991) Hepatocellular and biliary expression of HLA antigens in primary biliary cirrhosis before and after ursodeoxycholic acid therapy. Am. J. Gastroenterol. 86, 1194–1199.

Thijs, J.C., Bosma, A., Henzen-Logmans, S.C. et al. (1985) Post infantile giant cell hepatitis in a patients with multiple autoimmune features. Am. J. Gastroenterol. 80, 294–297.

Treichel, U., Poralla, T., Hess, G. et al. (1990) Autoantibodies to human asialoglycoprotein receptor in autoimmune-type chronic hepatitis. Hepatology 11, 606–612.

Tsurui, N., Komatsu, M., Yagisawa, H. et al. (1988) A case of lupoid hepatitis associated with glomerulonephritis – concerning the findings of renal lesion by immunofluorescence microscopy. Jap. J. Gastroenterol. 85, 1114–1118 (in Japanese).

Van de Water, Turchany, J., Leung. P.S.C. et al. (1993) Molecular mimicry in primary biliary cirrhosis. Evidence for biliary expression of a molecule cross-reactive with pyruvate dehydrogenase complex-E$_2$. J. Clin. Invest. 91, 2653–2664.

Van den Oord, J.J., Fevery, J., De Groote, J. et al. (1984) Immunohistochemical characterization of inflammatory infiltrates in primary biliary cirrhosis. Liver 4, 264–274.

Van den Oord, J.J., De Vos, R. and Desmet, V.J. (1990) HLA expression in liver disease. Prog. Liver Dis. 9, 373–388.

Vento, S. and Eddleston, A.L.W.F. (1987) Immunological aspects of chronic active hepatitis. Clin. Exp. Immunol. 68, 225–232.

Vento, S. and Eddleston, A. (1990) Autoimmunity and liver disease. Prog. Liver Dis. 9, 335–343.

Vento, S., Hegarty, J.E., Bottazzo, C. et al. (1984) Antigen specific suppressor cell function in autoimmune chronic active hepatitis. Lancet 1, 1200.

Vento, S., O'Brien, C.J., McFarlane, B.M. et al. (1986) T-lymphocyte sensitization to hepatocyte antigens in autoimmune chronic active hepatitis and primary biliary cirrhosis. Gastroenterology, 91, 810–817.

Vento, S., McFarlane, B.M., McSorley, C.G. et al. (1988) Liver autoreactivity in acute virus A, B and non A, non B hepatitis. J. Clin. Lab. Immunol. 25, 1–7.

Vento, S., Garofano, T., Di Perri G. et al. (1991) Identification of hepatitis A virus as a trigger for autoimmune chronic hepatitis type I in susceptible individuals. Lancet 337, 1183–1187.

Vyberg, M. (1989) Diverticular bile duct lesion in chronic active hepatitis. Hepatology 10, 774–780.

Wang, K.K. and Czaja, A.J. (1988) Hepatocellular carcinoma in corticosteroid-treated severe autoimmune chronic active hepatitis. Hepatology 8, 1679–1683.

Whittingham, S.F., Irwin, J., Mackay, I.R. et al. (1966) Smooth muscle autoantibody in 'autoimmune' hepatititis. Gastroenterology 51, 499–505.

Wiesner, R.H., Ludwig, J., Hoek, B.V. et al. (1991) Current concepts in cell-mediated hepatic allograft rejection leading to ductopenia and liver failure. Hepatology 14, 721–729.

Wu, P.C., Lai, C.L. and Chay, C. (1991) Neutrophils in chronic active hepatitis type B. Arch. Pathol. Lab. Med. 115, 930–933.

Yamada, G., Hyodo, I., Tobe, K. et al. (1986) Ultrastructural immunocytochemical analysis of lymphocytes infiltrating bile duct epithelia in primary biliary cirrhosis. Hepatology 6, 385–391.

Yonekura, T., Kuroda, H. and Tajima, J. (1989) Ultrastructural study of interlobular bile ductural disorganization in autoimmune liver diseases. Jap. J. Gastroenterol. 86, 1638–1644 (in Japanese).

Autoimmune Hepatitis
Edited by M. Nishioka, G. Toda and M. Zeniya
© *1994, Elsevier Science B.V. All rights reserved*

Chapter 7

Histopathology of autoimmune hepatitis

H.P. Dienes and F. Autschbach

Department of Pathology, University of Mainz, Langenbeckstrasse 1, D-55101 Mainz (Germany)

1. Introduction

Although, based on a putative common pathogenesis of autoimmune mechanisms, the entity of autoimmune hepatitis (AIH) seems to be rather heterogeneous and can be subdivided into several groups (Manns et al., 1987) by subtyping of autoantibodies. (For an extensive review of the clinical and immunological aspects, see the recent review of Meyer zum Büschenfelde et al. (1990).) Attempts to characterize the histopathology of the disease have been made that reflect the heterogeneity of the disease and so far pathognomonic features of AIH have not been found (Dienes et al., 1989; Korb, 1989). However, it is now being investigated whether the unifying concept of an autoimmune-mediated effector mechanism directed at the plasma membrane of hepatocytes is reflected in some basic histopathologic lesions that distinguish AIH from viral hepatitis (Dienes et al., 1991). This chapter is based on an analysis of a large cohort of patients cared for and examined in a center specialized in hepatic immunopathology as well as on the literature on this subject.

2. Light microscopy of AIH

In the majority of patients, the disease presents itself at first as an acute flare-up of chronic active hepatitis (CAH) or cirrhosis with CAH (about 70%) and only about 20% display chronic persistent hepatitis on their first admission to hospital. The remaining patients have chronic lobular hepatitis or acute hepatitis, and rather infrequently a hepatocellular carcinoma has already developed. The damaging pattern of the disease is only expressed during its active phase and may be obscure or absent in the persistent or latent stage.

In the following, characteristic histopathologic features will be described that have been observed by the authors and other investigators (Lefkowitch et al., 1984; Bianchi et al., 1987; Korb, 1989; Dienes, 1989; Dienes et al., 1991).

To begin with, no pathognomonic feature has been described so far.

Portal tracts and periportal areas present the focus of the necroinflammatory lesion with abundant lymphocytic infiltrates (Fig. 1). In the majority of patients, the bile ducts are inconspicuous or display only minor degenerative changes of the epithelia. However, there are cases of AIH that exhibit lesions almost indistinguishable from non-suppurative destructive chronic cholangitis (i.e., primary biliary cirrhosis (PBC)). Even epithelioid granulomas have been reported (Korb and Berg, 1990) in close vicinity to the bile ducts in up to 10% of biopsies (Fig. 2). These cases can be distinguished by taking into account the degree of inflammatory activity in the lobule. However, a true overlap syndrome does exist in some cases as reported (Klöppelet al., 1977; Carrougher et al., 1991) and only an exact immunoserologic analysis and a careful evaluation of the patient's history will help to elucidate the correct diagnosis. Portal lymph follicles

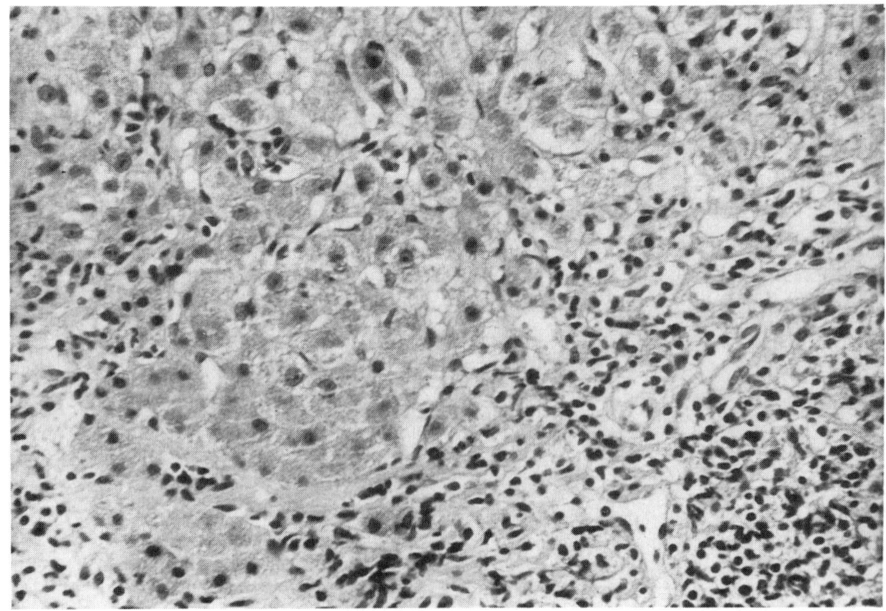

Fig. 1. Chronic active AIH: enlarged portal tracts are densely infiltrated by lymphocytes that spill over into the parenchyma in areas of piecemeal necrosis. Hematoxylin–eosin stain. × 240.

or pseudo-lymph follicles are less frequent than in chronic hepatitis C. As in this disease, they are mostly located close to altered bile ducts. DPAS-positive macrophages may be present in small groups during active periods of the disease, indicating the portal scavenger function of this cell population because of lymph drainage of the lobule into the portal tracts. Lymphocytes and macrophages constitute the predominant infiltrating cell population, whereas plasma cells are not a prominent feature of AIH, either in the portal or in the lobular infiltrates (Dienes, 1989). Fibrotic scarring in the portal tracts may be observed in long-standing disease after the inflammation has receded due to steroid therapy. The formation of active septa extending from the portal tracts into the surrounding parenchyma seems to be an early event in chronic AIH. The portal tracts assume a stellate-shaped appearance by this process.

The formation of piecemeal necroses (PMN) often results in the confluence of broad areas of collapse (Fig. 3). These zones of collapse localized preferentially in the periportal area, show thickening of the reticulin framework and contain scattered infiltrates of lymphocytes. The periportal parenchymal reacting area is the most active and progressing zone of the lobule in which acinar transformation or rosetting of hepatocytes (Fig. 4) starts to occur. The acinar arrangement of the hepatocytes often surrounds dilated bile canaliculi with cholestasis, although cholestasis is not a prominent feature in AIH. Another morphologic lesion that

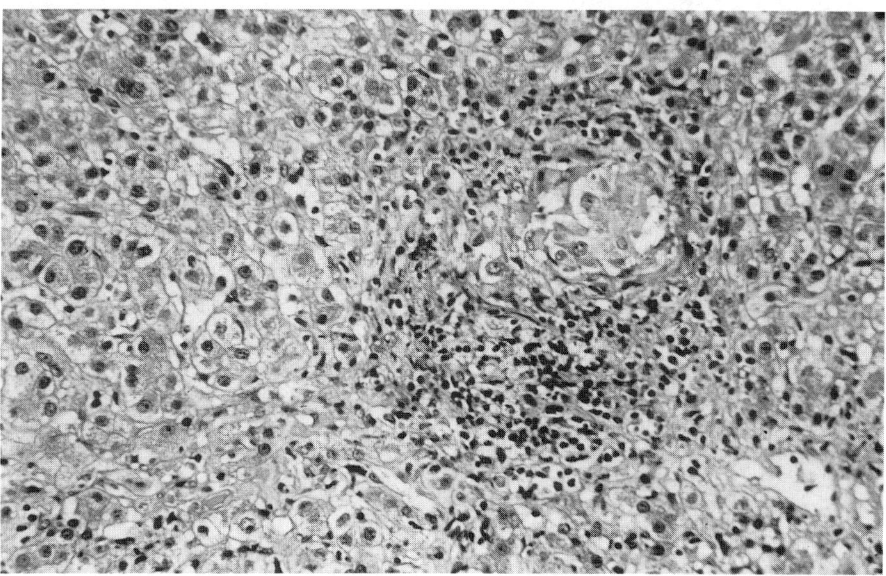

Fig. 2. Chronic active AIH: epithelioid granuloma located in an extended portal tract. Hema-toxylin–eosin stain × 180.

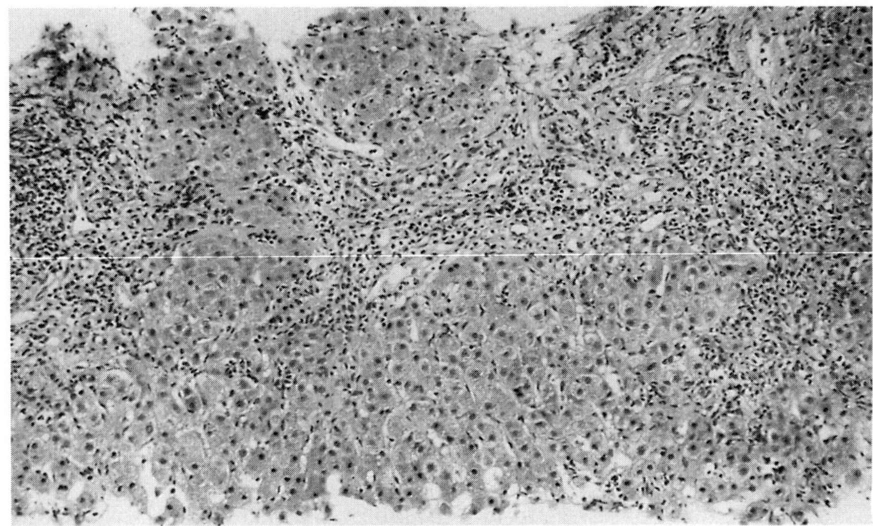

Fig. 3. Chronic active AIH displaying large areas of collapse. The portal and periportal predominance of lymphocytic infiltrates and necrotic inflammatory activity are evident. Hematoxylin–eosin stain. × 80.

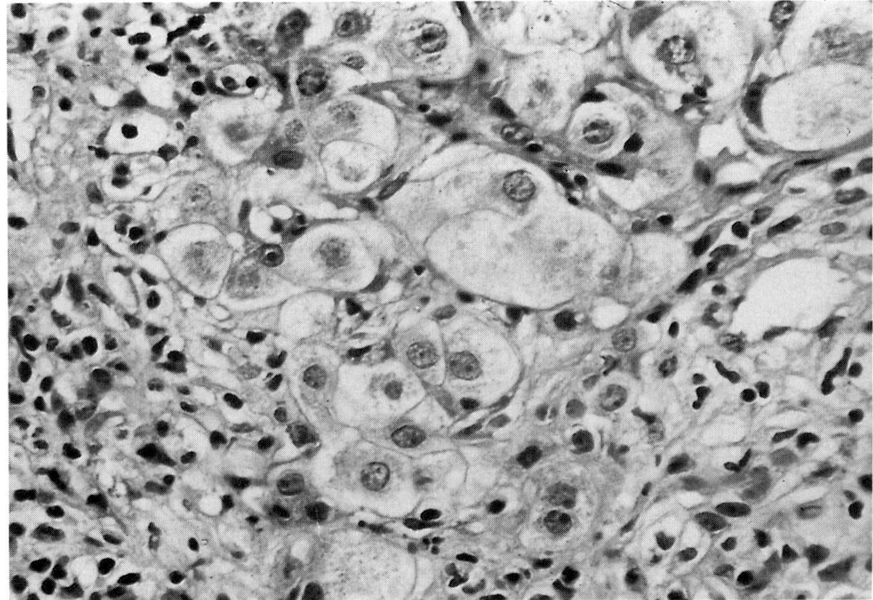

Fig. 4. Chronic active AIH: periportal area with microacinar transformation of hepatocytes flanked by piecemeal necrosis. Hematoxylin–stain. × 480.

can be observed in AIH and is also present in the viral type is the proliferation of ductules sometimes associated with mild cholangiolitis.

In the *lobules* the lytic pathway of necrosis is the predominant type, whereas the acidophilic bodies are less conspicuous than in viral hepatitis. Hydropic swelling and ballooning of hepatocytes, presumably a prestige of lytic necrosis, is abundant in AIH (Fig. 5) and especially pronounced in areas of microacinar transformation. Eosinophilic cell damage or cytoplasmic condensation is only secondary and less frequent. The inflammatory infiltrate in the lobule consists mainly of mononuclear cells as lymphocytes and Kupffer cells. Polymorphonuclear leucocytes and eosinophils are virtually absent. Plasma cells are not a constituent feature of AIH when compared to viral hepatitis. Emperipolesis of lymphocytes is a frequent phenomenon which supports the hypothesis of a lymphocytic-mediated cell necrosis in AIH (Eggink et al., 1982; Meuer and Dienes, 1989; Lohse et al., 1990; Meyer zum Büschenfelde et al., 1990). The lymphocytes spill over from the portal tracts into the lobules and are often arranged in an Indian file formation in the sinusoids (Fig. 1). The intra-lobular changes and the lymphocytic infiltrate bear a great similarity to experimental AIH induced by adaptive lymphocyte transfer (Lohse et al., 1990).

These histopathologic characteristic features do apply to all subgroups of AIH, rendering a histopathologic distinction of the different subgroups impossible.

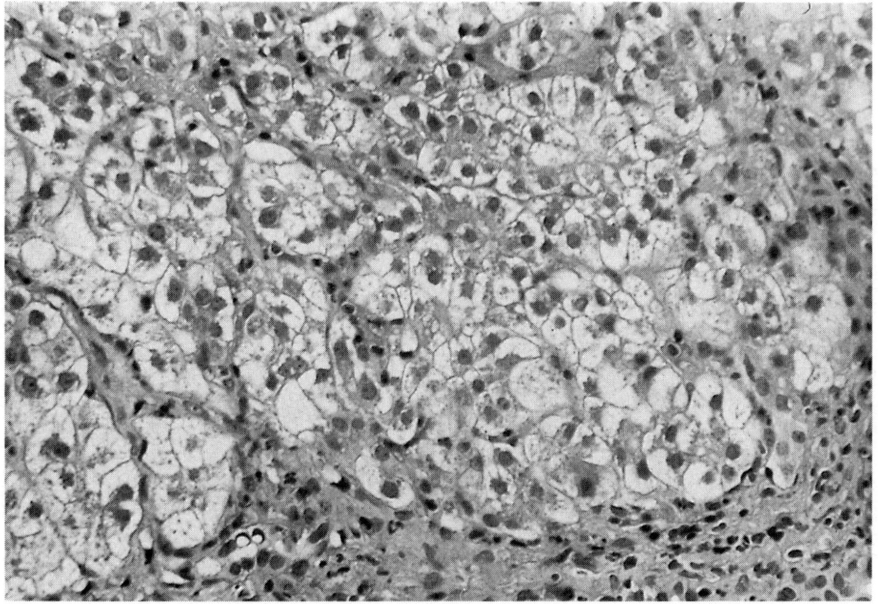

Fig. 5. Chronic active AIH: ballooning degeneration and lytic necrosis is the predominant type of cell lesion. Hematoxylin–eosin stain. × 240.

3. *Ultrastructural lesions in AIH*

At the electron microscopic level, likewise, there is no pathognomonic feature
distinguishing AIH from viral hepatitis. Cell damage in AIH mainly shows
hydropic swelling with dilation of the endoplasmic reticulum (ER) finally resulting in lytic necrosis (Fig. 6). The profiles are disarranged, sometimes forming
small vesicles. Ribosomes can be observed detached from the membranes of the
ER and a loss of glycogen indicates the degree of cell damage. The mitochondria
display no specific lesions. Some may show condensation or loosening of the
matrix (Fig. 7). Megamitochondria in AIH are the exception when compared to
viral hepatitis. The nuclei of these ballooned hepatocytes show rounding with
loosening of the karyoplasm. These cell alterations can be interpreted as a prestige of lytic necrosis of hepatocytes. Overt disruptures of the plasma membrane

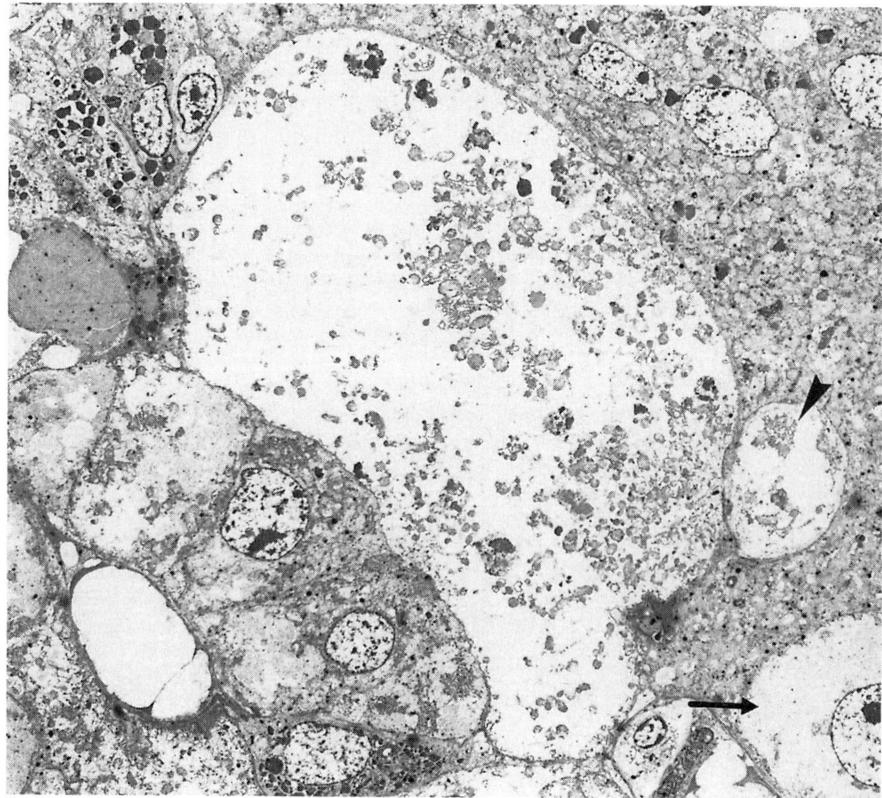

Fig. 6. Chronic active AIH: electron micrograph of a hepatocyte with ballooning degeneration
(arrow) and a lytic necrosis (arrowhead) spilling the cellular debris in a dilated sinusoid. × 1700.

are hardly seen since this event seems to be of a spurious time span only. During the active phase of the disease, alterations of the membrane are observed: flattening of the plasma membrane with loss of microvilli; and bleb formation into the space of Dissé. The ballooning type of degeneration is mostly encountered in the periportal zone of the lobule. The hepatocytes of this area are often arranged in a microacinar transformation (Fig. 7A). These rosettes of hepatocytes display a flattened plasma membrane at the outer circle of the rounded hepatocytes, whereas the inner surface is often arranged around a dilated bile canaliculus. The space of Dissé at the outer surface is often filled with basement-membrane-like material (Fig. 7B). The early rosetting of hepatocytes in AIH is remarkable and remains to be elucidated in its pathogenetic relevance. The phenomenon of lytic necrosis usually fails to arouse a conspicuous scenario of tissue damage since the debris of the necrotic cells is flushed away immediately and disappears (Fig. 6). Occasionally, swollen hepatic giant cells may be observed (Fig. 8).

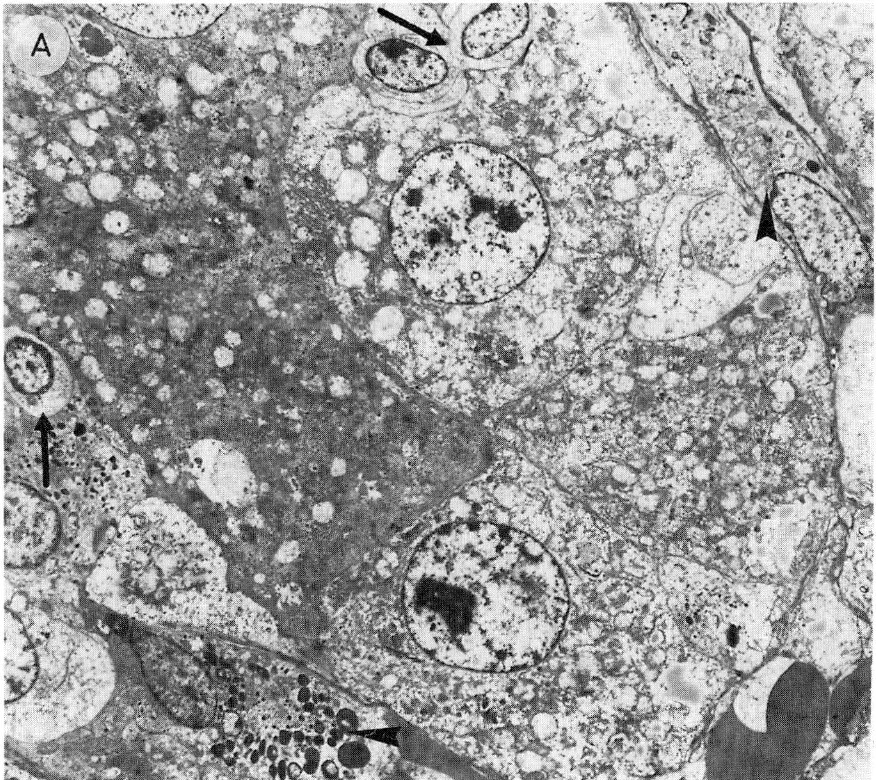

Fig. 7A.

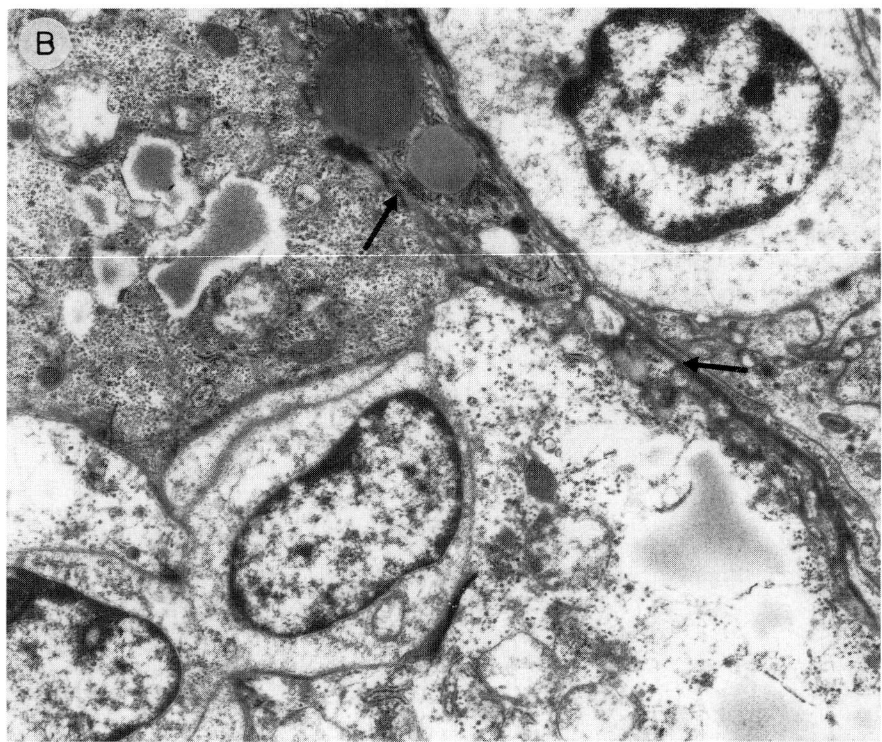

Fig. 7. Chronic active AIH: A: microacinar transformation of hepatocytes surrounded by inflammatory cells as lymphocytes (arrows) and Kupffer cells (arrowhead; × 1700). B: higher magnification of A (× 10,500) giving details of lymphocytes in emperipolesis and basement-like material (arrow) around the acinar transformation.

The other type of cell injury, acidophilic damage of hepatocytes, is less frequent in AIH than in viral hepatitis. The lesion starts with condensation of cytoplasmic organelles. The ER is compressed and profiles of the ER are shrunk to parallel mostly concentric bands.

Apoptotic bodies hardly discernible by light microscopy are infrequently distributed over the lobules containing condensed organelles of the cytoplasm. Either type of necrosis may be induced by T-cell-mediated cell injury (Ramadori et al., 1990) following different ways of target cell killing. Both mechanisms seem to be independent: the lytic type is induced by pore-forming mechanisms like perforin (Podack, 1985); whereas the apoptotic type of necrosis is brought about by endogenous nucleases triggering the target cell to commit programmed suicide (Ucker, 1987).

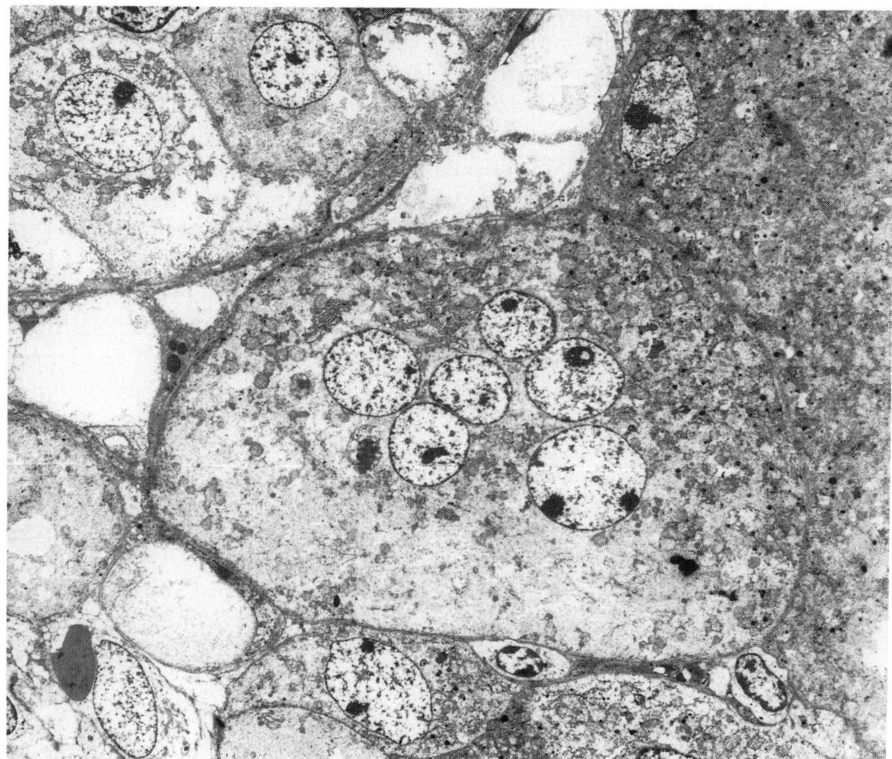

Fig. 8. Chronic active AIH with a hepatogenic giant cell displaying ballooning degeneration.

Affection of the bile ducts in AIH is variable, but can attain a high degree in the overlapping syndrome. The basement membrane may be fragmented or split with some dense deposits between the lamellae. So far, however, we have not been able to detect overt disrupture. The bile duct epithelia may show pycnosis and necrotic cells in some instances with the membrane lying bare.

In the later stages of the disease, the space of Dissé becomes clogged with basement-membrane-like material ('capillarization') and collagen fibrils start to develop. The process is most pronounced in the periportal area along the formation of the septa.

4. *The inflammatory infiltrate*

The dense mononuclear infiltrate is the hallmark of AIH, signifying that the underlying mechanism of tissue damage is immune mediated, probably T-cell dependent. The invasion of the cells seems to start from the portal tracts or active septa. Analysis of the different types of the mononuclear cells by light and electron microscopy shows a majority of lymphocytes, whereas plasma cells are not a constituting feature of AIH making up about 5–8% which is the same figure as in viral hepatitis. The term 'plasma cell hepatitis' should, therefore, be avoided. In the chronic B and C types, this population of inflammatory cells is at least as frequent as in AIH. Polymorphonuclear leucocytes constitute only a very small percentage of the infiltrating cells as do the eosinophils. The lymphocytes are most numerous in the sinusoids and in the space of Dissé, often in close contact with the hepatocytes. The invasion of the hepatocytes by lymphocytes is a common phenomenon, thus augmenting the interface between both cells resulting in a state of emperipolesis. By electron microscopy, a variable degree of cell damage of the hepatocytes can be described as flattening of the microvilli, focal cytoplas-

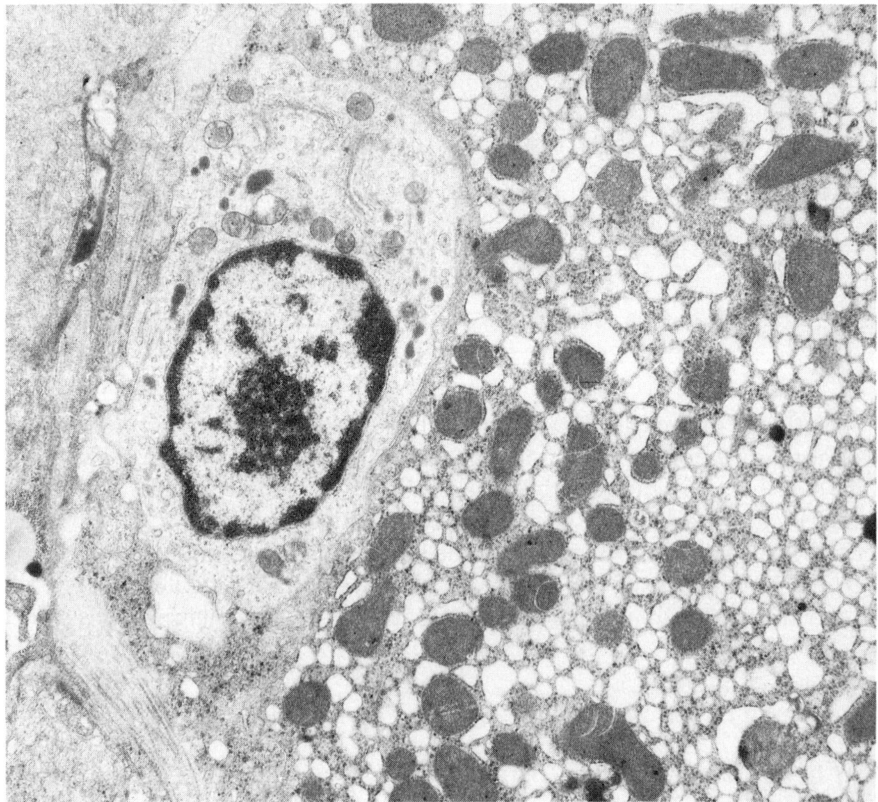

Fig. 9. Chronic active AIH: a cytotoxic lymphocyte with many organelles and dense granules in a state of emperipolesis. × 10,500.

mic degeneration or dilatation of the ER (Fig. 9). It is tempting to regard this feature as an effector–target cell interaction, but most hepatocytes do not show overt cell damage; disrupture of the plasma membrane as known from immune-mediated cell attack is hardly seen by electron microscopy.

The infiltrating lymphocytes display a different morphology when analyzed by electron microscopy. Many lymphocytes show a narrow rim of cytoplasm with few cell organelles. Among the lymphocytes in the space of Dissé, there is a large number with broad cytoplasm and many cell organelles as mitochondria and peroxisomes and membrane-bound dense granules (Fig. 9). These granules are regarded as indicators of a state of activation and presumably harbor the cytotoxic tools of the lymphocytes that can be induced by interleukins. Another type of cytotoxic lymphocytes recognizable by the presence of parallel tubular rays in the cytoplasm, and regarded as genuine killer cells, however, is rather infrequent. The role of Kupffer cells in the course of the disease as a factor in the immune response and their function as antigen-presenting cells or even as cytotoxic effector cells is poorly understood, and so far, few reports have been published on this subject. The Kupffer cells can make up to 40% of the inflammatory infiltrate which is about the same in viral and autoimmune hepatitis. Subtyping of the infiltrating cells by electron microscopy is a rather rough tool and does not give conclusive hints to the functional role of the cells which can be evaluated only by the immunostaining of relevant epitopes of the lymphocytes or by in vitro testing. Studies applying these techniques have shown that T-lymphocytes prevail with a CD4/CD8 ratio of about 1 : 1.5. The discussion of this subject, however, is beyond, the scope of this chapter.

References

Bianchi, L., Spichtin, H.-P. and Gudat, F. (1987) In R.N.M. MacSween, P.P. Anthony and P.J. Scheuer (Eds.), Pathology of the Liver. Churchill Livingstone, Edinburgh, pp. 310–341.

Carrougher, J.G., Shaffer, R.T., Canales, L.I. et al. (1991) Diagnostic problems in clinical hepatology – a 33-year-old woman with an autoimmune syndrome. Semin. Liver Dis. 11, 256–262.

Dienes, H.P. (1989) Viral and Autoimmune Hepatitis, Fischer, Stuttgart.

Dienes, H.P., Popper, H., Manns, M. et al. (1989) Histologic features in autoimmune hepatitis. Z. Gastroenterol. 27, 325–330.

Dienes, H.P., Autschbach, F. and Gerber, M.A. (1991) Ultrastructural lesion in autoimmune hepatitis and steps of the immune response in liver tissue. Semin. Liver Dis. 11, 197–204.

Eggink, H.F., Houthoff, H.J., Huitema, S. et al. (1982) Cellular and humoral immune reactions in chronic active liver diseases. I. Lymphocyte subsets in liver biopsies of patients with untreated idiopathic autoimmune hepatitis, chronic active hepatitis B and primary biliary cirrhosis. Clin. Exp. Immunol. 50, 17–24.

Klöppel, G., Seifert, G., Lindner, H. et al. (1977) Histopathologic features in mixed types of chronic aggressive hepatitis and primary biliary cirrhosis. Virchows Arch. A 373, 143–160.

Korb, G. (1989) Aktuelle Aspekte zur Morphologie der chronischen Hepatitis. Z. Klin. Med. 44, 357–360.

Korb, G. and Berg, P.A. (1990) The morphologic spectrum of autoimmune hepatitis (Abstract). Int. Acad. Pathol., Buenos Aires, 43.

Lefkowitch, J.H., Apfelbaum, T.F., Weinberg, L. et al. (1984) Acute liver biopsy lesions in early autoimmune ('lupoid') chronic active hepatitis. Liver 4, 379–386.

Lohse, A.W., Manns, M., Dienes, H.P. et al. (1990) Experimental autoimmune hepatitis: disease induction, time course and T-cell reactivity. Hepatology 11, 24–30.

Manns, M., Gerken, G., Kyriatsoulis, A. et al. (1987) Heterogeneity of autoimmune type chronic active hepatitis: characterization of a new subgroup of autoantibodies against soluble liver antigen. Lancet I, 292–294.

Meuer, S.C. and Dienes, H.P. (1989) Lymphocyte mediated cell lysis. Virchows Arch. B 57, 1–9.

Meyer zum Büschenfelde, K.-H., Lohse, A.W., Manns, M. et al. (1990) Autoimmunity and liver disease. Hepatology 12, 354–363.

Podack, E.R. (1985) The molecular mechanism of lymphocyte-mediated tumor cell lysis. Immunol. Today. 6, 21.

Ramadori, G., Moebius, C., Dienes, H.P. et al. (1990) Lymphocytes from hepatic inflammatory infiltrate kill rat hepatocytes in primary culture. Virchows Arch. B 59, 263–270.

Ucker, D.S. (1987) Cytotoxic T lymphocytes and glucocorticoids activate an endogenous suicide process in target cells. Nature 327, 62.

Section IV

Autoantibodies in Autoimmune Hepatitis

Autoimmune Hepatitis
Edited by M. Nishioka, G. Toda and M. Zeniya
© *1994, Elsevier Science B.V. All rights reserved*

Chapter 8

Anti-asialoglycoprotein receptor antibodies

Barbara M. McFarlane and Ian G. McFarlane

Institute of Liver Studies, King's College Hospital and School of Medicine and Dentistry,
Denmark Hill, London SE5 9RS (U.K.)

1. Background

The discovery that patients with chronic active hepatitis (CAH) have circulating autoantibodies that react with the galactose-specific hepatic asialoglycoprotein receptor (ASPG-R) arose out of studies on the characterization of the high-molecular-weight fraction of normal liver known as the 'liver-specific membrane lipoprotein' (LSP) complex (McFarlane et al., 1977). The latter was first described by Meyer zum Büschenfelde and Miescher (1972) in Germany and had been used for many years as a source of liver-specific antigens to study cellular and humoral autoreactions in liver disease (for review see McFarlane, 1984). Early in vitro studies had shown that patients with autoimmune CAH exhibit antibody-dependent (K-cell) cellular cytotoxic (ADCC) reactions against hepatocytes (Cochrane et al., 1976; Gonzales et al., 1979), and that these reactions were targeted at antigens in the LSP preparation – although it was not until 1978 that definitive proof of the existence of autoantibodies to this preparation was obtained (Jensen et al., 1978; Kakumu et al., 1979; Manns et al., 1980).

During this period, several investigators had been attempting to identify the target autoantigens in LSP by conventional techniques, but without success. However, in the early 1980s, evidence began to emerge suggesting that LSP is partly comprised of fragments of liver cell plasma membranes (DeKretser et al., 1980; Lebwohl and Gerber, 1980; Jensen et al., 1983). It seemed likely, therefore, that the LSP preparation should contain the ASGP-R, which had been extensively characterized biochemically and was known to be specific to hepatocytes and expressed in the plasma membrane (McFarlane, 1983; Schwartz, 1984). It was found that LSP does, indeed, contain the ASGP-R – which seems to be a highly immunogenic component of the preparation, in that animals immunized with LSP show an early, high titre, antibody response to ASGP-R (McFarlane et al., 1984a).

2. *The asialoglycoprotein receptor*

The ASGP-R participates in the binding and endocytosis of serum asialoglycoproteins bearing terminal galactose or *N*-acetyl-galactosamine (GalNAc) residues (McFarlane, 1983; Schwartz, 1984), and is distinct from other carbohydrate receptors, such as those on Kupffer cells, endothelial lining cells, or in plasma (Kolb-Bachofen et al., 1982; Lehrman and Hill, 1983; Roos et al.,1985; Taylor and Summerfield, 1986; Pfeffer, 1988). Binding to the receptor is highly dependent on the number and spatial arrangement of the terminal galactose residues in the oligosaccharide – ligands with the highest affinity having at least 3 terminal galactose residues (Baenziger, 1985; Spiess, 1990; Lodish, 1991). The ASGP-R is well preserved phylogenetically. It has been isolated from rabbit (Hudgin et al., 1974), human (Baenziger and Maynard, 1980), rat (Schwartz et al., 1981), and mouse (Hong et al., 1988; Sanford et al., 1988) livers, and a similar receptor has been described in avian species (Kawasaki and Ashwell, 1977; Loeb and Drickamer, 1987).

Calcium is essential for binding of asialoglycoprotein ligands to ASGP-R, which occurs only above pH 6.5 (Spiess, 1990). Optimal Ca^{2+} concentration is 0.1 mM for isolated hepatocytes (Weigel, 1980), 2.0 mM for isolated liver plasma membranes (Van Lenten and Ashwell, 1972), and 20 mM for the purified rabbit receptor (Andersen et al., 1982). Acidification or addition of chelating agents (e.g., EDTA) leads to rapid dissociation of prebound ligand (Andersen et al., 1982; Spiess, 1990). Purification of the receptor from liver involves affinity chromatography of Triton X-100 extracts of acetone powders of fresh tissue on immobilized asialoglycoprotein (usually asialo-orosomucoid) (Hudgin et al., 1974; Baenziger and Maynard, 1980), lactose (Treichel et al., 1990), or galactose (Halberg et al., 1987), in a Ca^{2+}-containing buffer at pH 7.8. The receptor bound to the column is then eluted with a Ca^{2+}-free buffer below pH 6.5 and Triton is removed by re-chromatography of the eluate in detergent-free buffer.

The purified receptor fulfils the criteria of a lectin, in that it is capable of inducing erythrocyte agglutination and lymphocyte mitosis in vitro (Stockert et al., 1974; Novogrodsky and Ashwell, 1977). For this reason, it was initially designated 'hepatic lectin', but the term has fallen into disuse because of a tendency for confusion with other animal and plant lectins.

2.1. Structure of the ASGP-R

The ASGP-R is itself a glycoprotein, with terminal carbohydrate sequences (-mannose/N-acetyl-glucosamine (GlcNac)/galactose/sialic acid) similar to those of the oligosaccharide moieties of other glycoproteins (Paulson et al., 1977). In aqueous solutions, the rabbit receptor has an apparent molecular weight (MW) of 500 kDa and a tendency to self-associate to form an oligomeric series bearing the integral proportions 1:2:3:4:5, but, in the presence of Triton X-100, a single monomeric species of approximately 250 kDa is obtained (Kawasaki and Ashwell, 1976a). The rabbit monomer is comprised of two subunits with MWs of 48 kDa (subunit A) and 40 kDa (subunit B) in a ratio of 1:2. Data from glycopeptide analysis (Kawasaki and Ashwell, 1976b) are consistent with the presence of two and three complex oligosaccharide moieties in subunits B (40 kDa) and A (48 kDa), respectively, with an additional 'polymannose' chain ($-[\text{Man}]_n$/GlcNac linked to asparagine) in subunit A.

It was initially presumed that the 250-kDa monomer constitutes two A and four B subunits (Kawasaki and Ashwell, 1976a). However, later estimations of the size of the monomer vary from 110 to 612 kDa, depending on the type of detergent employed, the presence or absence of Ca^{2+}, and the method of analysis (Steer et al., 1981; Andersen et al., 1982), and the question of the size of the functional receptor remains unresolved (see below).

Major advances in elucidating the structure of the ASGP-R have been made in recent years. It is now known that, in the rat, it is comprised of 3 subunits: a predominating form of approximately 42 kDa (R1) and two minor subunits of about 50 (R2) and 55 (R3) kDa (Tanabe et al., 1979; Schwartz et al., 1981; Halberg et al., 1987). Protein and cDNA sequence analyses have revealed that the amino acid sequences of R2 and R3 are identical, but differ from R1, and it is thought that R2 and R3 arise from a single mRNA and differ only in the extent of glycosylation and/or other post-translational modifications (Drickamer et al., 1984; Halberg et al., 1987; Sanford et al., 1988).

As prepared from liver, human ASGP-R appears to be a single polypeptide (H1) of either 41 kDa (Baenziger and Maynard, 1980) or 46 kDa (Schwartz and Rup, 1983), depending on the method of preparation (it is thought that the smaller form is a precursor species and the larger is the fully processed mature receptor (Schwartz and Rup, 1983)). However, cloning of the human ASGP-R has revealed a second receptor protein (H2) (Spiess and Lodish, 1985), which exists as two subspecies, H2A and H2B (Lodish, 1991). In Hep-G2 cells, 90% of H2 is in the form of H2B, which appears to be a spliced version of H2A with just 5 amino acids missing (Lederkremer and Lodish, 1991). Comparison of the amino acid sequences of the rat and human receptors reveals greater sequence homology between H1 and R1 than H1 and H2, and that H2 bears greater similarity to R2 than to H1. Mouse ASGP-R, like its rat counterpart, is also comprised of 3 subunits (42, 45 and 51 kDa) (Hong et al., 1988) and two genes homologous to

ASGP-R have been identified in the mouse genome on chromosome 11 (Sanford et al., 1988). To date, there are no cloning or sequencing data on the rabbit receptor.

When inserted in the plasma membrane, the ASGP-R has a transmembrane disposition, with an NH$_2$-terminal segment of about 40 amino acid residues on the cytosolic side of the membrane (Fig. 1), a short (19-residue) hydrophobic segment spanning the lipid bilayer, and the remainder (approximately 80%) of the molecule oriented on the external (mainly sinusoidal) surface of the hepatocyte (Chiacchia and Drickamer, 1984; Schwartz, 1984; Spiess and Handschin, 1987). The hydrophobic membrane-spanning segment contains the signal sequence that targets synthesis of the receptor to the endoplasmic reticulum (ER) and initiates its insertion in the ER membrane in the correct orientation (Spiess and Handschin, 1987). The externally oriented part of the molecule comprises an α-helical stalk of about 90 amino acids and the remaining 130, COOH-terminal,

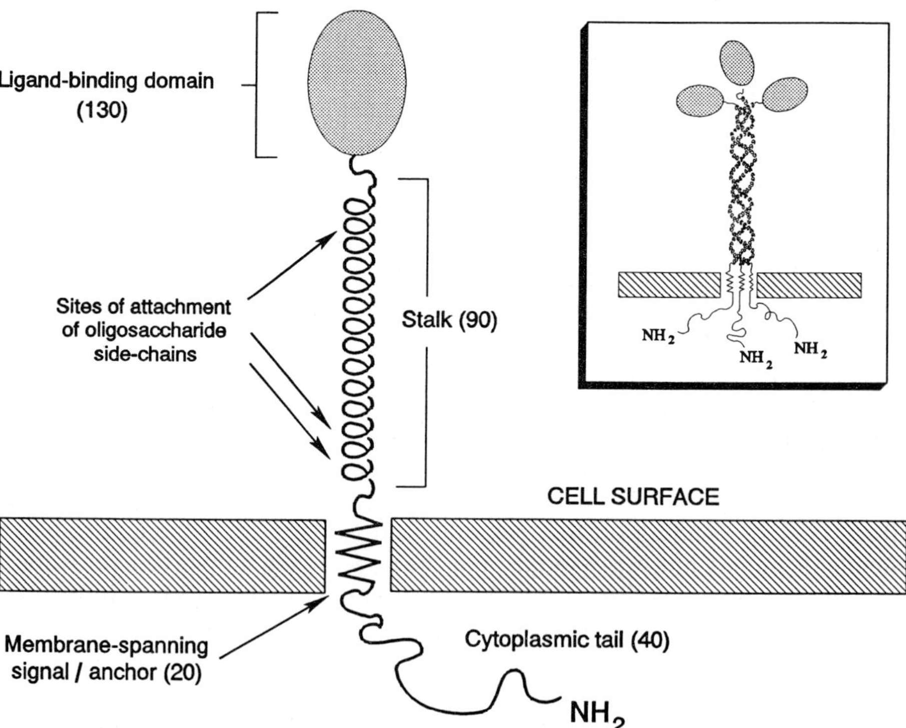

Fig. 1. Diagrammatic representation of the structure of the hepatic asialoglycoprotein receptor (ASGP-R). Numbers in brackets indicate approximate numbers of amino acid residues in each segment. Inset shows postulated arrangement of the ASGP-R as a trimer in the plasma membrane in vivo.

amino acid residues are thought to comprise a globular structure representing the ligand-binding domain of the receptor (Hsueh et al., 1986; Drickamer, 1987; Spiess, 1990), containing both the ligand-binding and the calcium-binding sites, which appear to be distinct from each other (Blomhoff et al., 1982). Recent evidence suggests that, when expressed on the cell surface, the ASGP-R exists as a hetero-oligomeric complex, probably at least a trimer (Drickamer, 1987; Lodish, 1991), with the stalk regions wound around each other to form an α-helical coiled-coil structure (Gould et al., 1991; Beavil et al., 1992) (Fig. 1).

2.2. Distribution of the ASGP-R

Biochemical (Tolleshaug et al., 1977) and electron microscopic autoradiographic (Hubbard et al., 1979) studies have confirmed the exclusivity of the ASGP-R to hepatocytes, and its liver-specificity has also been confirmed on immunochemical criteria (McFarlane et al., 1984a; McSorley et al., 1988; Sipos et al., 1989). Other studies have demonstrated the ASGP-R along the entire surface of the hepatocyte plasma membrane, but with some 90% of the surface-expressed receptor concentrated in clathrin-coated pits at the sinusoidal poles of the cells (Wall and Hubbard, 1981; Geuze et al., 1982). Estimates of the number of functional receptors on hepatocyte surfaces vary according to the method employed from about 30,000 to 500,000 per cell (Schwartz et al., 1980; Steer and Ashwell, 1980; Weigel, 1980; Zeitlin and Hubbard, 1982; Eisenberg et al., 1991).

In common with other proteins destined for the plasma membrane and/or for export, the polypeptide moiety of the receptor is initially inserted into the membrane of the rough ER and is then transported to the cell surface through a series of intermediate organelles (including the smooth ER and the Golgi apparatus) where it undergoes post-translational modifications (including glycosylation) (Schwartz and Rup, 1983; Kornfeld and Kornfeld, 1985; Hsueh et al., 1986). ASGP-R functionally and structurally identical to the plasma membrane receptor is also found in lysosomes, endocytic vesicles and other subcellular membranous organelles (Pricer and Ashwell, 1976; Herzig and Weigel, 1990) and, at any given time, between 40 and 90% of the ASGP-R in the liver may be present on various intra-cellular structures (Schwartz, 1984; Bischoff and Lodish, 1987). This substantial pool of intra-cellular ASGP-R is thus thought to represent, partly, nascent receptor en route to the plasma membrane and, partly, mature ASGP-R participating in cyclical endocytic functions.

The intra-cellular ASGP-R can be demonstrated by immunohistochemical staining of cryostat sections of frozen liver using specific antibodies, but careful attention has to be paid to the method of fixation of the tissue (Sipos et al., 1989). By this technique, it can be shown that all hepatocytes contain the receptor. However, studies of ligand uptake and perfusion studies with anti-ASGP-R antibodies indicate that, in vivo, the receptor is predominantly expressed on periportal hepatocytes (Fig. 2), with little or no cell surface expression in the

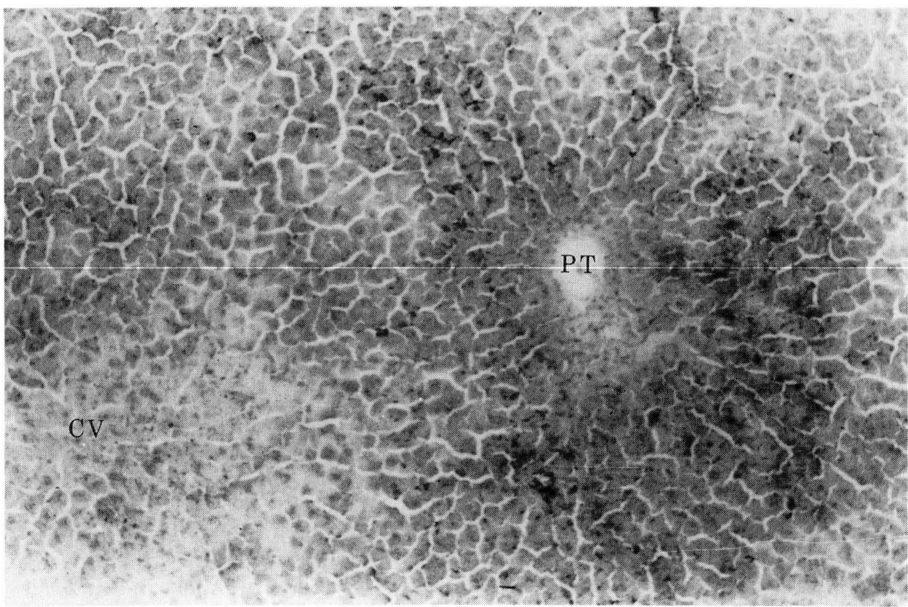

Fig. 2. Photomicrograph of rat liver following perfusion in situ with a murine monoclonal anti-human ASGP-R antibody and localization of the antibody by immunohistochemical staining with peroxidase-conjugated rabbit anti-mouse immunoglobulin. Note dense staining of periportal hepatocytes. Apparent cytoplasmic staining is due to spill-over of chromogen. Counterstained with Mayer's haemalum. PT, portal tract; CV, central vein. From McFarlane et al. (1990), with permission.

pericentral zone (Daniels et al., 1987; McFarlane et al., 1990). Thus the importance of the ASGP-R as an autoantigen in CAH derives not only from demonstrations of autoreactions against it (see below) but also from its organ-specificity and its preferential expression on the surfaces of those hepatocytes that are the main targets of tissue damage in this condition.

3. Detection of anti-ASGP-R autoantibodies

3.1. Methods

Anti-ASGP-R autoantibodies were first detected by a specific liquid phase radioimmunoassay (RIA), using purified rabbit ASGP-R labelled with ^{125}I by the lactoperoxidase method (David and Reisfeld, 1974) and *Staphylococcus aureus* (Newman D_2C strain) cells to precipitate [^{125}I]ASGP-R/anti-ASGP-R immune complexes (McFarlane et al., 1985). The assay is performed in a Ca^{2+}-free buffer with added EDTA, to avoid binding of carbohydrate residues in immuno-globulins to the receptor. This RIA is highly sensitive, but has the disadvantage that it cannot discriminate between different isotypes of specific antibodies, since the staphylococcal cells bind IgM, IgA_2, and IgG_1, IgG_2 and IgG_4 (Brunda et al., 1977). Later, Treichel et al. (1990) developed a solid-phase enzyme-linked immunoassay (ELISA) which seems to be somewhat less sensitive but has the potential for investigation of different anti-ASGP-R antibody isotypes. This assay is performed in phosphate-buffered saline without EDTA and there is, therefore, a theoretical possibility of false-positive reactions due to binding of immunoglobulins directly to the receptor via carbohydrate residues. However, this seems unlikely because addition of GalNAc to the system does not inhibit antibody binding (Treichel et al., 1990).

3.2. Anti-ASGP-R in chronic active hepatitis

The earliest report of circulating anti-ASGP-R documented the finding of antibodies against *rabbit* ASGP-R in 83% of patients with autoimmune CAH who had active disease at the time of testing by RIA (McFarlane et al., 1986). Titres of anti-ASGP-R correlated strongly with histologically assessed severity of disease, but not with biochemical parameters of liver injury nor with serum immunoglobulin concentrations or titres of other autoantibodies, and patients in complete remission on immunosuppressive therapy were all seronegative for anti-ASGP-R. That study also found a high frequency (73%) of anti-ASGP-R in

Table 1

Autoantibodies against rabbit ASGP-R in various liver disorders
Cumulative data from McFarlane et al. (1986), Vento et al. (1988), and
Bedlow et al. (1989).

	Percent positive by RIA
Autoimmune CAH	
Active	83
In remission	0
HBsAg-positive	
CAH	73
CPH	25
Chronic non-A, non-B hepatitis	14
Primary biliary cirrhosis	23
Primary sclerosing cholangitis	10
Acute viral hepatitis	
A	30
B	40
Non-A, non-B	5

CAH due to chronic hepatitis B virus (HBV) infection (HBV-CAH) (Table 1), but at significantly lower titres than in autoimmune CAH.

In the later (ELISA-based) study of Treichel et al. (1990), the species cross-reactivity of anti-ASGP-R antibodies was examined by testing sera on microtitre plates coated with human, rabbit or rat ASGP-R. Antibodies against *human* ASGP-R were found in 50% of patients with autoimmune CAH (titres were not reported). The highest frequency (88%) was seen in patients with histologically documented active disease – compared with 31% of those in clinical (but not necessarily biochemical or histological) remission. However, only 27% overall (42% in the subgroup with biopsy-proven active disease) had antibodies against *rabbit* ASGP-R and 40% had anti-*rat*-ASGP-R. In the majority (60%) of patients with anti-ASGP-R the antibodies reacted with human and either rat and/or rabbit ASGP-R, but 30% of these sera reacted only with the human receptor protein and 10% recognized exclusively rat or rabbit ASGP-R (Table 2). By contrast, in HBV-CAH, only 4% of patients studied had anti-*human* ASGP-R while 21% of the sera reacted with *rabbit* ASGP-R and almost all of these positive sera also reacted with *rat* ASGP-R.

The finding that almost all of the anti-ASGP-R antibodies in HBV-CAH patients, and a small proportion of those in autoimmune CAH, react exclusively with xenogeneic ASGP-R suggests that these patients had somehow become specifically sensitized to the rabbit or rat receptor, without producing antibodies that cross-react with human epitopes. This is very difficult to understand especially in view of the marked sequence homology, at both the amino acid and the genomic levels (see above), between ASGP-R molecules from different species. The ELISAs for antibodies against ASGP-R from the 3 species were essentially 3 distinct assays and one possibility that must be considered is that, although each was carefully standardized (Treichel et al., 1990), there might have been

Table 2

Species cross-reactivity of anti-ASGP-R autoantibodies in various liver disorders
Data from Treichel et al. (1990).

	Number tested	Percent of anti-ASGP-R-positive sera reactive vs ASGP-R from species shown		
		Human only	Human and rabbit or rat	Rabbit or rat only
Autoimmune CAH	49	31	59	10
HBsAg-positive CAH	17	0	12	88
Chronic non-A, non-B hepatitis	10	0	0	100
Primary biliary cirrhosis	22	18	23	59
Alcoholic liver disease	17	0	18	82
Acute viral hepatitis	5	0	20	80

subtle differences in binding of the antigens to the solid phase that could have influenced expression of conformational epitopes. Unfortunately, it was not reported whether absorption of sera with human ASGP-R abolished reactivity against rabbit or rat ASGP-R, which might have provided an answer to this question.

Because of the technical differences between the RIA and ELISA systems and also because of differences in categories of patients studied and in methods of reporting the data, direct comparisons between studies with the different assays cannot be made. Nevertheless, there is good overall agreement between the findings in the different laboratories, in that anti-ASGP-R seems to be particularly associated with histologically active CAH, independently of serum biochemical parameters and of the presence or absence of other autoantibodies, and seems to decline in titre and/or disappear with response to therapy (McFarlane et al., 1986; Johnson et al., 1990; Treichel et al., 1990).

3.3. Anti-ASGP-R in other liver disorders

3.3.1. Primary biliary cirrhosis
In primary biliary cirrhosis (PBC), antibodies reacting with rabbit ASGP-R have been found in 23% of patients by RIA and in 22% by ELISA (Bedlow et al., 1989; Treichel et al., 1990), and correlate with severity of periportal inflammation and piecemeal necrosis in the later stages of the disease (Bedlow et al., 1989). In addition, seropositivity for (and titres of) anti-ASGP-R appear to be influenced by inheritance of the HLA allotypes DR2 and DR3. Thus, the highest titres of these antibodies were found in patients who were DR3 + /DR2–, while all DR2 + patients (even if they also had DR3) were anti-ASGP-R-negative (Bedlow et al., 1989). DR3 in these patients was also associated with significantly higher, and DR2 with lower, serum IgG concentrations – independent of anti-ASGP-R. These findings suggest that, in PBC, DR2 and DR3 are associated with one or more genes that code, respectively, for down-regulation or for elevation of overall immunoresponsiveness, and it seems that production of anti-ASGP-R in PBC may be part of the background immunological 'noise' in this condition and may not be primarily related to hepatocellular injury, although the antibodies may contribute to this (Bedlow et al., 1989).

3.3.2. Primary sclerosing cholangitis
Anti-ASGP-R is rare in adults with primary sclerosing cholangitis (PSC). In the only study to date (Bedlow et al., 1989), only 10% of patients had anti-ASGP-R and the antibodies did not correlate with histological evidence of periportal inflammation and piecemeal necrosis. The situation is somewhat more complicated in children with PSC because the condition overlaps considerably with autoimmune CAH but, in one detailed study of liver autoreactivity in paediatric cases (Mieli-Vergani et al., 1989), only two of 8 patients had anti-ASGP-R and the

presence of the antibodies did not appear to correlate with any of the large number of clinical, histological and immunological parameters investigated.

3.3.3. Chronic non-A, non-B viral hepatitis

In common with other autoantibodies, anti-ASGP-R occurs infrequently (–15%) in patients who present with post-transfusion or sporadic (i.e., 'community-acquired') chronic non-A, non-B (NANB) hepatitis (McFarlane et al., 1986; Treichel et al., 1990). Since, until recently, the diagnosis of chronic NANB hepatitis was made by exclusion of other aetiological factors and the absence of autoantibodies, and since patients with autoimmune CAH can sometimes present without conventional autoantibodies (Czaja et al., 1990; Johnson et al., 1990), it was thought that the few chronic NANB patients with anti-ASGP-R may have been undiagnosed cases of autoimmune CAH. However, the situation in no longer clear.

Following the development of serological tests for antibodies against the hepatitis C virus (HCV) (Kuo et al., 1989) reports from Spain (Esteban et al., 1989) and from Italy (Lenzi et al., 1990), documented the finding of anti-HCV in a high proportion of type 1 (anti-nuclear antibody (ANA) or smooth muscle antibody (SMA)-positive) and type 2 (liver–kidney microsomal antibody (LKM-1)-positive) autoimmune CAH patients. Initial studies in our laboratories revealed a similarly high frequency of positive anti-HCV results among British patients with type 1 autoimmune CAH, but these seemed to be false-positive reactions (McFarlane et al., 1990).

That the original anti-HCV tests were prone to false-positivity is now well documented (for review see McFarlane, 1991). However, subsequent studies have revealed that there is an element of geographical heterogeneity with respect to the association between HCV infections and autoimmune CAH. A collaborative study of patients from the United Kingdom and Italy, using a new anti-HCV test (Hosein et al., 1991) that does not give false-positive reactions with autoimmune CAH sera, has confirmed that a high proportion of Italian patients who fulfil all of the current criteria (including anti-ASGP-R) for diagnosis of type 1 or type 2 autoimmune CAH do apparently have anti-HCV antibodies (53 and 88%, respectively, vs 13 and 0% in U.K. patients) (Lenzi et al., 1991). Furthermore, it has since been confirmed that the majority of the anti-HCV-positive type 2 Italian patients have chronic HCV infection, as determined by demonstration of HCV-RNA genomic material in their sera by the polymerase chain reaction (PCR) technique (Garson et al., 1991). Anti-HCV-positive type 1 patients were not tested by PCR in that study.

It is not clear whether these Italian patients represent a group with auto-immune CAH who have superimposed HCV infections or whether this is a subpopulation of chronic HCV patients with autoantibodies or, as has been suggested (Garson et al., 1991), HCV has induced autoimmune CAH in these cases. However, recent studies have shown that Italian patients with essential mixed cryoglobulinaemia also have a high frequency of apparent chronic HCV infections (McFarlane, 1992). Taken together, these findings suggest that individuals with immunological abnormalities may be more prone to develop chronic HCV following sporadic infections, i.e., that the HCV is secondary to the underlying condition, which might explain the high frequency of HCV in patients with immunological disorders in areas where the virus is endemic.

3.3.4. Other chronic liver disorders

In addition to the above categories, there is a group of patients with chronic active liver disease who are seronegative for ANA, SMA and LKM antibodies and in whom none of the known aetiological factors can be implicated. Some of these 'cryptogenic' cases are responsive to immunosuppressive therapy and, in this and other respects (apart from the absence of circulating ANA, SMA or LKM), are indistinguishable from patients with autoimmune CAH (Czaja et al., 1990; Gitnick, 1990; Johnson et al., 1990). It has been found that the majority of such patients (who may account for up to 30% of patients with steroid-responsive, presumed autoimmune, CAH) have anti-ASGP-R antibodies, and that titres fluctuate with response to therapy and in relation to disease activity (Fig. 3) in a manner similar to that seen in autoimmune CAH (Johnson et al., 1990).

Apart from the above, there have been no definitive studies of anti-ASGP-R in other chronic liver disorders, but Treichel et al. (1990) have reported that 26% of patients with alcoholic liver disease (ALD) have anti-rabbit-ASGP-R antibodies and similar findings have been obtained in our laboratories (Wojcicka-McFarlane, 1990). Whether these patients represent a particular subgroup of ALD is not yet known, but previous studies have shown that a similar proportion of ALD patients have anti-LSP antibodies and that these correlate with the histological picture of active cirrhosis (Perperas et al., 1981) – raising the possibility that auto-reactions against liver antigens may be involved in liver damage in some patients. Further studies of anti-ASGP-R in ALD are required to resolve this question.

3.3.5. Acute viral hepatitis

Anti-ASGP-R can be detected by RIA in up to 60% of patients with uncomplicated acute virus A (HAV) or B (HBV) hepatitis (Vento et al., 1988). Titres reach a peak within the first few weeks of onset and decline rapidly thereafter, with patients becoming negative during the recovery phase. In contrast, anti-ASGP-R occurs very rarely in acute NANB hepatitis – even in Italian patients (see above) (Vento et al., 1988). Treichel et al. (1990) have reported finding anti-rabbit ASGP-R antibodies in 36% of patients with acute viral hepatitis, but details of which viruses were involved and timing of testing were not given and serial studies were not performed.

In protracted acute virus A or B hepatitis, particularly those cases that progress to chronic hepatitis (McFarlane, 1991), anti-ASGP-R titres may remain elevated. During a prospective study of relatives of patients with autoimmune CAH, Vento et al. (1991) documented progression to type 1 autoimmune CAH in two of three previously healthy individuals who developed asymptomatic acute

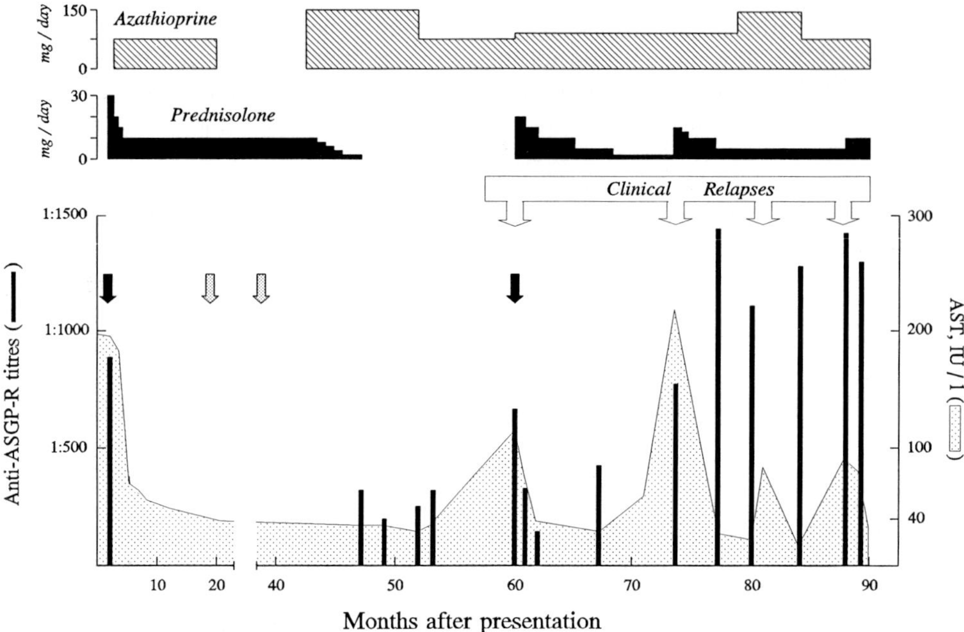

Fig. 3. Fluctuations in titres of anti-ASGP-R autoantibodies in relation to immunosuppressive therapy and disease activity in a patient with presumed autoimmune CAH who was seronegative for anti-nuclear, anti-smooth muscle and liver–kidney microsomal antibodies. Note increases in anti-ASGP-R titres at 51 and 67 months, preceding relapses, and persistently high titres from months 74 to 90 during subsequent multiple relapses. Solid arrows indicate histologically assessed moderate or severe disease activity, and shaded arrows mild or inactive disease, in liver biopsies.

virus A hepatitis. In all three, anti-ASGP-R antibodies appeared at the time of the first rise in serum alanine aminotransferase (ALT). One subject became negative for anti-ASGP-R within 6 weeks, coinciding with complete recovery (Fig. 4). In the other two, despite recovery from the acute infection (with disappearance of IgM anti-HAV antibodies and return of ALT to normal), anti-ASGP-R titres continued to rise. Six weeks later, serum ALT activities began to rise again and both patients became seropositive for ANA and SMA and, a fortnight after this, both patients presented with classical, acute onset, symptomatic type 1 autoimmune CAH which subsequently responded to corticosteroid therapy.

4. Clinical applications of anti-ASGP-R antibodies

It is well recognized that the standard biochemical liver tests do not correlate well with severity of hepatocellular damage in patients with chronic liver disease and

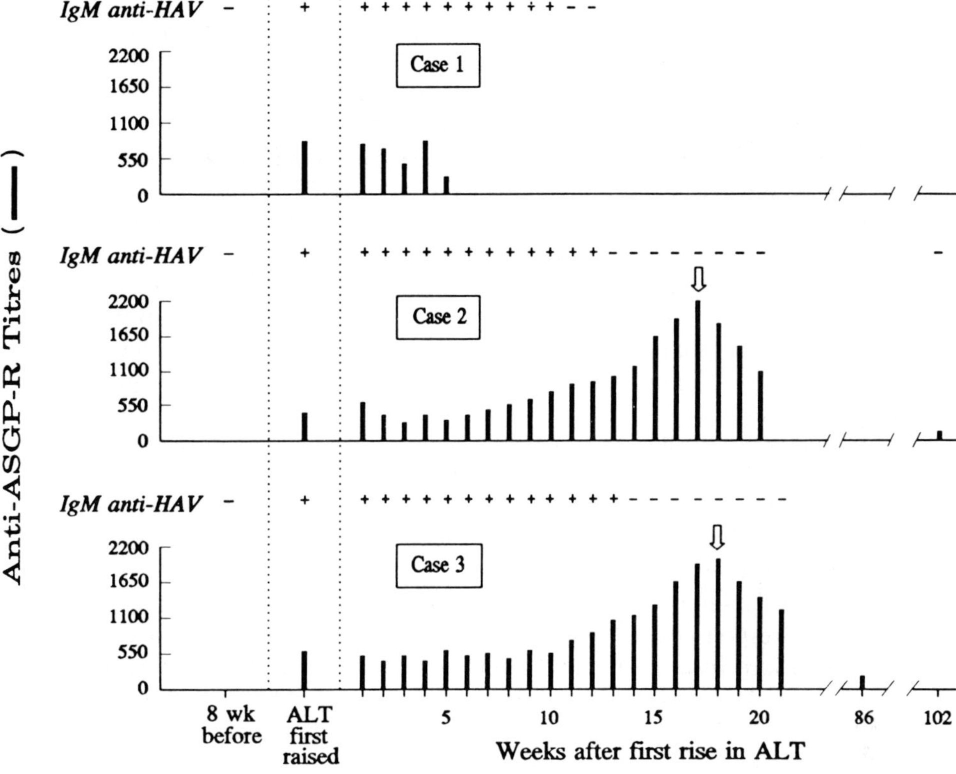

Fig. 4. Fluctuations in titres of anti-ASGP-R autoantibodies in 3 patients with acute hepatitis A, two of whom (cases 2 and 3) subsequently developed classical type 1 autoimmune CAH. Arrows indicate commencement of corticosteroid therapy. ALT, alanine aminotransferase. $+/-$, seropositivity/negativity for IgM anti-hepatitis A virus antibodies. Adapted from Vento et al. (1991).

that this can only be reliably assessed by histological examination of liver biopsies. Since anti-ASGP-R antibodies correlate with the histological finding of periportal inflammation and piecemeal necrosis, the most direct application of these antibodies in clinical hepatology is probably as a surrogate test in the diagnosis of CAH. The fact that anti-ASGP-R occurs not only in autoimmune CAH but also in HBV-CAH and in some patients with PBC does not present a problem because the latter conditions can usually be distinguished by the presence or absence of other serum markers (e.g., HBsAg in HBV-CAH). It is not known whether anti-ASGP-R will identify patients with the PBC-autoimmune CAH overlapping syndrome (Johnson et al., 1991) but, in the absence of a liver biopsy, anti-ASGP-R may be a useful indicant of underlying CAH in HBsAg carriers.

The difficulty in distinguishing between chronic NANB infections (particularly of the sporadic type) and autoimmune CAH is a major clinical problem at present because interferon therapy, which is proving effective in some cases of NANB hepatitis, is potentially hazardous in patients with underlying autoimmune conditions (Burman et al., 1989; Schultz et al., 1989; Vento et al., 1990). Although HCV can be implicated in a high proportion of cases of chronic NANB, it has become apparent that some individuals have ongoing HCV infections without anti-HCV antibodies in their sera (Villa et al., 1991) while, as noted above, in certain areas where HCV is endemic, a high proportion of patients who present with serum markers of autoimmune CAH and other immunological abnormalities have chronic HCV infections. Conversely, anti-ASGP-R is rare in patients who *present* with apparent NANB infections, but occurs in the majority of patients with type 1 or type 2 autoimmune CAH as well as in that group of cryptogenic cases who seem to have autoimmune CAH without ANA, SMA or LKM at presentation. Because of these uncertainties in diagnosis, the current policy in our Institute is to initially treat anti-ASGP-R-positive cryptogenic CAH patients with the standard regimen of corticosteroid therapy used for autoimmune CAH and, if there is no satisfactory response within 6 weeks, to then try interferon therapy.

Other potential clinical applications of anti-ASGP-R antibodies include the monitoring of responses to immunosuppressive therapy in autoimmune CAH. At present, there are insufficient data from serial studies to properly define the dynamics of the anti-ASGP-R response during treatment, but it is clear that the antibodies rapidly decrease in titre and disappear during induction of remission by corticosteroids (McFarlane et al., 1986; Johnson et al., 1990; Treichel et al., 1990). Also, it seems that titres rise in advance of relapses and that persisting high titres are associated with continuing relapses (see, e.g., Fig. 3). However, it is our impression that anti-ASGP-R is not as sensitive as anti-LSP for predicting exacerbations of the disease during reduction or withdrawal of immunosuppressive therapy (McFarlane et al., 1984b) – tending to re-appear and/or rise in titre rather later than anti-LSP in advance of relapses.

Since anti-ASGP-R antibodies in acute HAV and HBV normally disappear during recovery (Vento et al., 1988), and in view of the findings of Vento et al. (1991) (Fig. 4), measurement of these antibodies may be useful for monitoring patients with acute viral hepatitis to warn of impending progression to CAH. An additional use may be in patients with ALD. There have been consistent reports of various cellular and humoral autoreactions in about 25% of patients with ALD (Zetterman and Sorrel, 1981; MacSween, 1984; Johnson and Williams, 1986; Kaku et al., 1988; Laskin et al., 1990; Ishak et al., 1991), particularly in those with alcoholic hepatitis and 'active' cirrhosis (Galambos,1975; Zetterman and Sorrel, 1981; MacSween, 1984), and some ALD patients seem to benefit from corticosteroid therapy (Hofer and McMahon, 1991). In this regard, the findings of Treichel et al. (1990) that 26% of ALD patients have circulating anti-ASGP-R is interesting, for these antibodies might identify a subgroup of patients with progressive disease that may respond to corticosteroids.

5. *Mechanistic considerations*

The relevance of anti-ASGP-R antibodies extends beyond their putative role as a serological marker. T-lymphocytotoxicity against hepatocytes is not demonstrable in autoimmune CAH (Mieli-Vergani et al., 1979) and it seems likely that tissue damage in this condition may be mediated by ADCC reactions involving co-operation between non-T (K)-cells and anti-ASGP-R autoantibodies (McFarlane and Eddleston, 1989). The latter probably arise through T-cell induction of autoreactive B-cells, since patients with autoimmune CAH have circulating T-cells that recognize ASGP-R as well as similarly 'primed' T-cells sequestered in the liver (Vento et al., 1986; Lohr et al., 1990; Wen et al., 1990). In normal subjects, ASGP-R is recognized by a subpopulation of suppressor–inducer (CD4+) T-cells that appear to control autoreactions to this autoantigen, but patients with autoimmune CAH have a defect in this control mechanism (O'Brien et al., 1986; Vento et al. 1987, 1991). This *antigen-specific* T-cell (Ts)-defect is inherited in an autosomal, non-HLA-linked mode and seems to be disease-specific (i.e., for autoimmune CAH). In common with other autoimmune disorders, autoimmune CAH patients also have a generalized heightened immune responsiveness relating to an HLA-linked (A1-B8-DR3) *non*-antigen-specific suppressor cell defect (Nouri-Aria et al., 1985). However, whereas the latter can be corrected by corticosteroid therapy, the antigen-specific Ts defect cannot (Nouri-Aria et al., 1982; Vento et al., 1986).

ADCC reactions involving anti-ASGP-R antibodies might also lead to tissue damage in HBV-CAH, but via a different pathway. HBV-CAH patients show T-cell cytotoxicity against *autologous* hepatocytes (probably against viral determinants on the surfaces of the patients' own liver cells) but, in common with autoimmune CAH, non-T (presumably ADCC) lymphocytotoxic reactions against hepatocytes (Mieli-Vergani et al., 1982) and a *non*-antigen-specific Ts-defect (Nouri-Aria et al., 1982) can also be demonstrated. In contrast to autoimmune CAH, however, in HBV-CAH: (1) there is no ASGP-R-specific Ts-defect; (2) the *non*-antigen-specific Ts-defect is not linked to inheritance of any particular HLA allotype, nor is it correctable by corticosteroid therapy (Nouri-Aria et al., 1982); and (3) patients do not have circulating T-cells that recognize ASGP-R (McFarlane and Eddleston, 1989). Thus, it appears that the autoreactions seen in HBV-CAH are probably 'virus-driven' and that the anti-ASGP-R response is likely to be a consequence of HBV-induced activation of autoreactive B-cells. If so, this must be a rather specific mechanism because polyclonal activation would presumably lead to production of a wide range of antibodies (including other autoantibodies), which is not a marked feature of HBV-CAH.

6. Concluding remarks

Although the precise mechanisms are not yet fully understood, there is now considerable evidence that the ASGP-R is an important target of potentially tissue-damaging autoreactions in liver disease (McFarlane and Eddleston, 1989; McFarlane, 1991; Poralla et al., 1991). It is not necessarily the only target, but its uniqueness to hepatocytes and its preferential expression on the surfaces of liver cells in those areas of the liver lobule where the principal lesion of CAH occurs makes the ASGP-R a prime candidate and, theoretically, an immune reaction against a single target on a cell surface is sufficient to cause cellular injury.

From a more pragmatic point of view, it seems that anti-ASGP-R autoantibodies may provide a useful serological marker of underlying CAH of various aetiologies and, in idiopathic CAH, their presence might be considered an indication for immunosuppressive therapy. This is not to say that anti-ASGP-R necessarily predicts a favourable response to such therapy, for virtually all patients with autoimmune CAH have high titres of anti-ASGP-R at presentation – including the subgroup with steroid-unresponsive disease (Czaja et al., 1983). In view of the Italian experience (see above), it is possible that some of these steroid-unresponsive patients may have chronic infections with hepatitis C or other (as yet unidentified) viruses.

References

Andersen, T.T., Freytag, J.W. and Hill, R.L. (1982) Physical studies of the rabbit hepatic galactoside-binding protein. Effects of calcium and ligands. J. Biol. Chem. 257, 8036–8041.

Baenziger, J.U. (1985) The role of glycosylation in protein recognition. Am. J. Pathol. 121, 382–391.

Baenziger, J.U. and Maynard, Y. (1980) Human hepatic lectin. Physico-chemical properties and specificity. J. Biol. Chem. 255, 4607–4613.

Beavil, A.J., Edmeades, R.L., Gould, H.J. and Sutton, B.J. (1992) Alpha-helical coiled-coil stalks in the low affinity receptor for IgE ($Fc_\varepsilon RII$/CD23) and related C-type lectins. Proc. Natl. Acad. Sci. U.S.A. 89, 753–757.

Bedlow, A.J., Donaldson, P.T., McFarlane, B.M., Lombard, M., McFarlane, I.G. and Williams, R. (1989) Autoreactivity to hepatocellular antigens in primary biliary cirrhosis and primary sclerosing cholangitis. J. Clin. Lab. Immunol. 30, 103–109.

Bischoff, J. and Lodish, H.F. (1987) Two asialoglycoprotein receptor polypeptides in human hepatoma cells. J. Biol. Chem. 262, 11825–11832.

Blomhoff, R., Tolleshaug, H. and Berg, T. (1982) Binding of calcium ions to the isolated asialoglycoprotein receptor. Implications for receptor function in suspended hepatocytes. J. Biol. Chem. 257, 7456–7459.

Brunda, M.J., Minden, P., Sharpton, T.R., McClatchy, J.K. and Farr, R.S. (1977) Precipitation of radiolabelled antigen–antibody complexes with protein A-containing Staphylococcus aureus. J. Immunol. 119, 193–198.

Burman, P., Totterman, T.H., Oberg, K. and Karlsson, F.A. (1989) Thyroid autoimmunity in patients on long term therapy with leucocyte-derived interferon. J. Clin. Endocrinol. Metabol. 63, 1086–1090.

Cochrane, A.M.G., Thomson, A.D., Moussouros, A., Eddleston, A.L.W.F. and Williams, R. (1976) Antibody-dependent cell-mediated (K cell) cytotoxicity against isolated hepatocytes in chronic active hepatitis. Lancet i, 441–444.

Chiacchia, K.B. and Drickamer, K. (1984) Direct evidence for the transmembrane orientation of the hepatic glycoprotein receptors. J. Biol. Chem. 259, 15440–15446.

Czaja, A.J., Davis, G.L., Ludwig, J., Baggenstoss, A.H. and Taswell, H.F. (1983) Autoimmune features as determinants of prognosis in steroid-treated chronic active hepatitis of uncertain etiology. Gastroenterology 85, 713–717.

Czaja, A.J., Hay, J.E. and Rakela, J. (1990) Clinical features and prognostic implications of severe corticosteroid-treated cryptogenic chronic active hepatitis. Mayo Clin. Proc. 65, 23–30.

Daniels, C.K., Smith, K.M. and Schmucker, D.L. (1987) Asialoorosomucoid hepato-biliary transport is unaltered by the loss of liver asialoglycoprotein receptors in aged rats. Proc. Soc. Exp. Biol. Med. 186, 246–250.

David, G.S. and Reisfeld, R.A. (1974) Protein iodination with solid state lactoperoxidase. Biochemistry 13, 1014–1021.

DeKretser, T.A., McFarlane, I.G., Eddleston, A.L.W.F. and Williams, R. (1980) A species non-specific liver plasma membrane antigen and its involvement in chronic active hepatitis. Biochem. J. 186, 679–685.

Drickamer, K. (1987) Membrane receptors that mediate glycoprotein endocytosis: structure and biosynthesis. Kidney Int. 32 (Suppl. 23), S167–S180.

Drickamer, K., Mamon, J.F., Binns, G. and Leung, J.O. (1984) Primary structure of the rat liver asialoglycoprotein receptor: structural evidence for multiple polypeptide species. J. Biol. Chem. 259, 770–778.

Eisenberg, C., Seta, N., Appel, M., Feldmann, G., Durand, G. and Feger, J. (1991) Asialoglycoprotein receptor in human isolated hepatocytes from normal liver and its apparent increase in liver with histological alterations. J. Hepatol. 13, 305–309.

Esteban, J.I., Esteban, R., Viladomiu, L., Lopez-Talavera, J.C., Gonzalez, A., Hernandez, J.M., Roget, M., Vargas, V., Genesca, J., Buti, M., Guardia, J., Houghton, M., Choo, Q.L. and Kuo, G. (1989) Hepatitis C virus antibodies among risk groups in Spain. Lancet ii, 294–297.

Galambos, J.T. (1975) The course of alcoholic hepatitis. In: J.M. Khanna, Y. Israel and H. Kalent (Eds.) Alcoholic Liver Pathology. Addiction Research Foundation of Ontario, Toronto; pp. 91–112.

Garson, J.A., Lenzi, M., Ring, C., Cassani, F., Ballardini, G., Briggs, M., Tedder, R. and Bianchi, F.B. (1991) Hepatitis C viraemia in adults with Type 2 autoimmune hepatitis. J. Med. Virol. 34, 223–226.

Geuze, H.J., Slot, J.W., Strous, G.J.A.M., Lodish, H.F. and Schwartz, A.L. (1982) Immunocytochemical localization of the receptor for asialoglycoproteins in rat liver cells. J. Cell Biol. 92, 865–870.

Gitnick, G. (1990) Cryptogenic versus autoimmune chronic hepatitis: to split or to lump? Mayo Clin. Proc. 65, 119–121.

Gonzales, C., Cochrane, A.M.G., Eddleston, A.L.W.F. and Williams, R. (1979) Mechanisms responsible for antibody-dependent cell-mediated cytotoxicity to isolated hepatocytes in chronic active hepatitis. Gut 20, 385–388.

Gould, H.J., Sutton, B.J., Edmeades, R.L. and Beavil, A.J. (1991) CD23/Fc$_\varepsilon$RII: C-type lectin membrane proteins with a split personality? Monogr. Allergy 29, 28–49.

Halberg, D.F., Wager, R.E., Farrell, D.C., Hildreth, J., Quesenberry, M.S., Loeb, J.A., Holland, E.C. and Drickamer, K. (1987) Major and minor forms of the rat liver asialoglycoprotein receptor are independent galactose-binding proteins. J. Biol. Chem. 262, 9828–9838.

Herzig, M.C.S. and Weigel, P.H. (1990) Surface and internal galactosyl receptors and heterooligomers and retain this structure after ligand internalization or receptor modulation. Biochemistry 29, 6437–6447.

Hofer, T. and McMahon, L. (1991) Corticosteroids and alcoholic hepatitis. Hepatology 13, 199–201.

Hong, W., Le, A.V. and Doyle, D. (1988) Identification and characterization of a murine receptor for galactose-terminated glycoproteins. Hepatology 8, 553–558.

Hosein, B., Fang, T., Popovsky, M.A., Ye, J., Zhang, M. and Wang, C.Y. (1991) Improved serodiagnosis of hepatitis C virus infection with synthetic peptide antigen from capsid protein. Proc. Natl. Acad. Sci. U.S.A. 88, 3647–3651.

Hsueh, E.C., Holland, E.C., Carrera, G.M. and Drickamer, K. (1986) The rat asialoglycoprotein receptor polypeptide must be inserted into a microsome to achieve its active conformation. J. Biol. Chem. 261, 4940–4947.

Hubbard, A.L., Wilson, G., Ashwell, G. and Stukenbrok, H. (1979) An electron microscope autoradiographic study of the carbohydrate recognition systems in rat liver. I. Distribution of ^{125}I-ligand among the liver cell types. J. Cell Biol. 83, 47–64.

Hudgin, R.L., Pricer, W.E., Ashwell, G., Stockert, R.J. and Morell, A.G. (1974) The isolation and properties of a rabbit liver binding protein specific for asialoglycoproteins. J. Biol. Chem. 249, 5536–5543.

Ishak, K.G., Zimmerman, H.J. and Ray, M.B. (1991) Alcoholic liver disease: pathologic, pathogenetic and clinical aspects. Alcoholism Clin. Exp. Res. 15, 45–66.

Jensen, D.M., McFarlane, I.G., Portmann, B., Eddleston, A.L.W.F. and Williams, R. (1978) Detection of antibodies directed against a liver-specific membrane lipoprotein in patients with acute and chronic active hepatitis. N. Engl. J. Med. 299, 1–9.

Jensen, D.M., Hall, C. and Majewski, T. (1983) The plasma membrane origin of liver-specific protein (LSP). Liver 3, 213–219.

Johnson, P.J., McFarlane, I.G., McFarlane, B.M. and Williams, R. (1990) Autoimmune features in patients with idiopathic chronic active hepatitis who are seronegative for conventional autoantibodies. J. Gastroenterol. Hepatol. 5, 244–251.

Johnson, P.J., McFarlane, I.G. and Eddleston, A.L.W.F. (1991) The natural course and heterogeneity of autoimmune-type chronic active hepatitis. Semin. Liver Dis. 11, 187–196.

Johnson, R.D. and Williams, R. (1986) Immune responses in alcoholic liver disease. Alcohol. Clin. Exp. Res. 10, 471–486.

Kaku, I., Izumi, N., Hasumura, Y. and Takeuchi, J. (1988) Differences of liver membrane antibody frequency in alcoholic liver disease: detection of IgG and IgA classes using radioimmunoassay. Dig. Dis. Sci. 33, 845–850.

Kakumu, S., Arakawa, Y., Goji, H., Kashio, T. and Yata, K. (1979) Occurrence and significance of antibody to liver-specific membrane lipoprotein by double-antibody immunoprecipitation method in sera of patients with acute and chronic liver disease. Gastroenterology 76, 665–672.

Kawasaki, T. and Ashwell, G. (1976a) Chemical and physical properties of an hepatic membrane protein that specifically binds asialoglycoproteins. J. Biol. Chem. 251, 1296–1302.

Kawasaki, T. and Ashwell, G. (1976b) Carbohydrate structure of glycopeptides isolated from an hepatic membrane protein specific for asialoglycoproteins. J. Biol. Chem. 251, 5292–5299.

Kawasaki, T. and Ashwell, G. (1977) Isolation and characterization of an avian hepatic binding protein specific for *N*-acetylglucosamine terminated glycoproteins. J. Biol. Chem. 252, 6536–6543.

Kolb-Bachofen, V., Schlepper-Schafer, J., Vogell, W. and Kolb, H. (1982) Electron microscopic evidence for an asialoglycoprotein receptor on Kupffer cells: localization of lectin-mediated endocytosis. Cell 29, 859–866.

Kornfeld, R. and Kornfeld, S. (1985) Assembly of asparagine-linked oligosaccharides. Annu. Rev. Biochem. 54, 631–664.

Kuo, G., Choo, Q.L., Alter, H.J. Gitnick, G.L., Redeker, A.G., Purcell, R.H., Miyamura, T., Dienstag, J.L., Alter, M.J., Stevens, C.E., Tegtmeier, G.E., Bonino, G., Colombo, M., Lee, W.S., Kuo, C., Berger, K., Shuster, J.R., Overby, L.R., Bradley, D.W. and Houghton, M. (1989) An assay for circulating antibodies to a major etiologic virus of human non-A, non-B hepatitis. Science 244, 362–364.

Laskin, C.A., Vidins, E., Blendis, L.M. and Soloninka, C.A. (1990) Autoantibodies in alcoholic liver disease. Am. J. Med. 89, 129–133.

Lebwohl, N. and Gerber, M.A. (1980) Characterization and demonstration of human liver-specific protein (LSP) and apo-LSP. Clin. Exp. Immunol. 46, 435–442.

Lederkremer, G.Z. and Lodish, H.F. (1991) An alternatively spliced miniexon alters the subcellular fate of the human asialoglycoprotein receptor H2 subunit – endoplasmic reticulum retention and degradation or cell surface expression. J. Biol. Chem. 266, 1237–1244.

Lehrman, M.A. and Hill, R.L. (1983) Purification or rat liver fucose binding protein. Methods Enzymol. 98, 309–320.

Lenzi, M., Ballardini, G., Fusconi, M., Cassani, F., Seleri, L., Volta, U., Zauli, D. and Bianchi, F.B. (1990) Type 2 autoimmune hepatitis and hepatitis C virus infection. Lancet 335, 258–259.

Lenzi, M., Johnson, P.J., McFarlane, I.G., Ballardini, G., Smith, H.M., McFarlane, B.M., Bridger, C., Vergani, D., Bianchi, F.B. and Williams, R. (1991) Antibodies to hepatitis C virus in autoimmune liver disease: evidence for geographical heterogeneity. Lancet 338, 277–280.

Lodish, H. (1991) Recognition of complex oligosaccharides by the multi-subunit asialoglycoprotein receptor. Trends Biochem. Sci. 16, 374–377.

Loeb, J.A. and Drickamer, K. (1987) The chicken receptor for endocytosis of glycoproteins contains a cluster of N-acetylglucosamine-binding sites. J. Biol. Chem. 262, 3022–3029.

Lohr, H., Treichel, U., Poralla, T., Manns, M., Meyer zum Büschenfelde, K.H. and Fleischer, B. (1990) The human asialoglycoprotein receptor is a target antigen for liver-infiltrating T cells in autoimmune chronic active hepatitis and primary biliary cirrhosis. Hepatology 12, 1314–1320.

MacSween, R.N.M. (1984) Alcohol and liver injury: genetic and immunologic factors. Acta Med. Scand. Suppl. 703, 57–65.

Manns, M., Meyer zum Büschenfelde, K.H. and Hess, G. (1980) Autoantibodies against liver-specific membrane lipoprotein in acute and chronic liver diseases: studies on organ-, species- and disease-specificity. Gut 21, 955–961.

McFarlane, B.M., McSorley, C.G., McFarlane, I.G. and Williams, R. (1985) A radioimmunoassay for detection of circulating antibodies reacting with the hepatic asialoglycoprotein receptor protein. J. Immunol. Methods 77, 291–299.

McFarlane, B.M., McSorley, C.G., Vergani, D., McFarlane, I.G. and Williams, R. (1986) Serum autoantibodies reacting with the hepatic asialoglycoprotein receptor protein (hepatic lectin) in acute and chronic liver disorders. J. Hepatol. 3, 196–205.

McFarlane, I.G. (1983) Hepatic clearance of serum glycoproteins. Clin. Sci. 64, 127–135.

McFarlane, I.G. (1984) Editorial review: autoimmunity in liver disease. Clin. Sci. 67, 569–578.

McFarlane, I.G. (1991) Autoimmunity and hepatotropic viruses. Semin. Liver Dis. 11, 223–233.

McFarlane, I.G. (1992) Immunological abnormalities and hepatotropic virus infections. Clin. Exp. Immunol. 87, 337–339.

McFarlane, I.G. and Eddleston, A.L.W.F. (1989) Chronic active hepatitis. In: S. Targan and F. Shanahan (Eds.) Immunology and Immunopathology of the Liver and Gastrointestinal Tract, Igaku-Shoin, New York, pp. 281–304.

McFarlane, I.G., Wojcicka, B.M., Zucker, G.M., Eddleston, A.L.W.F. and Williams, R. (1977) Purification and characterization of human liver-specific membrane lipoprotein (LSP). Clin. Exp. Immunol. 27, 381–390.

McFarlane, I.G., McFarlane, B.M., Major, G., Tolley, P. and Williams, R. (1984a) Identification of the hepatic asialoglycoprotein receptor (hepatic lectin) as a component of liver-specific membrane lipoprotein (LSP). Clin. Exp. Immunol. 55, 347–354.

McFarlane, I.G., Hegarty, J.E., McSorley, C.G., McFarlane, B.M. and Williams, R. (1984b) Antibodies to liver specific protein predict outcome of treatment withdrawal in autoimmune chronic active hepatitis. Lancet ii, 954–956.

McFarlane, I.G., Smith, H.M., Johnson, P.J., Bray, G.P., Vergani, D. and Williams, R. (1990) Hepatitis C virus antibodies in chronic active hepatitis: pathogenetic factor or false-positive result? Lancet 335, 754–757.

McSorley, C.G., Isaac, J.E., McFarlane, B.M., McFarlane, I.G. and Williams, R. (1988) Production of murine monoclonal antibodies against a liver-specific, species-cross-reactive antigen in the human liver-specific lipoprotein (LSP) preparation. J. Immunol. Methods 114, 161–166.

Meyer zum Büschenfelde, K.H. and Miescher, P.A. (1972) Liver specific antigens, purification and characterization. Clin. Exp. Immunol. 10, 89–102.

Mieli-Vergani, G., Vergani, D., Jenkins, P.J., Portmann, B., Mowat, A.P., Eddleston, A.L.W.F. and Williams, R. (1979) Lymphocyte cytotoxicity to autologous hepatocytes in HBsAg-negative chronic active hepatitis. Clin. Exp. Immunol. 38, 16–21.

Mieli-Vergani, G., Vergani, D., Portmann, B., White, Y., Murray-Lyon, I., Marigold, J.H., Woolf, I., Eddleston, A.L.W.F. and Williams, R. (1982) Lymphocyte cytotoxicity to autologous hepatocytes in HBsAg-positive chronic liver disease. Gut 23, 1029–1036.

Mieli-Vergani, G., Lobo-Yeo, A., McFarlane, B.M., McFarlane, I.G., Mowat, A.P. and Vergani, D. (1989) Different immune mechanisms leading to autoimmunity in primary sclerosing cholangitis and autoimmune chronic active hepatitis of childhood. Hepatology 9, 198–203.

Nouri-Aria, K.T., Hegarty, J.E., Alexander, G.J.M., Eddleston, A.L.W.F. and Williams, R. (1982) Effect of corticosteroids on suppressor-cell activity in autoimmune and viral chronic active hepatitis. N. Engl. J. Med. 307, 1301–1304.

Nouri-Aria, K.T., Donaldson, P.T., Hegarty, J.E., Eddleston, A.L.W.F and Williams, R. (1985) HLA A1-B8-DR3 and suppressor cell function in first-degree relatives of patients with autoimmune chronic active hepatitis. J. Hepatol. 1, 235–241.

Novogrodsky, A. and Ashwell, G. (1977) Lymphocyte mitogenesis induced by a mammalian protein that specifically binds desialylated glycoproteins. Proc. Natl. Acad. Sci. U.S.A. 74, 676–678.

O'Brien, C.J., Vento, S., Donaldson, P.T., McSorley, C.G., McFarlane, I.G., Williams, R. and Eddleston, A.L.W.F. (1986) Cell-mediated immunity and discrete suppressor T-cell defects to liver-derived antigens in families of patients with autoimmune chronic active hepatitis. Lancet i, 350–353.

Paulson, J.C., Hill, R.L., Tanabe, T. and Ashwell, G. (1977) Reactivation of asialo-rabbit liver binding protein by resialylation with β-D-galactoside $\alpha 2 \rightarrow 6$ sialyl-transferase. J. Biol. Chem. 252, 8624–8628.

Perperas, A., Tsantoulas, D., Portmann, B., Eddleston, A.L.W.F. and Williams, R. (1981) Autoimmunity to a liver membrane lipoprotein and liver damage in alcoholic liver disease. Gut 22, 149–152.

Pfeffer, S.R. (1988) Mannose 6-phosphate receptors and their role in targeting proteins to lysosomes. J. Membr. Biol. 103, 7–16.

Poralla, T., Treichel, U., Lohr, H. and Fleischer, B. (1991) The asialoglycoprotein receptor as target structure in autoimmune liver diseases. Semin. Liver Dis. 11, 215–222.

Pricer, W.E. and Ashwell, G. (1976) Subcellular distribution of a mammalian hepatic binding protein specific for asialoglycoproteins. J. Biol. Chem. 251, 7539–7544.

Roos, P.H., Hartma, J.J., Schlepper-Schafer, J., Kolb, H. and Kolb-Bachofen, V. (1985) Galactose-specific receptors on liver cells: II. Characterisation of the purified receptor from macrophages reveals no structural relationship to the hepatocyte receptor. Biochim. Biophys. Acta 847, 115–121.

Sanford, J.P., Elliott, R.W. and Doyle, D. (1988) Asialoglycoprotein receptor genes are linked on chromosome 11 in the mouse. DNA 7, 721–728.

Schultz, M., Muller, R., von zur Muhlen, A. and Brabant, G. (1989) Induction of hyperthyroidism by interferon-alpha-2b. Lancet i, 1452.

Schwartz, A.L. (1984) The hepatic asialoglycoprotein receptor. C.R.C. Crit. Rev. Biochem. 16, 207–233.

Schwartz, A.L. and Rup, D. (1983) Biosynthesis of the human asialoglycoprotein receptor. J. Biol. Chem. 258, 11249–11255.

Schwartz, A.L., Rup, D. and Lodish, H.F. (1980) Difficulties in the quantification of asialoglycoprotein receptors on the rat hepatocyte. J. Biol. Chem. 255, 9033–9036.

Schwartz, A.L., Marshak-Rothstein, A. and Rup, D. (1981) Identification and quantification of the rat hepatocyte asialoglycoprotein receptor. Proc. Natl. Acad. U.S.A. 78, 3348–3352.

Sipos, J., McFarlane, B.M., McSorley, C.G., Gove, C.D., Williams, R. and McFarlane, I.G. (1989) Immunohistochemical demonstration of the asialoglycoprotein receptor in rat liver by a sensitive avidin–biotin technique. J. Pathol. 158, 247–252.

Spiess, M. (1990) The asialoglycoprotein receptor: a model for endocytic transport receptors. Biochemistry 29, 10009–10018.

Spiess, M. and Handschin, C. (1987) Deletion analysis of the internal signal-anchor domain of the human asialoglycoprotein receptor H1. EMBO J. 6, 2683–2691.

Spiess, M. and Lodish, H. (1985) Sequence of a second human asialoglycoprotein receptor: conservation of two receptor genes during evolution. Proc. Natl. Acad. Sci. U.S.A. 82, 6465–6469.

Steer, C.J. and Ashwell, G. (1980) Studies on a mammalian hepatic binding protein specific for asialoglycoproteins. Evidence for receptor recycling in isolated rat hepatocytes. J. Biol. Chem. 255, 3008–3013.

Steer, C.J., Kempner, E.S. and Ashwell, G. (1981) Molecular size of the hepatic receptor for asialoglycoproteins determined in situ by radiation inactivation. J. Biol. Chem. 256, 5851–5856.

Stockert, R.J., Morell, A.G. and Scheinberg, I.H. (1974) Mammalian hepatic lectin. Science 186, 365–366.

Tanabe, T., Pricer, W.E. and Ashwell, G. (1979) Subcellular membrane topology and turnover of a rat hepatic binding protein specific for asialoglycoproteins. J. Biol. Chem. 254, 1038–1043.

Taylor, M.E. and Summerfield, R.A. (1986) Mammalian mannose-binding proteins. Clin. Sci. 70, 539–546.

Tolleshaug, H., Berg, T., Nilsson, M. and Norum, K.R. (1977) Uptake and degradation of ^{125}I-labelled asialo-fetuin by isolated rat hepatocytes. Biochim. Biophys. Acta 499, 73–84.

Treichel, U., Poralla, T., Hess, G., Manns, M. and Meyer zum Büschenfelde, K.H. (1990) Autoantibodies to human asialoglycoprotein receptor in autoimmune-type chronic hepatitis. Hepatology 11, 606–612.

Van Lenten, L. and Ashwell, G. (1972) The binding of desialylated glycoproteins by plasma membrane of rat liver. J. Biol. Chem. 247, 4633–4640.

Vento, S., O'Brien, C.J., McFarlane, B.M., McFarlane, I.G., Eddleston, A.L.W.F. and Williams, R. (1986) T-lymphocyte sensitization to hepatocyte antigens in autoimmune chronic active hepatitis and primary biliary cirrhosis: evidence for different underlying mechanisms and different antigenic determinants as targets. Gastroenterology 91, 810–817.

Vento, S., O'Brien, C.J., McFarlane, I.G., Williams, R. and Eddleston, A.L.W.F. (1987) T-cell inducers of suppressor lymphocytes control liver-directed autoreactivity. Lancet i, 886–887.

Vento, S., McFarlane, B.M., McSorley, C.G., Ranieri, S., Giuliani-Piccari, G., Dal Monte, P.R., Verucchi, G., Williams, R., Chiodo, F. and McFarlane, I.G. (1988) Liver autoreactivity in acute virus A, B and non-A, non-B hepatitis. J. Clin. Lab. Immunol. 25, 1–7.

Vento, S., Di Perri, G., Garofano, T., Cosco, L., Concia, E., Ferraro, T. and Bassetti, D. (1990) Hazards of interferon therapy for HBV-seronegative chronic hepatitis. Lancet ii, 926 (letter).

Vento, S., Garofano, T., Di Perri, G., Dolci, L., Concia, E. and Bassetti, D. (1991) Identification of hepatitis A virus as a trigger for autoimmune chronic hepatitis type 1 in susceptible individuals. Lancet 337, 1183–1187.

Villa, E., Ferretti, I., De Palma, M., Melegari, M., Scaglioni. P.P., Trande, P., Vecchi, C., Fratti, N. and Manenti, F. (1991) HCV-RNA in serum of asymptomatic blood donors involved in post-transfusion hepatitis (PTH). J. Hepatol., 13, 256–259.

Wall, D.A. and Hubbard, A.L. (1981) Galactose-specific recognition system of mammalian liver: receptor distribution on the hepatocyte cell surface. J. Cell Biol. 90, 687–696.

Weigel, P. (1980) Characterization of the asialoglycoprotein receptor on isolated rat hepatocytes. J. Biol. Chem. 255, 6111–6120.

Wen, L., Peakman, M., Lobo-Yeo, A., McFarlane, B.M., Mowat, A.P., Mieli-Vergani, G. and Vergani, D. (1990) T-cell-directed hepatocyte damage in autoimmune chronic active hepatitis. Lancet 336, 1527–1530.

Wojcicka-McFarlane, B.M. (1990) The Asialoglycoprotein Receptor as an Autoantigen. PhD Thesis, University of London.

Zeitlin, P.L. and Hubbard, A.L. (1982) Cell surface distribution and intracellular fate of asialoglycoproteins: a morphological and biochemical study of isolated rat hepatocytes and monolayer cultures. J. Cell Biol. 92, 634–647.

Zetterman, R.K. and Sorrell, M.F. (1981) Immunologic aspects of alcoholic liver disease. Gastroenterology 81, 616–624.

Autoimmune Hepatitis
Edited by M. Nishioka, G. Toda and M. Zeniya
© *1994, Elsevier Science B.V. All rights reserved*

Chapter 9

Relevance of cytoplasmic autoantigens in autoimmune hepatitis

Michael Peter Manns

*Department of Gastroenterology and Hepatology, Zentrum Innere Medizin, Medizinische Hochschule
Hannover, Konstanty Gutschow Str. 8, D–30625 Hannover (Germany)*

1. Introduction

A loss of tolerance against autologous liver tissue is regarded as the principal
pathogenetic mechanism in autoimmune liver diseases. Autoimmune hepatitis
(AIH), primary biliary cirrhosis (PBC) and primary sclerosing cholangitis (PSC)
are the 3 major autoimmune liver diseases. While the primary target of tissue
destruction in AIH is the hepatocyte, biliary tract epithelia are destroyed in PBC
and PSC. In general, autoimmune syndromes are chronic inflammatory diseases
usually of unknown cause characterized by a female predominance, a genetic
predisposition, a good response to immunosuppressive drugs and characteristic
autoantibodies. Extra-hepatic autoimmune syndromes such as arthritis,
thyroiditis, inflammatory bowel disease, etc. are frequently associated with autoimmune liver diseases, including autoimmune chronic active hepatitis (CAH).
In contrast to PBC and PSC, immunosuppression increases life expectancy for
patients with AIH. T-lymphocytes are major components of the cellular infiltrate.
Therefore, they are believed to mediate tissue destruction. In recent years,
intensive research has focussed on cellular immune reactions. However, our
knowledge of the mechanisms responsible for tissue destruction in autoimmune
liver diseases is still limited. An interesting experimental approach is the application of molecular biological techniques to identify the structures recognized by
disease-specific autoantibodies. This chapter tries to provide the reader with an
updated knowledge of the recent advances made in the identification and
characterization of autoantibodies and their cytoplasmic antigens, especially
those associated with autoimmune CAH.

2. Classification of autoimmune hepatitis on the basis of circulating autoantibodies

AIH is characterized by histological changes compatible with CAH, a female predominance, hypergammaglobulinemia, an immunogenetic background, response to corticosteroid treatment, an association with extra-hepatic auto-immune syndromes, and characteristic autoantibodies. On the basis of different autoantibody specificities, at least 3 serologically distinct subgroups of AIH can be distinguished (Table 1) (Manns et al., 1987). Anti-nuclear antibodies (ANA) characterize classical autoimmune type 'lupoid' hepatitis. In this subgroup of AIH, also called type 1, smooth muscle antibodies (SMA) and liver membrane autoantibodies (LMA) are frequently detectable. ANAs are routinely detected by indirect immunofluorescence. However, they are very heterogeneous and almost all subtypes that occur in rheumatological disorders are found in 'lupoid' hepatitis, including antibodies to double-stranded DNA. Classical AIH, type 1, was first described in the early 1950s: young females with hypergamma-globulinemia showing a good response to corticosteroids.

AIH type 2 is serologically characterized by liver–kidney microsomal (LKM-1) antibodies. In about 50% of patients, AIH type 2 starts in childhood while in the other 50%, the disease starts between the age of 35 and >60 years (Table 1) (Homberg et al., 1987; Michel et al., 1992). Usually ANAs and SMAs are negative in this autoimmune liver disease. However, thyroid microsomal, thyro-globulin, and parietal cell antibodies are frequently detected. Extra-hepatic syndromes (Table 2) are frequently observed in the younger patient group of

Table 1

Heterogeneity of HBsAG-negative chronic hepatitis

ANA, anti-nuclear antibodies; LKM-1, liver–kidney microsomal antibodies against cytochrome P-450-IID6; SLA antibodies against soluble liver antigens; SMA, smooth muscle antibodies; AMA, anti-mitochondrial antibodies; HCV, hepatitis C virus; UDCA, ursodeoxycholic acid.

	ANA	LKM-1	SLA	SMA	AMA	Anti-HCV	Anti-GOR	Therapy
Chronic hepatitis C	−	−	−	−	−	+	+	Interferon
Autoimmune hepatitis								
Type 1	+	−	−	+	−	−	−	Immunosuppression
Type 2a	−	+	−	−	−	−	−	Immunosuppression
Type 2b	−	+	−	−	−	+	+	?
Type 3	−	−	+	+/−	+/−	−	−	Immunosuppression
Type 4	−	−	−	+	−	−	−	Immunosuppression
Primary biliary cirrhosis	−	−	−	−	+	−	−	UDCA etc.

Table 2
Extra-hepatic syndromes associated with LKM-1-positive AIH

Vitiligo
Thyroid disorders
Insulin-dependent diabetes mellitus
Autoimmune hemolytic anemia
Idiopathic thrombocytopenic purpura
Pernicious anemia
Rheumatoid arthritis
Ulcerative colitis
Chronic glomerulonephritis
Fibrosing alveolitis
Multi-organ vascular dysplasia
Celiac disease
Nail dystrophy
Alopecia

autoimmune hepatitis type 2, but are less common in the older patient population. This older patient population presents with serological hepatitis C virus (HCV) infection while such markers of HCV infection are absent in the younger and corticosteroid-responsive group (see below). Furthermore, AIH type 2 is characterized by low IgA levels, and hypergammaglobulinemia is less prominent. Female predominance is around 60% (Homberg et al., 1987). The disease may start with an episode of acute hepatitis in 30–40% of the patients. Rapid progression to cirrhosis is common in the young patient population. The prevalence of AIH type 2 is estimated to be from 5–10 cases per million population. This may differ geographically. However, the disease does occur worldwide.

A third subgroup of AIH, type 3, is associated with soluble liver antigen autoantibodies (anti-SLA). These antibodies react with liver cytokeratins. In the initial study, the picture of AIH type 3 was described in 23 patients (Manns et al., 1987). The female predominance was 90% and the mean age at onset was 37 years. Hypergammaglobulinemia was evident in most patients with a mean of 3.2 g/l and response to immunosuppressive treatment was good. Anti-SLA antibody titers decline during therapy when disease activity regresses. In 25% of anti-SLA antibody-positive patients, no other autoantibodies are found. Therefore, this marker is important in distinguishing this subgroup of AIH from anti-HCV-negative non-A, non-B hepatitis.

It may be that high titer SMAs directed against F-actin characterize a fourth subgroup of AIH which is frequently observed in young children (Table 1) (Odievre et al., 1983).

Autoantibodies are important diagnostic markers for the differentiation of chronic hepatitis (Manns, 1989). Therefore, we discuss in the following recent progress concerning autoantibodies and their cytoplasmic antigens in AIH.

2.1. Anti-nuclear antibodies

ANA were the first autoantibodies that had been described in chronic hepatitis. The association of AIH type 1 with ANA led to the term 'lupoid' hepatitis (Mackay et al., 1956). So far no subtype of ANA has been claimed to be specific for 'lupiod' hepatitis. The detection of ANA by indirect immunofluorescence on Hep-2 cells is the appropriate test in clinical diagnosis.

2.2. Smooth muscle antibodies

Autoantibodies reacting with vessel walls in immunofluorescence were termed SMA and may be found in high titers in patients with AIH. They frequently occur together with ANA in AIH type 1, but they may represent the only serological marker for this subgroup (Table 1). The main antigen of SMAs in autoimmune liver disease is F-actin. F-actin is in close anatomic association with the liver plasma cell membrane.

2.3. Autoantibodies against microsomal antigens

The advent of immunoblotting made significant progress towards the molecular identification of autoantigens, since they could be defined according to their molecular weight. When LKM-1-positive sera were tested against solubilized human liver microsomes, 3 microsomal antigens at 50, 55 and 64 kDa were recognized (Manns et al., 1989). One LKM-1-positive serum reacting at a high titer with the 50- and 64-kDa antigen was chosen to screen a λ-GT11 human liver cDNA library (Manns et al., 1989). Autoantibodies, affinity purified on recombinant protein derived from isolated immunopositive cDNA clones, reacted only with the 50- but not with the 64- or 55-kDa antigens. The sequence analysis of isolated immunopositive cDNA clones revealed that the 50-kDa antigen is human cytochrome P-450-db1 nowadays termed P-450-IID6. The 50-kDa LKM-1 antigen in liver and kidney was found to be immunologically identical. Zanger and coworkers (Zanger et al., 1988) were able to immunopurify P-450-IID6 with LKM-1-positive serum and then demonstrated specific inhibition of enzyme function by these sera. Cytochrome P-450-IID6 is a drug-metabolizing enzyme and is responsible for the metabolism of more than 25 commonly used drugs, among them β-blockers, anti-arrhythmic drugs, anti-depressants, and anti-hypertensive drugs like debrisoquine. The immunodominant B-cell epitope of P-450-IID6 has been localized on human cytochrome P-450-IID6 and consists of a linear sequence of 8 amino acids (Manns et al., 1991a). The sequence of this epitope is highly conserved for class

IID P-450s. LKM-1 antibodies are restricted to the subclasses IgG-1 and IgG-4 which differs from the IgG-3 restriction seen for anti-mitochondrial antibodies (AMA) in PBC (Weber et al., 1988). Interestingly, the overall IgG subclass distribution is normal for patients with LKM-1-positive hepatitis, whereas the proportion of IgG-3 subclass is increased in patients with PBC. The 55- and 64-kDa antigens have not yet been identified at the molecular level.

The application of recombinant DNA technology proved to be of particular relevance for the identification of microsomal autoantigens (Table 3). Although 90% of LKM sera from patients with AIH recognize the 50-kDa cytochrome P-450-IID6, 10% react with a 50-kDa microsomal protein different from P-450-IID6. Thus, the minority of LKM sera in AIH reacts with 50-kDa microsomal proteins that differ from P-450-IID6. One such antigen has been identified as cytochrome P-450-IA2. This P-450-IA2 was recognized in serum from a patient with chronic hepatitis, alopecia, vitiligo, and nail dystrophy (Manns et al., 1990a; Sacher et al., 1990). A similar patient has recently been described. In immuno-fluorescence, anti-P-450-IA2 serum predominantly stains perivenous hepatocytes (Bourdi et al., 1990). Cytochrome P-450-IA2 is a liver-specific antigen. Prednisolone therapy in this patient led to normalization of transaminases and liver histology. Furthermore, antibody titers had disappeared after 1 year of treatment when liver histology became normal (Sacher et al., 1990). Anti-IA2 antibodies inhibit enzyme function in vitro. In man, P-450-IA2 is responsible for the metabolism of phenacetin. Cytochrome P-450-IA2 antibodies have also been decribed in patients with dihydralazine-induced hepatitis (Bourdi et al., 1990). Since dihydralazine reduced the metabolism of ethoxyresurofin in isolated human liver microsomes, it was concluded that dihydralazine may be metabolized by P-450-IA2. The authors then proposed a mechanism for anti-P-450-IA2 autoantibody formation by this drug similar to the one suggested for LKM-2 antibody formation (Beaune et al., 1987).

Table 3
Diagnostic significance of recombinant LKM-1 (P-450-IID6) antigen (LKM-R)
AIH, autoimmune hepatitis; PBC, primary biliary, cirrhosis.

	No.	LKM-IF	Western blot (50 kDa)	LKM-R (P-450-IID6)
AIH ANA-positive ('lupoid')	20	–	–	–
AIH LKM-positive	46	46	28	40
AIH SLA-positive	10	–	–	–
Acute hepatitis (A, B, C, non-A, non-B)	51	–	–	–
PBC	20	–	–	–
Extra-hepatic cholestasis	10	–	–	–
Malignancies	20	–	–	–
Immunopathies	20	3	–	–
Controls	20	–	–	–

Anti-microsomal antibodies in a form of hepatitis caused by the diuretic drug ticrynafen were termed LKM-2 antibodies (Table 4). The LKM-2 antigen was the first to be identified as a cytochrome P-450 protein: P-450-IIC9. Beaune et al. (1987) proposed the following mechanism for LKM-2 autoantibody formation: a drug, i.e., ticrynafen, is metabolized by P-450-IIC9 and the reactive metabolite binds to the P-450 protein which then becomes antigenic.

An Italian group of investigators reported that sera from 10% of patients with chronic hepatitis D (δ) virus infection react with the cytoplasm of human liver and kidney tissue (Crivelli et al., 1983). They termed these autoantibodies LKM-3. The antigen has not yet been characterized. Interestingly, additional autoantibodies have been reported in hepatitis D virus (HDV) infection (Zauli et al., 1984; Amengueal et al; 1989), such as basal layer cell antibodies and antibodies against thymic cells. Recently, antibodies against the nuclear envelope proteins lamin A and C were reported in hepatitis D.

All cytochrome P-450 autoantibodies (Table 4) inhibit the function of their cognitive antigens in vitro. Furthermore, P-450-IID6 and P-450-IIC9 are genetically polymorphic. The molecular basis of the genetic polymorphism of P-450-IID6 is a consequence of erroneously spliced P-450-IID6 messenger RNAs (mRNA). LKM-2 antibodies were used to study the polymorphic drug metabolism of mephenytoin. It was suggested that a functionally altered cytochrome P-450 enzyme causes the deficiency for P-450-IIC9 (Meier and Meyer, 1987). A genetic polymorphism is also suggested for P-450-IA2 since the metabolism of phenacetin may vary up to 40% between different individuals.

We were able to study P-450-IID6 protein expression in the livers of patients, the in vivo phenotype for P-450-IID6 catalyzed drug metabolism as well as inhibition of P-450-IID6 function in isolated human liver microsomes by LKM-1 sera in vitro (Manns et al., 1990b). All LKM-1 sera inhibited P-450-IID6-mediated 2-dehydrospartein formation in isolated human liver microsomes. All patients with LKM-1-postitive AIH type 2 were extensive metabolizers for cytochrome P-450-IID6-mediated drug metabolism in vivo. We concluded from these experiments that patients with LKM-1-positive liver disease express func-

Table 4

Microsomal autoantigens in liver diseases – 1992

n.n, not nominated.

MW (kDa)	Nomenclature	Biochemical definition	Disease association
50	LKM-1	P450-db1 (IID6)	AIH
50	LKM-2	P450-meph (IIC9)	Drug-induced hepatitis (tienilic acid)
?	LKM-3	?	Chronic hepatitis D
50	LM	P450-IA2	AIH, dihydralazine hepatitis
55	n.n	?	AIH
64	n.n	?	AIH

tionally intact autoantigen in their livers since the antibody does not sufficiently penetrate through the intact liver cell membrane. To my knowledge, in these studies, the function of an autoantigen has been studied for the first time in vivo. Possibly a functionally intact autoantigen is necessary for the manifestation of the disease, since we have not found a single LKM-1-positive poor metabolizer for P-450-IID6.

It is debatable whether cytoplasmic and in particular cytochrome P-450 autoantigens are expressed on the surface of hepatocytes. We were able to show that patients with AIH type 2 are extensive metabolizers for P-450-IID6. This means that the inhibitory LKM-1 antibodies do not sufficiently penetrate the liver cell membrane to inhibit enzyme function in vivo. However, tissue destruction may be mediated by binding of antibodies to P-450 antigens expressed on the surface of hepatocytes. A French group of investigators has provided data indicating that all P-450s identified as autoantigens are expressed on the surface of human hepatocytes (Loeper et al., 1990). Furthermore, the cellular expression of autoantigens may be modulated by cytokines secreted by tissue-infiltrating lymphocytes. Interestingly, we found that the cellular expression of cytochrome P-450-IID6 (LKM-1 antigen) is decreased by acute-phase mediators such as interleukin-1 (IL-1), IL-6, and tumor necrosis factor (TNF) (Trautwein et al., 1992). So far, we have not identified cytokines that up-regulate the expression of P-450-IID6. We have identified P-450-IID6-specific T-lymphocyte clones from liver biopsies of patients with AIH type 2. However, only 5 out of 189 T-cell clones proved to be antigen-specific for P-450-IID6 (Löhr et al., 1991). Therefore, it is obvious that the other T-lymphocytes have a different antigen specificity or are just bystander T-cells which secrete cytokines that modulate the immune response.

2.4. Autoantibodies against cytosolic components

We observed several cases with chronic hepatitis and hypergammaglobulinemia responding well to corticosteroids that were negative for ANA, LMA, SMA, LKM-1 and hepatitis B surface antigen (HBsAg). These patients had no history of blood transfusion or drug abuse. In addition, they were shown to be anti-HCV-negative. Anti-SLA antibodies were recognized by an inhibitory radioimmunoassay (Manns et al., 1987). The major target of these antibodies seems to be liver cytokeratins 8 and 18 (Wächter et al., 1990). The clinical characteristics of this subgroup of AIH type 3, characterized by anti-SLA antibodies have been described above. Furthermore, it was shown that SLA antigen expression is up-regulated by cytokines (Manns et al., 1988). For these experiments, two hepatoma cell lines were used. One HBsAg-negative (MzHep) and one HBsAg-positive (PLC/PRF5) were treated with recombinant α- and γ-interferons, TNF-α and IL-2. All these cytokines up-regulated the cellular expression of SLA antigen.

Autoantibodies against further cytoplasmic antigens of possible similar diagnostic significance, like anti-SLA, have been described by complement fixation technique. Since they react with an antigen of liver and pancreas they were termed anti-LP (Berg and Stechemesser, 1981). Furthermore, Meliconi et al. (1987) found autoantibodies against a fraction of 100,000-g supernatants of liver homogenates which is called LP-2. Martini et al. (1988) using immunodiffusion techniques defined anti-liver-cytosol antibody type 1 (anti-LC-1) (Martini et al., 1988). All 21 sera positive for anti-LC-1 antibodies were from patients with idiopathic CAH. Seven out of 21 anti-LC-1-positive sera were negative for other autoantibodies, whereas in 14 sera anti-LC-1 occurred together with anti-LKM-1. Sera monospecific for anti-LC-1 show a characteristic immunofluorescence staining of the cytoplasm of periportal hepatocytes. They spare the cellular layer around the central veins of mouse and rat liver. Further work is necessary to define the LC-1 antigen at the molecular level.

2.5. Anti-mitochondrial antibodies in CAH

AMA are specific and sensitive diagnostic markers for PBC as will be described below. In a proportion of patients with clinical and histological signs of chronic hepatitis showing a good response to immunosuppressive treatment, AMA are found. Such patients are regarded as having a clinical overlap syndrome CAH–PBC. However, the mitochondrial antigen specificity of these AMA is not different from that of AMA seen in classical PBC.

3. Immunogenetics and the serological heterogeneity of AIH

In classical AIH type 1, the association with the HLA-haplotype A1-B8-DR3 is well established for Caucasians (Donaldson et al., 1991). In Japan, a significant increase in DR4 has been described for AIH type 1 (Zeniya et al., 1990). HLA-DR4 was also increased in the DR3-negative population reported from the United Kingdom (Donaldson et al., 1991). In addition, a significant increase of null alleles for complement component C4 (C4A-QO) has been reported in AIH type 1 (Briggs et al., 1987). While there are no HLA data available for AIH type 3, we have recently reported that HLA DR3 and C4A-DQ alleles are increased in AIH type 2, predominantly in the young patient population which is anti-HCV-negative (Manns et al., 1991b).

4. Hepatotropic viruses and AIH

Several of the major hepatotropic viruses have been accused of inducing AIH. Recently, Italian scientists have reported that classical autoimmune 'lupoid' CAH developed after acute hepatitis A virus infection.

There has been an intensive and controversial discussion on the role of HCV in autoimmune liver diseases. The initial high percentage of positive results with the first-generation anti-HCV test were due to false-positive results caused by hypergammaglobulinemia. The application of second-generation anti-HCV tests revealed that the association of HCV infection with autoimmune liver diseases was limited to AIH type 2, which is associated with LKM-1 autoantibodies. While in Italy 80% of LKM-1-positive cases seem to be HCV associated, in England less than 10% of these patients are anti-HCV-positive (Lenzi et al., 1992).

In contrast, 50% of patients with AIH type 2 are anti-HCV-positive in Germany (Michel et al., 1992) and France (Lunel et al., 1991). The anti-HCV-positive population of AIH type 2 consists mainly of older individuals above the age of 40 years, the disease is slowly progressive, the female predominance is less profound and extra-hepatic syndromes are rarely observed. The response to corticosteroids is limited. The role of HCV for this group of patients is supported by the detection of anti-GOR, an HCV-specific autoimmune reaction against a hitherto poorly defined intra-cellular autoantigen and by the detection of HCV-RNA in the serum of several of these cases. The anti-HCV-negative group of AIH type 2 consists predominantly of females, the disease often starts in childhood and disease activity is significant. When untreated, rapid progression is frequently observed. However, patients usually show a good response to corticosteroids but face rapid progression to cirrhosis when untreated. Extra-hepatic clinical autoimmune syndromes are frequently observed. Interestingly, all patients with anti-HCV-negative AIH type 2 have serological signs of HSV-1 infection. The immediate early protein, IE 175 of HSV exhibits a highly significant sequence homology with the B-cell epitope of LKM-1 antigen, i.e., cytochrome P-450-IID6 (Manns et al., 1991a).

Acknowledgement

This research is presently supported by the Deutsche Forschungsgemeinschaft SFB 244.

References

Amengueal, M.J., Catalfana, M., Pujol, A. et al. (1989) Autoantibodies in chronic delta virus infection recognize a common protein of 46 kD in forestomach basal cell layer and stellate thymic epithelial cells. Clin. Exp. Immunol. 78, 80–84.

Beaune, P.H., Dansette, P.M. Mansuy, D. et al. (1987) Human anti-endoplasmic reticulum autoantibodies appearing in a drug-induced hepatitis A directed against a human liver cytochrome P450 that hydroxylates the drug. Proc. Natl. Acad. Sci. U.S.A. 84, 551–555.

Berg, P.A. and Stechemesser, E. (1981) Hypergammaglobulinamische chronisch aktive Hepatitis mit Nachwieis konplememntbindender partiell leberspezifischer Antikorper. Verh. Dtsch. Ges. Inn. Med. 87, 921.

Bourdi, M., Larrey, D., Nataf, J. et al. (1990) Anti-liver endoplasmic reticulum autoantibodies are directed against human cytochrome P-450 IA2. J. Clin. Invest. 85, 1967–1973.

Briggs, D.C., Donaldson, P.T., Hayes, P. et al. (1987) A major histocompatibility complex class III allotype (C4B2) associated with primary biliary cirrhosis (PBC). Tissue Antigens 29, 141–145.

Crivelli, D., Lavarini, C., Chiaberge, E. et al. (1983) Microsomal autoantibodies in chronic infections with HBsAg associated delta agent. Clin. Exp. Immunol. 54, 232.

Donaldson, P.T., Doherty, D.G., Hayllar, K.M., et al. (1991) Susceptibility to autoimmune chronic active hepatitis: human leucocyte antigens DR4 and A1-B8-DR3 are independent risk factors. Hepatology 13, 701–705.

Homberg, J.C., Abuaf, N., Bernard, Q. et al. (1987) Chronic active hepatitis associated with anti-liver/kidney microsome autoantibody type I: a second type of 'autoimmune' hepatitis. Hepatology 1, 1333–1339.

Lenzi, M., Johnson, P.J., McFarlane, I.G. et al. (1992) Antibodies to hepatitis C virus in autoimmune liver disease: evidence for geographical heterogeneity. Lancet 338, 277–280.

Loeper, J., Descatoire, V., Maurice, M. et al. (1990) Presence of cytochrome P-450 on human hepatocyte plasma membrane. Recognition by several autoantibodies (Abstract) Hepatology 12, 909.

Löhr, H., Manns, M., Trautwein, C. et al. (1991) Clonal analysis of liver infiltrating T cells in patients with chronic active hepatitis (AI-CAH). Clin. Exp. Immunol. 84, 297–302.

Lunel, F., Maismeuve, P., Marcellin, P. et al. (1991) Relationship between anti-HCV antibodies measured by a quantitative RIBA assay and response to interferon in patients with chronic non-A, non-B hepatitis. J. Hepatol. 13 (Suppl. 2), S47.

Mackay, I.R., Taft, C.O. and Cowly, D.S. (1956) Lupoid hepatitis. Lancet 2, 1323–1326.

Manns, M. (1989) Autoantibodies and antigens in liver diseases – updated. J. Hepatol. 9, 272–280.

Manns, M., Gerken, G., Kyriatsoulis, A. et al. (1987) Characterization of a new subgroup of autoimmune chronic active hepatitis by autoantibodies against a soluble liver antigen. Lancet 1, 292–294.

Manns, M., Lamprecht, E., Gerken, G. et al. (1988) Influence of recombinant human alpha and gamma interferon on the expression of hepatocellular autoantigens in hepatoma cell lines. J. Hepatol. 7 (Suppl. 1), 557.

Manns, M., Johnson, E.F., Griffin, K.J. et al. (1989) The major target antigen of liver and kidney microsomal autoantibodies in idiopathic autoimmune hepatitis is cytochrome P-450 dbl. J. Clin. Invest. 83, 1066–1072.

Manns, M.P., Griffin, K.J., Quattrochi, L.C. et al. (1990a) Identification of cytochrome P-450 IA2 as a human autoantigen. Arch. Biochem. Biophys. 280, 229–232.

Manns, M., Zanger, U., Gerken, G. et al. (1990b) Patients with type II autoimmune hepatitis express functionally intact cytochrome P-450 db1 that is inhibited by LKM-1 autoantibodies in vitro but not in vivo. Hepatology 12, 127–132.

Manns, M.P., Griffin, K.J., Sullivan, K.F. et al. (1991a) LKM-1 autoantibodies recognize a short linear sequence on P-450-IID6, a cytochrome P450 monooxygenase. J. Clin. Invest. 88, 1370–1378.

Manns, M., Scheuchter, S., Jentzsch, M. et al. (1991b) Genetics in autoimmune hepatitis type 2. Hepatology, 14, 60A.

Martini, E., Nisen, A., Cavalli, F. et al. (1988) Antibody to liver cytosol (anti-LC1) in patients with autoimmune chronic active hepatitis type 2. Hepatology, 8, 1662–1666.

Meier, U.T. and Meyer, U.A. (1987) Genetic polymorphism of human cytochrome P-450 (S)-mephenytoin-4-hydroxylase. Studies with human autoantibodies suggest a functionally altered cytochrome P450 isoenzyme as cause of the genetic deficiency. Biochemistry 26, 8466–8474.

Melliconi, R., Facchini, A., Miglio, F. et al. (1987) Antibodies to liver cytoplasmic protein complex in chronic hepatitis disease (Letter). Lancet 1, 683.

Michel, G., Ritter, A., Gerken, G. et al. (1992) Anti-GOR and hepatitis C virus in autoimmune liver disease. Lancet 339, 267–269.

Odievre, A.M., Maggiore, G., Homberg, J.C. et al. (1983) Seroimmunologic classification of chronic hepatitis in 57 children. Hepatology 3, 407–409.

Sacher, M., Blumel, P., Thaler, H. et al. (1990) Chronic active hepatitis associated with vitiligo nail dystrophy alopecia and a new variant of LKM antibodies. J. Hepatol. 10, 364–369.

Trautwein, C., Ramadori, G., Gerken, G. et al. (1992) Regulation of cytochrome P-450 IID by acute phase mediators in C3H/HeJ mice. Biochem. Biophys. Res. Commun. 182, 617–623.

Wächter, B., Kyriatsoulis, A., Lohse, A.W. et al. (1990) Characterization of liver cytokeratin as a major target antigen of anti-SLA antibodies. J. Hepatol. 11, 232–239.

Weber, M., Lohse, A.W., Manns, M. et al. (1988) IgG subclass distribution of autoantibodies to glomerular basement membrane in Goodpasture's syndrome compared to other autoantibodies. Nephron 49, 54–57.

Zanger, U.M., Hauri, H.P., Loeper, J. et al. (1988) Antibodies against human cytochrome P-450 db1 in autoimmune hepatitis type II. Proc. Natl. Acad. Sci. U.S.A. 27, 8256–8260.

Zauli, D., Fuscon, M., Crespi, C. et al. (1984) Close correlation between basal cell layer autoantibodies and hepatitis B virus associated chronic delta infection. Hepatology 4, 1103–1106.

Zeniya, M., Takahashi, H., Aizawa, Y. et al. (1990) Reevaluation of liver specific protein and immunogenetic analysis of the pathogenesis of autoimmune hepatitis. In Sixth Int. Congress on Mucosal Immunology, July 22–27, Tokyo.

Autoimmune Hepatitis
Edited by M. Nishioka, G. Toda and M. Zeniya
© 1994, Elsevier Science B.V. All rights reserved

Chapter 10

Anti-nuclear antibodies in autoimmune hepatitis

Soichiro Terada, Syed Ahmed Morshed and Mikio Nishioka

Third Department of Internal Medicine, Kagawa Medical School, Kagawa, 761-07 (Japan)

1. Introduction

Antibodies specific for nuclear macromolecules (ANA) are frequently observed in sera from patients with autoimmune hepatitis (AIH), as well as collagen diseases. A considerable amount of information is now available as to the nuclear autoantigens seen in collagen diseases (Tan, 1989), but little is known about nuclear proteins reacted with sera from patients with liver disease. This chapter will present ANA profiles of AIH on the basis of immunofluorescent studies and Western blot analysis.

2. Anti-nuclear antibody appearance in autoimmune hepatitis

ANA were detected by indirect immunofluorescence (IF) using mouse liver as a substrate. In recent years, the substrates used in the IF method have changed. Nowadays, HEp-2 cells are most frequently used. In this case, the incidence of ANA are high and the fluorescent pattern of ANA can be clearly analyzed. Fig. 1 is typical of immunofluorescent patterns of ANA seen in sera from AIH patients.

The fluorescent patterns of ANA are known to be varied, such as homogeneous, speckled, centromere, peripheral/rim, nuclear dots and others. Recently, ANA have been classified by the Center for Disease Control (CDC) (Tan et al., 1988) as shown in Table 1.

In our study of 17 Japanese patients with AIH (Table 2) (Terada et al., 1990), the most common patterns were homogeneous (59%). Speckled patterns were found in 29%, centromere in 12%, peripheral in 12% and nuclear dots in 6% of AIH. Homogeneous patterns of ANA seem to be more common in AIH (Table 2).

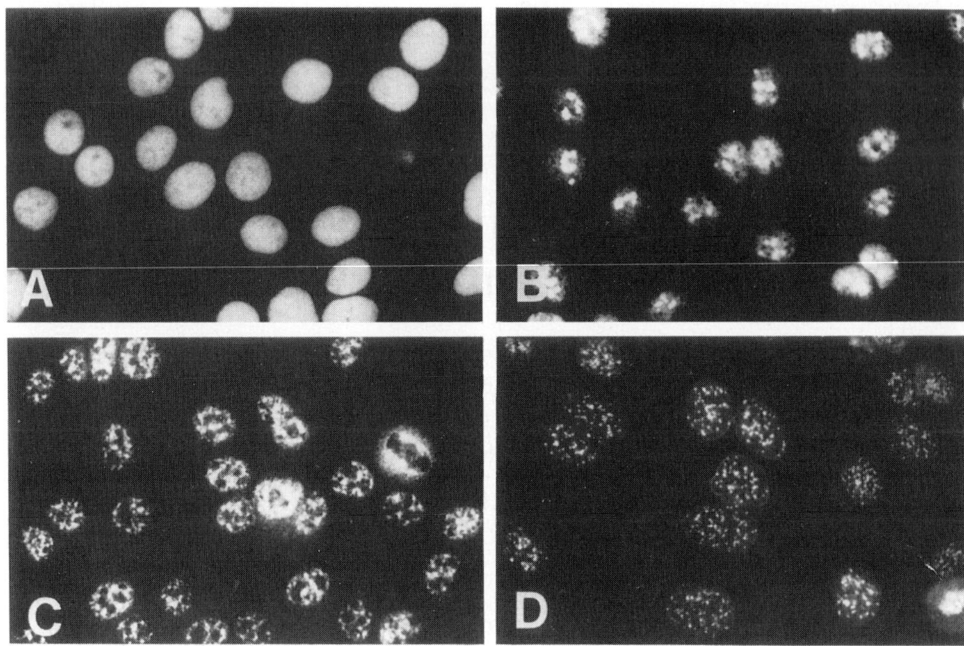

Fig. 1. Immunofluorescent patterns common in autoimmune hepatitis. A: homogeneous pattern.
B: nuclear dots pattern. C: speckled pattern. D: centromere pattern.

Table 1
Reference anti-nuclear antibodies (ANA) available
From Tan et al., 1988.

Reagent	Immunologic features
AF/CDC-1	Homogeneous-pattern ANA (doubles as anti-native DNA)
AF/CDC-2	Anti-La (SS-B)
AF/CDC-3	Speckled-pattern ANA
AF/CDC-4	Anti-U1 RNP (U1 small nuclear ENP)
AF/CDC-5	Anti-Sm (U1, U2, U5, U4/6, small nuclear RNP)
AF/CDC-6	Nucleolar-pattern ANA
AF/CDC-7	Anti-Ro (SS-A)
AF/CDC-8	Centromere-pattern ANA
AF/CDC-9	Anti-Scl-70 (DNA topoisomerase I)
AF/CDC-10	Anti-Jo-1 (histidyl-transfer RNA synthetase)

Bernstein et al. (1984) also reported the high frequency of homogeneous patterns in patients with HBs-negative chronic active hepatitis (CAH). They did not notice the presence of centromere pattern in HBs-negative and -positive CAH patients. However, in our studies, a centromere pattern, which is a diagnostic marker for scleroderma was found in 12% of AIH patients. It is notable that the centromere pattern of ANA was present in sera of patients with AIH and primary biliary cirrhosis (PBC) as well as scleroderma. The occurrence of other types of antibodies such as antibodies to SS-A, SS-B, Scl-70, Sm and U1-RNP detected by routine laboratory tests are very rare in sera from patients with AIH.

It is tempting to evaluate the clinical relevance of ANA patterns in AIH patients. Clinical characteristics of our patients with AIH are described in relation to fluorescent patterns of ANA as seen in Table 3. Patients with a homogeneous pattern of ANA had an acute onset of the disease, compared with the other patterns of ANA. On the other hand, patients with anti-centromere

Table 2

Fluorescent patterns of ANA in patients with AIH

Characteristics	AIH
	17
Homogeneous	10 (59%)
Speckled	5 (29%)
Nuclear dot	1 (6%)
Centromere	2 (12%)
Nucleolar	0 (0%)
Peripheral	2 (12%)

Table 3

Characteristics in patients with AIH in relation to ANA
Homo, homogeneous nuclear; Sp, speckled nuclear; Cent, anti-centromere; RA, rheumatoid arthritis; PSS, progressive systemic sclerosis.

	Homo	Sp	Cent
Sex (F:M ratio)	7:2	3:1	2:0
Age at onset (years)	40	52	47
Acute onset (cases)	4	0	1
Duration of disease (years)	3	4	13
Complications (cases)			
Renal disease	0	1	0
RA	1	2	1
Sjögren's syndrome	2	1	0
PSS	0	1	0
CREST syndrome	1	0	1
Dermatitis	3	1	1
Gall stone	2	1	0

antibody had a mild course and a long duration of disease after the onset, when compared with other groups. They had a good prognosis, because of the long duration of the disease. The complication of other autoimmune diseases is known in patients with AIH. Golding et al. reported that as many as 63% of patients with AIH had diseases of at least one organ other than the liver (Golding et al., 1973). In our study, about half of the patients with AIH were also complicated by some other autoimmune disease. Patients positive for homogeneous ANA are often complicated by rheumatoid arthritis (RA), Sjögren's syndrome and/or dermatitis, but further observations are necessary to help understand the relationship between the clinical characteristics and fluorescent patterns of ANA in the sera of these patients.

3. Analysis of ANA by utilizing immunoblotting

Immunofluorescent assay for the detection of ANA is an easy and rapid method in the clinical laboratory. However, the existence of the ANA does not mean the ultimate existence of particular antibodies. Immunodiffusion and double immunodiffusion methods for the detection of ANA subtypes have been replaced by more reliable enzyme immunoassay methods with the advent of recombinant DNA technology. However, the Western blot is the most suitable method for detecting the peptides according to their molecular size, but it still remains at the research level, particularly in the field of liver diseases. For the purpose of estimating the molecular weights of peptides as well as the specificity of nuclear antigens in liver diseases, the Western blot method was undertaken in our study.

3.1. Western blot analysis

Purified nuclear fractions from HeLa cells were prepared by the method of Penner et al. (1985). Nuclear fractions were analyzed by electrophoresis on 4–20% sodium dodecyl sulfate gradient polyacrylamide gel (SDS–PAGE). After electrotransfer to nitrocellulose (NC) membrane using a semi-dry electroblotter, the remaining protein-binding sites of the NC membrane were blocked with blotto buffer (3% non-fat dry milk in phosphate-buffered saline). The NC strips were incubated with sera from patients with AIH as well as sera from normal healthy individuals at a dilution of 1/100 in blotto buffer. Bound ANA were eluted on the NC- membrane according to the instructions of the Stravegen kit (Biogenex Lab., San Ramon, CA) using the Strept–Avidin–Biotin method, then visualized with 3-amino-9-ethylcarbazole (AEC).

3.2. Characterization of autoantigen

Nuclear proteins of various molecular weights were found in the present study. These data showed a considerable heterogeneity of the nuclear antigens which were reacted by ANA from AIH, even by the ANA that show a similar fluorescent pattern. Similar findings have been reported in the sera from patients with connective tissue diseases (Tan, 1982). In the sera with the homogeneous ANA pattern, 9 bands of 33–100 kDa nuclear proteins were detected (Fig. 2a). In the speckled pattern, there were 4 bands of 50–80 kDa (Fig. 2b). In the patients with the centromere pattern, 7 bands of 17–140 kDa were detected (Fig. 2c) and in patients with peripheral patterns, 3 bands of 70–100 kDa were observed (Fig. 2d). A 17-kDa peptide was found specifically in all the patients positive for the anti-centromere antibody. The molecular weights observed by this Western blot method using sera from AIH patients are summarized in Table 4.

Previous studies showed that immunoblotting can distinguish several antigens including a 200-kDa polypeptide (Lassoued et al., 1988a) lamin B (68 kDa), lamin C (60 kDa) (Lassoued et al., 1988a), and pore complex glycoproteins. It is becoming clear that antibodies against the 200-kDa polypeptide provide good markers for PBC with an incidence of 26–53% of cases (Ruffati et al., 1985; Lassoued et al., 1988a; Lozano et al., 1988). It remains to be elucidated whether similar type(s) of autoantibodies may be present in AIH, although the antibody to the 200-kDa polypeptide was not detected in 17 sera from our AIH patients as well as the sera from Penner et al.'s patients (Penner et al., 1985). Further large-scale screening is necessary using sera from patients with AIH. Penner and colleagues (Wesierka-Gader et al., 1988) have found antibodies to lamins A and C in patients with active classical AIH, but not in patients in remission. However, these anti-lamin antibodies have also been observed in other connective tissue disorders including acute or chronic hepatitis (McKeon et al., 1983; Ruffati et al., 1985; Reeves et al., 1987; Lassoued et al., 1988b). They have also shown that 12 out of 51 patients (24%) were positive for anti-lamin antibodies (Wesierka-Gader et al., 1988). Interestingly, in their study, antibodies to lamins solely occurred in active lupoid hepatitis (75%). In the present study, antibodies to 70- and 60-kDa polypeptides are seen in sera with peripheral, homogeneous and speckled ANA, but whether this polypeptide is identical to lamins A and C is unclear. The clinical significance of anti-lamin antibodies is not well established. It seems likely that this antibody is a marker of autoimmune disease associated with AIH and PBC. The clinical association with these antibodies, in particular in regard to therapy and prognosis, remains to be clarified in further studies.

In the present study, AIH sera also reacted with low-molecular-weight poly-peptides such as 17, 25, 30, 33, 36 and 50 kDa. They may be target antigens of anti-U1-RNP. Anti-U1-RNP recognizes unique proteins of 33 and 22 kDa of the U1 small ribonucleoprotein. Anti-Sm antibodies are capable of recognizing the small nuclear ribonucleic acid U1-6 and two proteins of 25 and 13 kDa (Lerner and Sleig, 1979). These antibodies are known to be involved in the splicing of precursor mRNA. On the other hand, antibodies to La antigen recognize a 48 kDa protein involved in the termination of RNA polymerase-III transcription, and the La antigen has recently been identified as part of the nucleic acid-dependent ATPase/dATPase (Bachmann et al., 1990). Antibody to La antigen

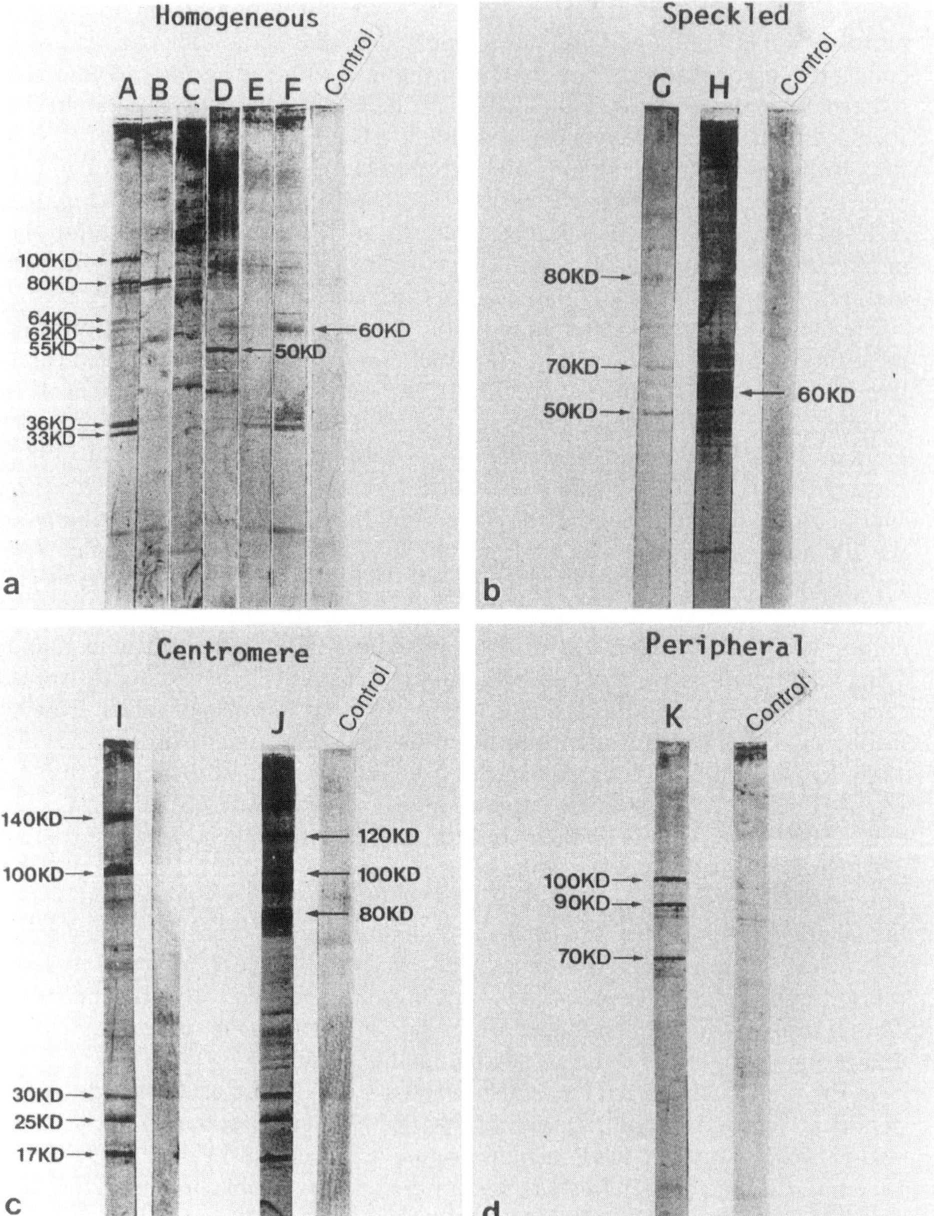

Fig. 2. The patterns of ANA as demonstrated by Western blotting using nuclear fractions derived from HeLa cells. From A to K shows bands with sera from the patients with autoimmune hepatitis. Control, reacted with sera from normal controls. a: homogeneous pattern. b: speckled pattern. c: centromere pattern. d: peripheral pattern.

Table 4
Molecular weights of target peptides of various types of ANA

Pattern of ANA	Target peptide (kDa)
Homogeneous	33, 36, 50, 55, 60, 62, 64, 80, 100
Speckled	50, 60, 70, 80
Centromere	17, 25, 30, 80, 100, 120, 140
Peripheral	70, 90, 100

was also present in 4% of AIH patients, but was absent in all PBC patients (Szostecki et al., 1987). Again by Western blot, 13% of AIH and 11% of PBC cases were positive for La antibody (Penner et al., 1985). In one out of our 17 patients, antibody to SS-A/Ro was found and the patient had the complication of Sjögren's syndrome. Detection of this autoantibody may be helpful for early diagnosis of complications of other autoimmune diseases such as Sjögren's syndrome. We have also found a unique antibody specific for transfer (t) RNA in AIH patients (Shirai et al., 1991).

ANA of the speckled pattern are preferentially found in AIH (53%) and PBC (34%), but have been described in up to one-third of all other types of liver disease (Szostecki et al., 1987). ANA of the speckled pattern in AIH reacted to 50-, 60-, 70-, and 80-kDa nuclear antigens. The characteristics and functions of these nuclear proteins are under investigation.

According to our and others immunoblotting results, there was a heterogeneity among the antigens specific for ANA in patients with AIH (Table 4). The present results suggest that the apparent target peptides of ANA common to AIH were the proteins of 25 (doublet), 33 (doublet), 55, 60, 80, 100 and 140-kDa as shown in Table 5. Peptides of 55 and 60 kDa were the nuclear proteins. A 140-kDa peptide has been thought to belong to the nuclear matrix. Proteins of 25-, 33-, 80-, and 100-kDa are composed of unknown nuclear portions, whereas peptides of 60 and 70 kDa could be anti-lamin antibodies. It is unclear how the antibodies relate to

Table 5
Apparent target peptides of ANA common to autoimmune hepatitis

Target peptide (kDa)
25 (doublet)
33 (doublet)
55, 60 (nuclear protein)
140 (nuclear matrix)
80, 100

the pathogenesis, but these antibodies may serve as valuable probes for the characterization of some nuclear antigens as well as being diagnostic markers in AIH patients.

References

Bachmann, M., Pfeifer, K. et al. (1990) Characterization of the antigen La as a nucleic acid-dependent ATPase/dATPase with melting properties. Cell 60, 85–93.

Berstein, R.M., Neuberger, J.M. et al. (1984) Diversity of autoantibodies in primary biliary cirrhosis and chronic active hepatitis. Clin. Exp. Immunol. 55, 553–560.

Golding, P.L., Smith, M. et al. (1973) Multisystemic involvement in chronic liver disease. Studies of the incidence and pathogenesis. Am. J. Med. 55, 772–782.

Lassoued, K., Guilly, M.N. et al. (1988a) Antinuclear antibodies specific for lamins. Characterization and clinical significance. Ann. Intern. Med. 108, 829–833.

Lassoued, K., Guilly, M.N. et al. (1988b) Autoantibodies to 200 KD polypeptide(s) of the nuclear envelope: a new serological marker of primary biliary cirrhosis. Clin. Exp. Immunol. 74, 283–288.

Lerner, M.R. and Sleig, J.A. (1979) Antibodies to small nuclear RNAs complexed with proteins are produced by patients with systemic lupus erythematosis. Proc. Natl. Acad. Sci. U.S.A. 7, 5495–5499.

Lozano, F., Pares, A. et al. (1988) Autoantibodies against unclear envelope-associated proteins in primary biliary cirrhosis. Hepatology 8, 930–938.

McKeon, F.D., Tuffanelli, D.K.L. et al. (1983) Autoimmune response directed against conserved determinants of nuclear envelope proteins in a patient with linear scleroderma. Proc. Natl. Acad. Sci. U.S.A. 80, 4374–4378.

Penner, E., Kindas-Mugge, I. et al. (1985) Nuclear antigens recognized by antibodies present in liver disease sera. Clin. Exp. Immunol. 63, 428–433.

Reeves, W.H., Chaudhary, N. et al. (1987) Lamin B autoantibodies in sera of certain patients with systemic lupus erythematosis. J. Exp. Med. 165, 750–762.

Ruffati, A., Arslan, P. et al. (1985) Nuclear membrane-staining antibody in patients with primary biliary cirrhosis. J. Clin. Immunol. 5, 357–361.

Shirai, M., Watanabe, S. et al. (1991) Autoantibody specific for transfer ribonucleic acid in patients with autoimmune chronic active hepatitis and primary biliary cirrhosis. Hepato-Gastroenterology 3, 468–469.

Szostecki, C., Krippner, H. et al. (1987) Autoimmune sera recognize a 100 KD nuclear protein antigen (sp-100). Clin. Exp. Immunol. 68, 108–116.

Tan, E.M. (1982) Autoantibodies to nuclear antigen (ANA): their immunology and medicine. Adv. Immunol. 33, 167–240.

Tan, E.M. (1989) Antinuclear antibodies. Diagnostic markers for autoimmune diseases and probes for cell biology. Adv. Immunol. 44, 93–151.

Ten, E.M., Feltamp, T.E.W. et al. (1988) Reference reagents for antinuclear antibodies. Arthritis Rheum. 31, 1331.

Terada, S., Hong, H.N. et al. (1990) Analysis of antinuclear antibodies (ANA) in autoimmune hepatitis. In M. Tsutiya (Ed.), Frontiers of Mucosal Immunology, Vol. 2, Elsevier, Amsterdam, pp. 39–42.

Wesierka-Gader, J., Penner, E. et al. (1988) Antibodies to nuclear lamins in autoimmune liver disease. Clin. Immunol. Immunopathol. 49, 107–115.

Autoimmune Hepatitis
Edited by M. Nishioka, G. Toda and M. Zeniya

Chapter 11

Cytoskeleton antibodies

Pekka Kurki

Department of Clinical Research, Sandoz Pharma Ltd and Department of Bacteriology and Immunology, University of Helsinki, Haartmaninkatu 3, SF-00290 Helsinki (Finland)

1. Introduction

The term cytoskeleton defines a group of structures that are thought to have a 'skeletal role' in cellular locomotion and subcellular organization (Lazarides, 1980; Porter, 1984). These structures form the skeleton that remains when the cell is extracted with detergents removing the cell membrane as well as the bulk of the cytoplasmic and nuclear constituents (Brown et al., 1976). There is a cytoplasmic and a nuclear skeleton. The cytoplasmic skeleton consists mainly of 3 types of filaments and fibers: microfilaments, intermediate-sized filaments and microtubules.

The cell nucleus also contains a skeletal structure, the nuclear matrix. It can be subdivided into nuclear pore complexes, nuclear lamina, residual nucleoli and a fibrogranular network. The main protein components of the nuclear matrix are lamins that are related to cytoplasmic intermediate filaments (McKeon et al., 1986; Bibor-Hardy et al., 1991). Almost all components of the cytoskeleton have been shown to be targets for autoantibodies – cytoskeleton antibodies.

Of all cell types, muscle cells have the most extensive cytoskeletal structure owing to their contractile function. Antibodies binding to smooth muscle of rat stomach were first described by Johnson et al. (1965) while screening for anti-nuclear antibodies by indirect immunofluorescence. The term smooth muscle antibodies (SMA) was introduced by Whittingham et al. (1966) who also confirmed the association of these antibodies with chronic active hepatitis (CAH), especially with its 'lupoid' subset. The term SMA proved to be somewhat unfortunate since the antibodies were shown to react with ubiquitous tissue components, such as actin-containing microfilaments, microtubules and intermediate filaments (Gabbiani et al., 1973; Kurki et al., 1977, 1979; Mead et al.,

1980). Thus, smooth muscle antibodies were the first antibodies that were assigned to the large group of antibodies reacting with the cytoskeleton.

2. Cytoskeleton of the hepatocyte

The cytoskeleton of the hepatocyte (Fischer and Phillips, 1979) may undergo significant changes in proliferating and transformed hepatocytes. This change is very prominent in the actin-containing microfilaments (Farrow et al., 1971). In the resting hepatocyte, microfilaments are concentrated around the bile canaliculi, whereas in proliferating hepatocytes the thick bundles of actin filaments, 'stress fibers', are clearly visible. Actin filaments are connected to the cell membrane through an apparatus containing α-actinin, talin and vinculin (Obrink, 1986). These proteins are associated with transmembrane proteins that mediate the attachment of the cells to the extra-cellular matrix and to the neighboring cells. Another prominent feature of this membrane–cytoskeleton complex is transmembrane signalling. Microfilaments can be disrupted with cytochalasins, whereas phalloidin causes an irreversible actin polymerization (Cooper, 1987).

Microtubules are composed of α- and β-tubulins as well as of the τ-protein, dynein and the microtubule-associated proteins (MAPs). Microtubules form a fine network in the interphase cells. Microtubules originate and radiate from centrioles. During mitosis, microtubules will form the mitotic spindle that separates the daughter chromosomes. Microtubules are associated with chromosomes via kinetochores. Microtubules are disrupted by colchicine and related drugs. Vinblastine will not only disrupt the cytoplasmic microtubules, but also induces the formation of tubulin paracrystals (Bensch and Malawista, 1968).

As an epithelial cell, the hepatocyte also has a network of intermediate-sized filaments – cytokeratin filaments. Cytokeratin filaments are composed of heterodimers of two different types of cytokeratins. Certain toxic agents like alcohol can disrupt the intermediate filament network and induce the pathological accumulation of filaments, the Mallory bodies (Denk et al., 1981). The macrophage-like sinusoidal cells express another filament type – vimentin filaments. In contrast to the cytokeratin filaments, the vimentin filament system is sensitive to the microtubule-disrupting drugs that collapse the cytoplasmic filament network and induce the formation of juxtanuclear vimentin filament bundles (Goldman and Knipe, 1972).

3. Cytoskeleton antibodies

The cytoskeleton antibodies can be classified into two categories: the (cytoplasmic) cytoskeleton antibodies and nucleoskeleton antibodies (Fig. 1). Antibodies to nucleoskeleton belong to the group of anti-nuclear antibodies (ANA) and are

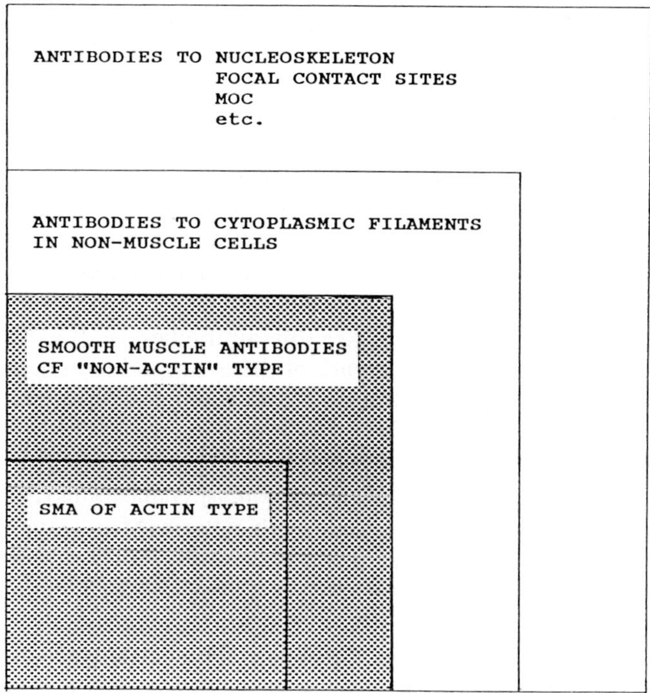

Fig. 1. Classification of cytoskeleton antibodies.

reviewed in Chapter 10. Antibodies to the cytoplasmic skeleton can be further classified by recognizing the subcellular structures that are the targets for autoantibodies (Kurki and Virtanen, 1984; Toh, 1979).

4. Diagnostic significance of cytoskeleton antibodies of anti-smooth muscle type

4.1. Smooth muscle antibodies in liver diseases

SMA are found in 50–70% of patients with autoimmune (type 1) CAH and in about 80% of its 'lupoid' subset. The highest titers of SMA are found in this patient category. Patients with drug-induced CAH may also have high titers of SMA (Lindberg et al., 1975). In other forms of CAH, in primary biliary cirrhosis (PBC, 50%) and in alcoholic liver disease (49%), SMA are less common and the titers tend to be low (Doniach et al., 1966; Whittingham et al., 1966; Galbraith et al., 1974; Lindberg et al., 1975; Husby et al., 1977; Kurki, 1979; Gluud et al., 1981; Mackay et al., 1985). It is possible that patients with a high IgG SMA titer but devoid of other auto-antibodies belong to a special subset of CAH (Manns, 1989; Odievre et al., 1983). There is a subgroup of autoimmune CAH characterized by cholestatic features. SMA in this patient group tend to have IgM class SMA (Kurki et al., 1980). The diagnostic specificity of SMA is poor since these antibodies are frequently found in healthy individuals and non-hepatic diseases (Kurki, 1979; Toh, 1979). An occult finding of circulating SMA does not predict the development of a liver disease (Jorde et al., 1987).

4.2. *Smooth muscle antibodies in viral infections and malignant disease*

The diagnostic specificity of cytoskeleton antibodies of the SMA type is hampered by the widespread occurrence of these antibodies in acute infections and in chronic inflammatory conditions. SMA occur frequently in viral hepatitis (Farrow et al., 1971; Andersen et al., 1976; Pedersen et al., 1981, 1982). SMA of IgM class also appear transiently after other acute viral (Holborow et al., 1973; Linder et al., 1979; Mead et al., 1980) and mycoplasma infections (Biberfeld et al., 1976; Bretherton and Toh, 1981). Patients with malaria (Mortazavi-Milani et al., 1984), schistosomiasis (Boehme et al., 1989) and cryptosporidiosis also have circulating SMA (Boonpucknavig and Bunyaratvej, 1988). Tubulin antibodies have been demonstrated in parasitic infections (Howard et al., 1987). Cytoskeleton antibodies are associated with chronic inflammation, such as rheumatoid arthritis and other connective tissue diseases as well as uveitis (Doniach et al., 1966; Kurki et al., 1983; Senécal et al., 1985; Murray, 1986).

Several studies have demonstrated the presence of cytoskeletal antibodies in cancer patients (see Kurki, 1986 for references). Occasionally, the monoclonal antibodies in lymphoproliferative disorders have anti-cytoskeleton activity (Dellagi et al., 1982; Dighiero et al., 1983). Thus, in cases of a very high cytoskeleton antibody titer it is reasonable to exclude the presence of monoclonal component.

5. *Classification and specificity of cytoskeleton antibodies*

5.1. *Classification at the tissue level*

Cytoskeleton antibodies of SMA type react with ubiquitous tissue components that are well exposed in smooth muscle cells and in certain non-muscle cells. The first attempt to classify cytoskeleton antibodies by indirect immunofluorescent microscopy were based on different staining patterns (Table 1). SMA that bind to non-muscle cells have been called 'glomerulus antibodies' and 'bile canalicular antibodies' depending on the tissue substrate. These antibodies are typical for type 1 CAH and can be neutralized by actin (Whittingham et al., 1966; Kurki et al., 1978, 1980). The identification of anti-actin antibodies by recording the

Table 1
Classification of SMA at the tissue level
From Bottazzo et al. (1976) and Kurki et al. (1980). V, blood vessel; G, glomerulus; T, renal tubule.

	Staining of			Staining of bile canaculi
	Renal vessels	Glomeruli	Peritubular fibers	
SMA-V	+	−	−	−
SMA-G[a]	+	+	−	−
SMA-T[a]	+	+	+	+

[a] Neutralized by actin.

differential binding of SMA to rat kidney and/or rabbit liver can be used to improve the diagnostic specificity of SMA (Bottazzo et al., 1976; Kurki et al., 1978, 1980). Recently, this classification has been complemented by an immunofluorescence assay using phalloidin-treated liver tissue as substrate (Fusconi et al., 1990).

5.2. Classification at the subcellular level

Cytoskeleton antibodies can also be classified at a subcellular level by using cultured cells as substrate (Figs. 2 and 3). It has been found that cytoskeleton antibodies of SMA type can react not only with actin-containing microfilaments (Gabbiani et al., 1973) but also with intermediate sized filaments (Kurki et al., 1977) and with microtubules (Kurki et al., 1979; Mead et al., 1980). The differentiation of cytoskeleton antibodies is facilitated by the treatment of cultured cells with vinblastine prior to the fixation (Kurki and Virtanen, 1984; Fig. 3). CAII, PBC and alcoholic liver disease have different profiles of antibodies to these cytoplasmic filamentous/fibrillar structures (Kurki et al., 1983). The requirements for the demonstration of cytoskeleton antibodies vary. In general, cells that are anchored to the substratum are preferred because they display a large cytoplasmic domain with well-developed cytoplasmic structures. However, vinblastine-treated peripheral blood mononuclear cells have also been used (Zauli et al., 1985). Actively spreading cells such as fibroblasts are suitable to study the locomotive part of the cytoskeleton − including microfilaments and sites of cell–substratum adhesion. On the other hand, confluent monolayers may be useful in observing the sites for cell–cell contacts.

5.3. Specificity of microfilament antibodies

Cytoskeleton antibodies in CAH react typically with microfilaments (Gabbiani et al., 1973; Fig. 2). The main component of microfilaments is actin. However,

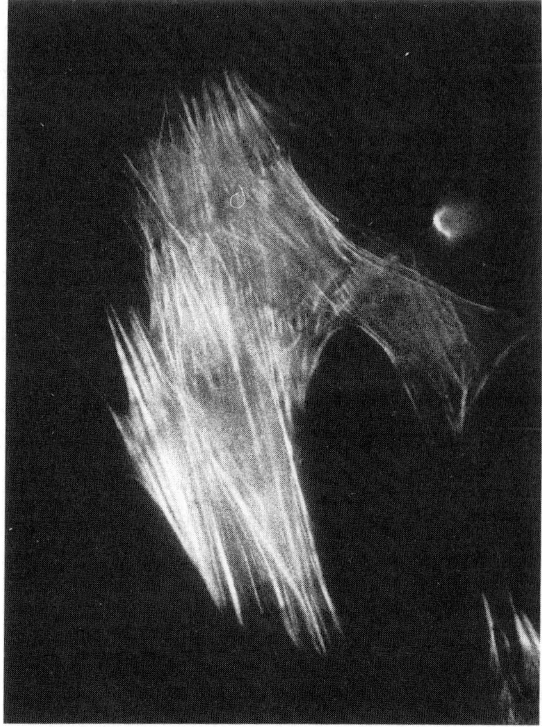

Fig. 2. Indirect immunofluorescent staining of a cultured fibroblast with human smooth muscle antibodies of anti-actin type. Note the staining of the parallel actin-containing microfilaments.

there are other components, such as tropomyosin and troponin. Most sera with high titers of microfilament antibodies react with actin. Antibodies to other 'contractile' proteins, such as myosin (31.5%), tropomyosin (34%) and troponin (11%) are also found in type 1 CAH (Dighiero et al., 1990) but may also occur in other diseases (Mayet et al., 1990). Patients with chronic hepatitis frequently have antibodies to α-actinin (Kurki and Vuoristo, unpublished results).

5.4. *Actin antibodies*

Actin type SMA seem to be the major type of cytoskeleton antibodies in CAH (Gabbiani et al., 1973; Lidman et al., 1976; Dighiero et al., 1990) whereas cytoskeleton antibodies in other diseases mainly belong to the 'non-actin' category (Andersen et al., 1976; Kurki et al., 1978; Kurki, 1979; Fusconi et al., 1990). The wide species cross-reactivity demonstrates that human actin antibodies react with well conserved determinants of actin. There are 3 isoforms of actin from which α-actin is present both in striated and smooth muscle, whereas β- and γ-actins are found in non-muscle tissue. The wide tissue cross-reactivity of human

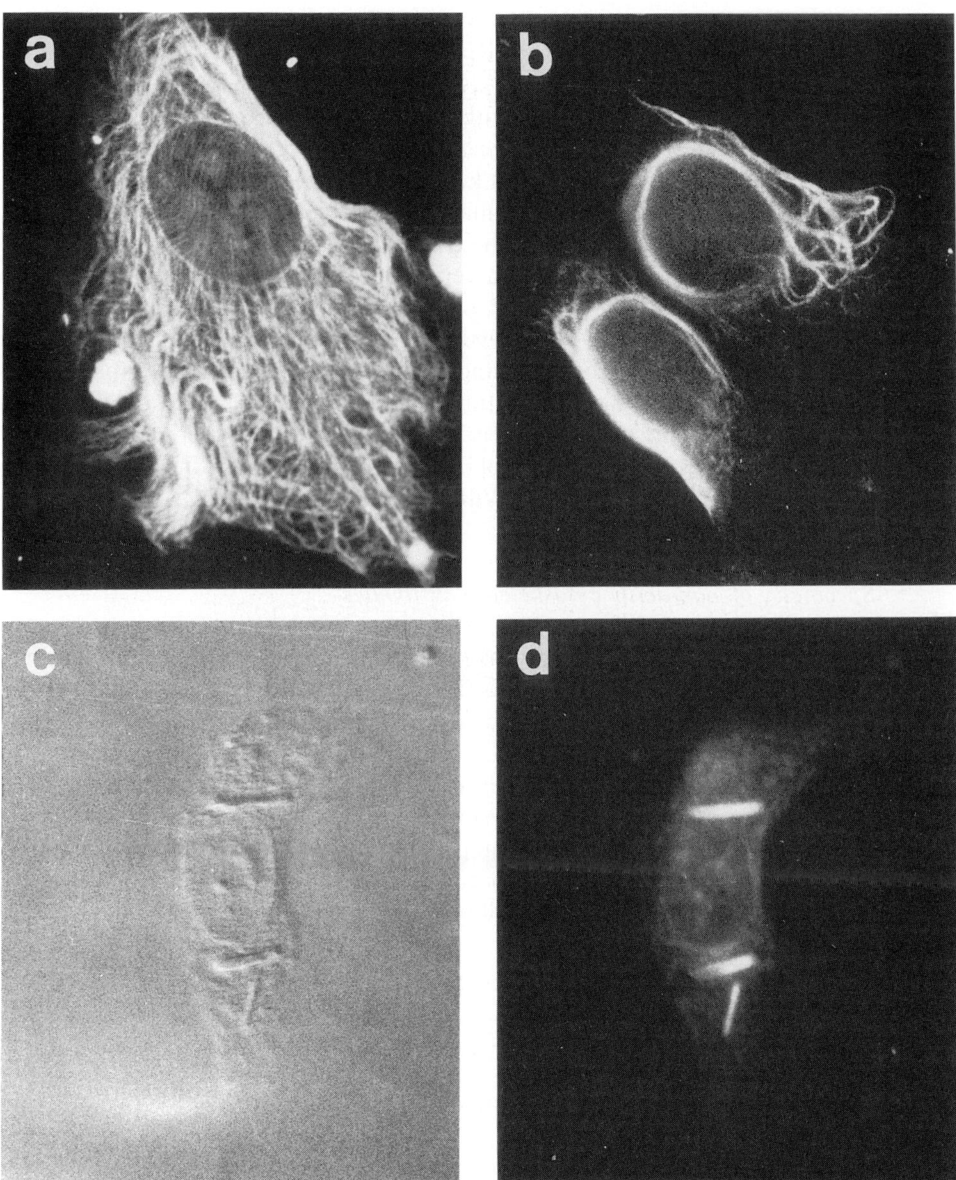

Fig. 3. Indirect immunofluorescence (a, b, d) and phase contrast (c) microscopy of cultured fibro-blasts. Cells in b, c and d were treated with vinblastine sulfate that collapses the intermediate filaments into juxtanuclear bundles (b) and induces the formation of tubulin paracrystals that are visible by phase contrast microscopy (c) and by indirect immunofluorescence microscopy (d). The cells were stained with human smooth muscle antibodies of either anti-intermediate filament (a, b) or anti-microtubulus (d) types.

actin antibodies suggests that the epitopes are shared with all 3 isoforms. The epitopes for human actin antibodies are present both in the polymerized (F-) and depolymerized (G-) forms of actin (Kurki et al., 1978; Thorstensson et al., 1981). If cells are labeled with human actin antibodies, only F-actin is seen by indirect immunofluorescence (IFL). This suggests that the antigenic determinants are covered by actin-binding proteins that keep actin in the monomeric form. Such blocking factors are also present in human serum (Norberg et al., 1979). Experimental actin antibodies can readily be assayed by solid-phase immunoassay whereas human actin antibodies give a very weak signal (Kurki 1978). Furthermore, actin antibodies demonstrated by solid-phase immunoassays are not specific for type 1 CAH (Mayet et al., 1990). Anti-actin-positive sera (as defined by indirect IFL) rarely give a strong labeling of the actin band by immunoblotting. Thus, the epitope of human anti-actin may be composed of discontinuous sequences accessible only in the native actin molecule. The interference of serum actin-binding proteins must also be kept in mind, since they may bind to the same epitopes as human actin antibodies (Williams and Lennon, 1986; Mejean et al., 1987).

5.5. Specificity of 'non-actin' cytoskeleton antibodies

SMA of intermediate filament type have been shown to react with the subunit protein vimentin in cultured fibroblasts (Dellagi et al., 1984; Senécal et al., 1985; Alcover et al., 1985; Fig. 3). Vimentin antibodies are prevalent in PBC and HBsAg-positive CAH (Pedersen et al., 1982; Kurki et al., 1983). In addition, a subgroup of intermediate filament antibodies react with desmin filaments in muscle cells (Kurki et al., 1989). Occasionally, vimentin antibodies cross-react with other intermediate filament subunit proteins including cytokeratins (Dellagi et al., 1984). Cytokeratin antibodies occur frequently in alcoholic liver disease (Kurki et al., 1984). Microtubulus antibodies react at least with tubulin (Mead et al., 1980; Fig. 3).

6. Mechanisms of cytoskeleton antibody production

6.1. Special features of cytoskeleton antibodies

The production of human cytoskeleton antibodies is intriguing for two reasons: because of the different disease associations and because of the antigenic epitopes involved. Actin antibodies can serve as an illustrative example for these questions. High titers of IgG-class actin-type SMA are found in type 1 CAH, but not in other liver diseases. Thus, this antibody response is not due to simple polyclonal hypergammaglobulinemia. Neither is it due to the liberation of actin from injured cells (Li et al., 1977). Actin is not an immunologically sequestered antigen since circulating actin is present in normal blood (Mejean et al., 1987). For these reasons, the production of actin type SMA must be intimately associated with the etiology of the type 1 CAH.

The second feature of anti-actin autoantibody that differs from a normal immunization process is the selection of antigen epitope(s). Actin autoantibodies react with conserved epitopes in actin whereas experimental actin antibodies tend to react with epitopes that are 'foreign' to the host. The conserved epitopes are likely to be functionally important. For instance, these domains may be responsible for attachment of microfilament-associated proteins or viral proteins. The involvement of these conserved 'active sites' has also been implicated in the production of ANA (Tan et al., 1988).

6.2. Germ-line genes encode for cytoskeleton antibodies

It is evident that genes coding for various cytoskeleton antibodies, such as actin, tubulin and vimentin antibodies, belong to the germ-line repertoire (Underwood et al., 1985). This explains the existence of M-components with SMA activity (Dellagi et al., 1982; Dighiero et al., 1983) as well as the finding of low levels of cytoskeleton antibodies in normal sera (Guilbert et al., 1982). It is known that a particular subset of B-cells, CD-5-positive B-cells, are prone to autoantibody production. Chronic lymphatic leukemia is characterized by a clonal expansion of CD-5-positive B-cells. These cells produce antibodies that are frequently directed against cytoskeletal components. A feature of these antibodies is the wide cross-reactivity with other autoantigens (Dighiero et al., 1990). However, the reasons for the occurrence of high titer cytoskeleton antibodies in certain diseases still need to be defined.

6.3. Cytoskeleton antibodies, viral infections and drug reactions

The fact that relatives of patients with CAH have a high prevalence of SMA may suggest that the production of such antibodies may be under genetic control (Galbraith et al., 1974). However, environmental factors may also play a role (Krawitt et al., 1987). Circulating cytoskeleton antibodies are transiently appearing during various acute infections. It has been demonstrated that monoclonal antibodies against viral and bacterial antigens cross-react with antigens in the cytoskeleton (Fujinami et al.,1983; Dale and Beachey, 1985; Kraus et al., 1989). It is also known that viruses can bind to the cytoskeleton and may alter its structure (Sharpe et al., 1982; Anomasiri et al., 1990). The altered cytoskeleton with associated viral antigens may induce an immune reaction according to the T-lymphocyte bypass concept. Cytoskeleton antibodies may be induced by drugs, such as oxyphenisatin, nitrofurantoin, clometacin, fenofibrate and paraverin (Lindberg et al., 1978; Homberg et al., 1985). Although such drugs may act as haptens there is an alternative explanation. Drugs will associate with enzymes

                    P. Kurki

during their metabolism. Such complexes may stimulate T-cells and become immunogenic, as in the case of tienilic acid (Homberg et al., 1985). This reaction is not irreversible since most drug-induced antibodies disappear upon discontinuation of the drug treatment.

6.4. The anti-cytoskeleton reaction may be (auto)antigen- and cytokine-driven

It is also possible that the germ-line genes of the cytoskeleton antibodies are the genes from which neutralizing antimicrobial antibodies are developed by recombination and point mutations. High titers of cytoskeleton antibodies might be produced when the immune reaction is maturing towards autoantigens instead of microbial antigens. Antibody against an exogenous antigen may undergo a change in specificity towards autoantigens after a single point mutation (see Eilat (1990) for references). In this situation, the immune reaction may become autoantigen- driven. This hypothesis is supported by the fact that an individual patient may have antibodies to several epitopes within the same cytoskeletal structure (Dighiero et al., 1990). In chronic inflammatory conditions, such as rheumatoid arthritis and chronic hepatitis, the excess production of cytokines, such as interleukins and interferons may be a facilitating factor for autoantibody production. It is not known whether the production of cytokines is due to the continuous stimulation of T-cells by antigen-presenting cells or whether the cytokines are produced as a result of inappropriate T-cell stimulation, such as superantigens. Interestingly, α-interferon therapy of viral or autoantibody-negative chronic B hepatitis is associated with a transient production of SMA and ANA (Mayet et al., 1989; Fattovich et al., 1991).

7. Conclusions

There are several types of cytoskeleton antibodies that can be distinguished by simple techniques. Cytoskeleton antibodies of anti-smooth muscle type (SMA) react with cytoplasmic filaments that are differentially expressed in non-muscle tissues. This fact can be used for the classification of SMA. The classification of SMA is aimed at distinguishing actin antibodies that are typical for auto-immune/idiopathic CAH from other types of SMA. The selectivity of this autoantibody response in CAH still needs to be explained. The solution of this problem may lead us closer to the clue of autoimmune liver disease.

Acknowledgements

The skilful secretarial assistance of Ms. Helena Noor is gratefully acknowledged. This study was supported by the Sigrid Juselius Foundation.

References

Alcover, A., Hernandez, C. and Avila, J. (1985) Human vimentin autoantibodies preferentially interact with a peptide of 30 kD mol WT, located close to the aminoterminal of the molecule. Clin. Exp. Immunol. 61, 24–30.

Andersen, P., Small, J.V. and Sobieszek, A. (1976) Studies on the specificity of smooth-muscle antibodies. Clin. Exp. Immunol. 26, 57–66.

Anomasiri, W.T., Tovell, D.R. and Tyrrell, D.L.J. (1990) Paramyxovirus membrane protein enhances antibody production to new antigenic determinants in the actin molecule: a model for virus-induced autoimmunity. J. Virol. 64, 3179–3184.

Bensch, K.G. and Malawista, S. (1968) Microtubule crystals: A new biophysical phenomenon induced by vinca alkaloids. Nature 218, 1176–1177.

Biberfeld, G. and Sterner, G. (1976) Smooth muscle antibodies in mycoplasma pneumoniae infection. Clin. Exp. Immunol. 24, 287–291.

Bibor-Hardy, V., LeMyre, A., Sakr, F. and Bernard, M. (1991) Expression nuclear matrix proteins in rat liver tissue. Exp. Cell Res. 192, 550–556.

Boehme, M.W.J., Kataaha, P.K. and Holborow, E.J. (1989) Autoantibodies to intermediate filaments in sera of patients with Schistosoma mansoni infection. Clin. Exp. Immunol. 77, 230–233.

Boonpucknavig, S. and Bunyaratvej, S. (1988) Detection of smooth muscle antibodies in patients with cryptosporidiosis. J. Clin. Lab. Immunol. 27, 153.

Bottazzo, G.F., Florin-Christensen, A., Fairfax, A., Swana, G., Doniach, D. and Gröschel-Stewart, U. (1976) Classification of smooth muscle autoantibodies detected by immunofluorescence. J. Clin. Pathol. 29, 403–410.

Bretherton, L. and Toh, B.H. (1981) IgM autoantibody to intermediate filaments in infectious mononucleosis. J. Clin. Lab. Immunol. 5, 7–10.

Brown, S., Levinson, W. and Spudich, J. (1976) Cytoskeletal elements of chick embryo fibroblasts revealed by detergent extraction. J. Supramol. Struct. 5, 119–130.

Cooper, J.A. (1987) Effects of cytochalasin and phalloidin on actin. J. Cell Biol. 105, 1473–1478.

Dale, J.B., Beachey, E.H. (1985) Epitopes of streptococcal M proteins shared with cardiac myosin. J. Exp. Med. 162, 583–591.

Dellagi, K., Brouet, J.C., Perreau, J. and Paulin, D. (1982) Human monoclonal IgM with autoantibody activity against intermediate filaments. Proc. Natl. Acad. Sci. U.S.A. 79, 446–450.

Dellagi, K., Brouet, J.C. and Seligmann, M. (1984) Anti-vimentin autoantibodies in angio-immunoblastic lymphadenopathy. N. Engl. J. Med. 310, 215–218.

Denk, H., Franke, W.W., Eckerstorfer, R., Schmid, E., Kerjaschki, D. (1979) Formation and involution of Mallory bodies (alcoholic hyalin) in murine and human liver revealed by immunofluorescence microscopy with antibodies to prekeratin. Proc. Natl. Acad. Sci. USA 76, 4112–4116.

Dighiero, G., Guilbert, B., Fernand, J.P., Lymberi, P., Danon, F. and Avrameas, S. (1983) Thirty-six human monoclonal immunoglobulins with antibody activity against cytoskeleton proteins, thyroglobulin, and native DNA. Immunological studies and clinical correlations. Blood 62, 264–270.

Dighiero, G., Lymberi, P., Monot, C. and Abuaf, N. (1990) Sera with high levels of anti-smooth muscle and anti-mitochondrial antibodies frequently bind to cytoskeleton proteins. Clin. Exp. Immunol. 82, 52–56.

Doniach, D., Roitt, I.M., Walker, J.G. and Sherlock, S. (1966) Tissue antibodies in primary biliary cirrhosis and other liver diseases and their clinical implications. Clin. Exp. Immunol. 1, 237–262.

Eilat, D. (1990) The role of germline gene expression and somatic mutation in the generation of autoantibodies to DNA. Mol. Immunol. 27, 203–210.

Farrow, L.J., Holborow, E.J. and Brighton, W.D. (1971) Reaction of human smooth muscle antibody with liver cells. Nature New Biol. 232, 186–187.

Fattovich, G., Betterle, C., Brollo, L., Pedini, B., Giustina, G., Realdi, G., Alberti, A. and Ruol, A. (1991) Autoantibodies during α-interferon therapy for chronic hepatitis Br. J. Med. Virol. 34, 132–135.

Fischer, M.M. and Phillips, M.J. (1979) Cytoskeleton of the hepatocyte. Prog. Liver Dis. 6, 105–121.

Fujinami, R.S., Oldstone, M.B.A., Wroblewska, Z., Frankel, M.E. and Koprowski, H. (1983) Molecular mimicry in virus infection: crossreaction of measles virus phosphoprotein or of herpes simplex virus protein with human intermediate filaments. Proc. Natl. Acad. Sci. U.S.A. 80, 2346–2350.

Fusconi, M., Cassani, F., Zauli, D., Lenzi, M., Ballardini, G., Volta, U. and Bianchi, F.B. (1990) Anti-actin antibodies: a new test for an old problem. J. Immunol. Methods 130, 1–8.

Gabbiani, G., Ryan, G.B., Lamelin, J.-P., Vassalli, P., Majno, G., Bouvier, C.A., Cruchaud, A. and Lüscher, E.F. (1973) Human smooth muscle autoantibody. Its identification as antiactin antibody and a study of its binding to 'nonmuscular' cells. Am. J. Pathol. 72, 473–488.

Galbraith, R.M., Smith, M., Mackenzie, R.M., Tee, D.E., Doniach, D. and Williams, R. (1974) High prevalence of seroimmunologic abnormalities in relatives of patients with active chronic hepatitis or primary biliary cirrhosis. New Engl. J. Med. 290, 63–69.

Gluud, C., Tage-Jensen, M., Bahnsen, M., Dietrichson, O. and Svejgaard, A. (1981) Autoantibodies, histocompatibility antigens and testosterone in males with alcoholic liver cirrhosis. Clin. Exp. Immunol. 44, 31–37.

Goldman, R.D. and Knipe, D.M. (1972) Functions of cytoplasmic fibres. Gold Spring Harbor Symp. Quant. Biol. 37, 523–534.

Guilbert, M., Dighiero, G. and Avrameas, S. (1982) Naturally occurring antibodies against nine common antigens in human sera. I. Detection, isolation and characterization. J. Immunol. 128, 2779–2787.

Holborow, E.J., Hemsted, E.H. and Mead, S.V. (1973) Smooth muscle antibodies in infectious mononucleosis. Br. J. Med. 3, 323–325.

Homberg, J.C., Abuaf, N., Helmy-Khalil, S., Biour, M., Poupon, R., Islam, S., Darnis, F., Levy, V.G., Opolon, P., Beaugrand, M. et al. (1985) Drug-induced hepatitis associated with anticytoplasmic organelle autoantibodies. Hepatology 5, 722–727.

Howard, M.K., Gull, K. and Miles, M.A. (1987) Antibodies to tubulin in patients with parasitic infection. Clin. Exp. Immunol. 68, 78–85.

Husby, G., Skrede, S., Blomhoff, J.P., Jakobsen, C.D., Berg, K., Gjone, E. (1977) Serum immunoglobulins and organ non-specific antibodies in diseases of the liver. Scand. J. Gastroenterol. 12, 297–304.

Johnson, G.D., Holborow, E.J. and Glynn, L.E. (1965) Antibody to smooth muscle in patients with liver disease. Lancet 2, 878–879.

Jorde, R., Skogen, B. and Rekvig, O.P. (1987) A reexamination of patients with previously detected autoantibodies to smooth muscle. Acta Med. Scand. 222, 471–475.

Kraus, W., Ohyama, K., Snyder, D.S. and Beachey, E.H. (1989) Autoimmune sequence of streptococcal M protein shared with the intermediate filament vimentin. J. Exp. Med. 169, 481–492.

Krawitt, E.D., Kilby, A.E., Albertini, R.J., Schanfield, M.S., Chastenay, B.F., Harper, P.C., Mickey, R.M. and McAuliffe, T.L. (1987) Immunogenetic studies of autoimmune chronic active hepatitis: HLA, immunoglobulin allotypes and autoantibodies. Hepatology 7, 1305–1310.

Kurki, P. (1979) Human Smooth Muscle Antibodies. Thesis, Helsinki University. ISBN 951-99193-7-6.

Kurki, P. (1986) Autoantibodies to cytoskeleton in malignancy. Cancer Rev. 4, 79–90.

Kurki, P. and Virtanen, I. (1984) the detection of human antibodies against cytoskeletal components. J. Immunol. Methods 67, 209–223.

Kurki, P. Virtanen, I., Stenman, S. and Linder, E. (1977) Human smooth muscle antibodies reacting with intermediate (100 Å) filaments. Nature 268, 240–241.

Kurki, P., Linder, E., Miettinen, A. and Alfthan, O. (1978) Smooth muscle antibodies of actin and 'non-actin' specificity. Clin. Immunol. Immunopathol. 9, 443–453.

Kurki, P., Virtanen, I., Stenman, S. and Linder, E. (1979) Smooth muscle antibodies reacting with microtubular antigens. Protides of the Biological Fluids 26, 629–632.

Kurki, P., Miettinen, A., Linder, E., Pikkarainen, P., Vuoristo, M. and Salaspuro, M. (1980) Different types of smooth muscle antibodies in chronic active hepatitis and primary biliary cirrhosis: their diagnostic and prognostic significance. Gut 21, 878–884.

Kurki, P., Miettinen, A., Salaspuro, M., Virtanen, I. and Stenman, S. (1983) Cytoskeleton antibodies in chronic active hepatitis, primary biliary cirrhosis and alcoholic liver disease. Hepatology 3, 297–302.

Kurki, P., Karjalainen, J., Hautanen, A. and Virtanen, I. (1989) Desmin antibodies in acute infectious myopericarditis. APMIS 97, 527–532.

Lazarides, E. (1980) Intermediate filaments as mechanical integrators of cellular space. Nature 283, 249–256.

Li, A.K.C., Trenchev, P.S., Holborow, E.J., Newsome, C. and Wynne, A.T. (1977) Experimental smooth muscle antibodies. Clin. Exp. Immunol. 27, 273–277.

Lidman, K., Biberfeld, G., Fagraeus, A., Norberg, R., Thorstenson, R., Utter, G. Carlsson, L., Luca and Lindberg, U. (1976) Anti-actin specificity of human smooth muscle antibodies in chronic active hepatitis. Clin. Exp. Immunol. 24, 266–272.

Lindberg, J., Lindholm, A., Lundin, P. and Iwarson, S. (1975) Trigger factors and HLA-A-antigens in chronic active hepatitis. Br. Med. J. 4, 77–79.

Lindberg, J., Lindholm, A. and Iwarson, S. (1978) Outcome of chronic active hepatitis: Influence of histocompatibility antigens and triggering factors. J. Infect. Dis. 137, 189–193.

Linder, E., Kurki, P. and Andersson, L.C. (1979) Autoantibody to "intermediate filaments" in infectious mononucleosis. Clin. Immunol. Immunopathol. 14, 411–417.

Mackay, I.R., Frazer, I.H., Toh, B.-H., Pedersen, J.S. and Alter, H.J. (1985) Absence of autoimmune serological reactions in chronic non A, non B viral hepatitis. Clin. Exp. Immunol. 61, 39–43.

Manns, M. (1989) Autoantibodies and antigens in liver disease – updated. J. Hepatol. 9, 272–280.

Mayet, W.J., Hess, G., Gerken, G. and Felde, K.-H. (1989) Treatment of chronic type B hepatitis with recombinant α-interferon induces autoantibodies not specific for autoimmune chronic hepatitis. Hepatology 1, 24–28.

Mayet, W.J., Press, A.G., Herrman, E., Moll, R., Manns, M., Ewe, K. and Meyer zum Büschenfelde, K.H. (1990) Antibodies to cytoskeletal proteins in patients with Crohn's disease. Eur. J. Clin. Invest. 20, 516–524.

McKeon, F.D., Kirschner, M.W. and Caput, D. (1986) Homologies in both primary and secondary structure between nuclear envelope and intermediate filament proteins. Nature 319, 463–468.

Mead, G.M., Cowin, P. and Whitehouse, J.M.A. (1980) Antitublin antibody in healthy adults and patients with infectious mononucleosis and its relationship to smooth muscle antibody (SMA). Clin. Exp. Immunol. 32, 328–336.

Mejean, C., Roustan, C., Benyamin, Y. (1987) Anti-actin antibodies. Detection and quantitation of total and skeletal muscle actin in human plasma using a competitive ELISA. J. Immunol. Meth. 99, 129–135.

Mortazavi-Milani, S.M., Badakere, S.S. and Holborow, E.J. (1984) Antibody to intermediate filaments of cytoskeleton in the sera of patients with acute malaria. Clin. Exp. Immunol. 55, 177–182.

Murray, P. (1986) Serum autoantibodies and uveitis. Br. J. Ophthalmol. 70, 266–268.

Norberg, R., Thorstensson, R., Utter, G. and Fagraeus, A. (1979) F-actin depolymerizing activity of human serum. Eur. J. Biochem. 100, 575–583.

Obrink, B. (1986) Epithelial cell adhesion molecules. Exp. Cell Res. 163, 1–21.

Odievre, A.M., Maggiore, G., Homberg, J.C. et al. (1983) Seroimmunologic classification of chronic hepatitis in 57 children. Hepatology 3, 407–409.

Pedersen, J.S., Toh, B.H., Locarnini, S.A., Gust, I.D., Shyamala, G.N. (1981) Autoantibody to intermediate filaments in viral hepatitis. Clin. Immunol. Immunopathol. 21, 154–161.

Pedersen, J.S., Toh, B.H., Mackay, I.R., Tait, B.D., Gust, I.D., Kastelan, A. and Hadzic, N. (1982) Segregation of autoantibody to cytoskeletal filaments, actin and intermediate filaments with two types of chronic active hepatitis. Clin. Exp. Immunol. 48, 527–532.

Porter, K.R. (1984) The cytomatrix: a short history of its study. J. Cell Biol. 99, 3s–12s.

Senécal, J.C., Oliver, J.M. and Rothfield N.F. (1985) Anticytoskeletal autoantibodies in the connective tissue diseases. Arthritis Rheum. 8, 889–898.

Sharpe, A.H., Chen, L.B. and Fields, B.N. (1982) The interaction of mammalian reoviruses with the cytoskeleton of monkey kidney CV-1 cells. Virology 120, 399–411.

Tan, E.M., Chan, E.K.L., Sullivan, K.F. and Rubin, R.L. (1988) Antinuclear antibodies (ANAs): diagnostically specific immune markers and clues toward understanding of systemic autoimmunity. Clin. Immunol. Immunopathol. 47, 121–141.

Thorstensson, R., Utter, G., Norberg, R. and Fagraeus, A. (1981) A radioimmunoassay for determination of anti-actin antibodies. J. Immunol. Methods 45, 15–26.

Toh, B.H. (1979) Smooth muscle autoantibodies and autoantigens. Clin. Exp. Immunol. 38, 621–628.

Underwood, J.R., Pedersen, J.S., Chalmers, P.J. and Toh, B.H. (1985) Hybrids from normal, germfree, ude and neonatal mice produce monoclonal antibodies to eight different intracellular structures. Clin. Exp. Immunol. 60, 417–426.

Whittingham, M.B., Mackay, I.R. and Irwin J. (1966) Autoimmune hepatitis. Immunofluorescence reactions with cytoplasm of smooth muscle and glomerular cells. Lancet 1, 1333–1335.

Williams, C.L. and Lennon, V.A. (1986) Thymic B-lymphocyte clones from patients with myasthenia gravis secrete monoclonal striational autoantibodies reacting with myosin, α-actinin, or actin. J. Exp. Med. 164, 1043–1059.

Zauli, D., Crespi, C., Bianchi, F.B. and Pisi, E. (1985) Immunofluorescent detection of anti-cytoskeleton antibodies using vinblastine-treated mononuclear cells. J. Immunol. Methods. 82, 77–82.

Section V

Immunological Aspects of Autoimmune Hepatitis

Autoimmune Hepatitis
Edited by M. Nishioka, G. Toda and M. Zeniya
© *1994, Elsevier Science B.V. All rights reserved*

Chapter 12

Immunological aspects of autoimmune hepatitis. General aspects, including clinical and overlapping syndromes

P.J. Johnson

Department of Clinical Oncology, Chinese University of Hong Kong, Shatin, NT (Hong Kong)

1. Introduction

In 1964, Sherlock noted that 'Chronic hepatitis is a very difficult condition to define. Different observers have quite differing viewpoints' (Sherlock, 1964). Internationally agreed criteria for the histological diagnosis were made over the next decade (Bianchi et al., 1977), but from the point of view of aetiological classification the situation remains difficult. The 1976 Fogarty meeting on classification of liver disease recognized only two subgroups of chronic active hepatitis (CAH) – hepatitis B surface antigen (HBsAg) seropositive and seronegative (Leevy et al., 1976). Since then distinct aetiologies for many of the HBsAg-negative cases have been recognized (Table 1), but when all of these have been excluded, a group remains which is classified as 'idiopathic' or 'cryptogenic' CAH. Within this group, those exhibiting high titres of organ-non-specific autoantibodies and high serum concentrations of γ-globulin are generally classified as suffering from 'autoimmune' chronic active hepatitis (AI-CAH).

Until recently, this definition has proved satisfactory and has formed the basis for most of the clinical and immunological studies into the disease. However, the two factors are now tending to blur what previously appeared to be clear-cut diagnostic boundaries. Firstly, the detection of antibodies to the hepatitis C virus (HCV) infection in a significant number of patients previously classified as suffering from AI-CAH. Secondly, there is an increasing realization that, whilst it is useful from a clinical point of view to exclude from the heading of AI-CAH any of the other causes of CAH, autoimmunity may well still be involved in their pathogenesis.

Table 1
Causes of, and diseases associated with, chronic active hepatitis
Reactions associated with therapeutic drugs closely resemble,
and are sometimes categorized with, the autoimmune type.

Hepatitis B virus and δ-infection
Non-A, non-B viral infections, including hepatitis C
Wilson's disease
Alcoholic liver disease
α_1-Antitrypsin deficiency
Drugs
   α-Methyldopa
   Oxyphenisatin
   Nitrofurantoin
   Isoniazid
   Tienylic acid
Autoimmune hepatitis
   Type 1
   Type 2
Cryptogenic hepatitis[a]

---

[a] The distinction between autoimmune and cryptogenic types is
not always made (see text).

The aim of this review is to summarize the role of immunological features used
in the classification of AI-CAH, the extent to which there is overlap with other
liver conditions, and the role of immunological mechanisms in pathogenesis.

2. Diagnosis and subclassification of autoimmune chronic active hepatitis

Hyperglobulinaemia, due mainly to elevated serum IgG concentrations, high
titres of organ-non-specific autoantibodies, together with female preponderance
and responsiveness to corticosteroid therapy, are the most constant yardstick for
diagnosing AI-CAH. In this chapter, the current practice of subclassifying
AI-CAH on the basis of autoantibody profile (Manns, 1989) is followed although
it should be recognized that response to immunosuppression is similar between
the groups and that there is little evidence that the subgroups so defined are
aetiologically distinct (Maddrey, 1987).

2.1. Type 1 or 'classical', autoimmune chronic active hepatitis

This form corresponds most closely with the early descriptions (Waldenstrom,
1950; Kunkel et al., 1954; Bearn et al., 1956) and with 'lupoid' hepatitis (Joske and

King, 1955; Mackay et al., 1956). Patients are required to have high titres of smooth muscle antibodies (SMA) and/or anti-nuclear antibodies (ANA) ($> 1:40$). It is now clear that only a minority of patients, perhaps 10–15%, have detectable lupus erythematosus (LE) cells and that such patients have no distinctive clinical or histological features (Soloway et al., 1972) and do not fall within the spectrum of systemic lupus erythematosus (SLE).

The patient is classically (although no longer typically) a young woman who presents with either an acute hepatitic or a chronic, rumbling, illness characterized by lethargy, arthralgia, oligomenorrhoea and fluctuating jaundice. Cushingoid appearance with striae, hirsutism and acne were also emphasized in early descriptions. Particularly in those with a more protracted onset of symptoms, cutaneous manifestations of chronic liver disease and signs of cirrhosis may be prominent. Other 'autoimmune' diseases such as hyperthyroidism and Coomb's-positive haemolytic anaemia may also be present. Laboratory investigations reveal hepatitic features with aspartate aminotransferase activity more than 10 times greater than the upper limit of the reference range and the γ-globulin concentration is grossly raised, often in the range 50–100 g/l. The latter is polyclonal in nature and largely accounted for by immunoglobulin G. Institution of corticosteroid therapy in moderate doses (less than 40 mg/day of prednisolone) leads to a rapid disappearance (within 3 months) of symptoms and normalization of liver biochemistry, but the disease usually relapses rapidly when treatment is withdrawn.

Increasingly, patients are being detected asymptomatically during routine laboratory screening (Hay et al., 1989) and in older age groups, to the extent that a second peak in the age distribution, above the age of 40 years, is becoming more prominent (Cattan et al., 1957). It was also a classical feature that, untreated, the disease was rapidly fatal (Mistilis et al., 1968), but this is not necessarily the case among patients seen today. Indeed, the necessity of treatment for those with milder disease, where bridging necrosis is not a feature, is being questioned (Cooksley et al., 1986) and the 'classical' form of the disease, as described above, appears to be getting less common, or at least to form a smaller proportion of the spectrum of AI-CAH.

2.1.1. Anti-nuclear antibodies

ANA are found in the sera of about 70% of cases at the time of presentation. Although useful diagnostic markers for AI-CAH, ANA are a very heterogeneous group of antibodies (Tan et al., 1988) that are also detectable in other liver disorders (Wood et al., 1986; Konikoff et al., 1989) and among apparently healthy subjects who, despite prolonged follow-up, do not appear to develop liver disease (Yadin et al., 1989). Most frequently, ANAs in AI-CAH patients give a 'homogeneous' pattern of immunofluorescent staining on tissue sections, similar to that seen with ANA in patients with SLE. However, in the latter group the reactivity is clearly directed against double-stranded DNA (dsDNA), whereas there is now general agreement that antibodies to dsDNA are very seldom detected in patients with AI-CAH when specific assays are used (Smeenk et al., 1982; Gurian et al., 1985; Legget et al., 1987). In SLE, the epitopes involved are the backbone phosphate groups or compound backbone bases (Mackworth-Young and Schwartz, 1988) whereas in AI-CAH they are less clearly defined but appear to include nuclear histones (Tan, 1989).

2.1.2. Smooth muscle antibodies

SMA were first described by Whittingham et al. (1966) and the target antigen(s) were subsequently identified as actin or other cytoskeletal proteins including vimentin and tubulin (Gabbiani et al., 1973; Toh, 1973). IgM class antibodies are well recognized in normal subjects, but high titres ($> 1:80$) of IgG class SMA with anti-actin specificity are much more specific for AI-CAH than ANA and clearly distinguish this condition from SLE in which they are not detected. However, similarly high titres of IgG class anti-actin antibodies have been reported in up to 20% of SMA-positive patients with primary biliary cirrhosis (PBC) (Kurki et al., 1980) and other liver diseases (Diederichsen and Riisom, 1980; Hamlyn and Berg, 1980). Furthermore, in only half the cases of AI-CAH are the antibodies directed at actin, either solely or also with other anti-cytoskeletal protein antibodies, and in the remaining half the target antigen of the SMA cannot be identified (Dighiero et al., 1990).

2.2. Type 2 autoimmune chronic active hepatitis

The presence of circulating anti-liver–kidney microsomal antibody (anti-LKM-1) has been used to define a separate subgroup of AI-CAH, 'type 2'. Similar antibodies only occur in a small minority of patients with non-hepatic auto-immune diseases (Smith et al., 1974; Homberg et al., 1987; Manns et al., 1989). Anti-LKM-1-positive cases appear to be less frequent than ANA/SMA-positive AI-CAH and have been described most often in continental Europe although even here the frequency is considerably less than that of PBC. The disease conforms in many respects to 'classical' AI-CAH, with a marked female predominance, bimodal age distribution, hypergammaglobulinaemia and steroid sensitivity. On the other hand, there are certain distinctive features including a tendency to present in the paediatric age group (Odievre et al., 1983) and the more common association with other 'autoimmune' disorders such as insulin-dependent diabetes, autoimmune thyroid disease and vitiligo (Table 2). The presentation is often acute, even fulminant, with severe histologic features and a marked propensity to progress rapidly to cirrhosis. These features are noteworthy in view of the recently reported association with antibodies to HCV (see below), particularly in the older age group (Lunel et al., 1991).

In the European cases of type 2 AI-CAH, it is characteristic that ANA and SMA are invariably absent, but some organ-specific antibodies, such as those

Table 2

Comparison of the clinical and immunological features of type 1 and type 2 autoimmune chronic active hepatitis

Adapted from Homberg et al. (1987). For comparison analogous data for Manns et al. (1987) is given, where available for the soluble liver antigen (SLA) group.

	Type 1 (Anti-actin)	Type 2 (Anti-LKM)	Anti-SLA
Age at presentation (years)	10–25 and 45–70	Less than 15	Mean 37
Associated disorders (%)	10	17	
Immunoglobulins (g/l)			
γ-globulins	37 ± 11	23 ± 8	Mean 32.2
			Range 1.8–5.2
IgG	37 ± 16	25 ± 10.4	
IgA	$3.7 \pm$	1.8 ± 0.9	
IgM	1.7 ± 1.1	2.4 ± 1.5	
Autoantibodies (%)			
Anti-SMA	100	0	34
ANA	33	2	0
AMA	8	0	22
Progression to cirrhosis after 3 years (%)	43	82	

reacting with gastric parietal cells, are frequently detected. This tends to also be true of adult patients in the U.K., but, in our experience, U.K. children with LKM-1 very often also have ANA and/or SMA.

2.2.1. *Liver–kidney microsomal autoantibodies*

This group of antibodies (anti-LKM), first described by Rizzetto and colleagues (1973), comprises a group of at least 3 distinct antibodies. Anti-LKM-1 reacts with cytochrome P-450-db1 (now termed P-450-IID6) (Manns et al., 1989), while anti-LKM-2 (associated with tienilic acid induced hepatitis) reacts with cytochrome P-450-8 (Beaune et al., 1987) and anti-LKM-3 (found in about 10% of chronic δ-virus infections) recognizes a third, as yet unidentified, microsomal antigen (Crivelli et al., 1983).

The factors influencing the titre of these organ-non-specific antibodies and the extent to which they reflect disease activity have received little attention, probably because of the difficulty in standardizing the assay and avoiding intra- and inter-assay variation. However, in the case of anti LKM-1 antibodies the titre was closely correlated with the serum γ-globulin concentration (Homberg et al., 1987). With the identification of target antigens for many of the autoantibodies, more specific assays will become available and will, no doubt, reveal a marked heterogeneity within autoantibody types as assessed by immunofluorescence.

2.3. *Anti-SLA antibody-positive autoimmune chronic active hepatitis*

Manns et al. (1987) described a new subgroup of AI-CAH characterized by the presence of antibodies, detectable only by radioimmunoassay, against a soluble liver antigen (SLA). The latter is a cytosolic liver protein that is also present in kidney and (at lower concentrations) in a wide range of other tissues, and SLA has since been identified as cytokeratins types 8 and 18 (Wachter et al., 1990). Anti-SLA was originally described in a small group of CAH patients who were seronegative for ANA and LKM antibodies. However, 30% of the group had SMA and 45% had liver membrane antibody (LMA), rheumatoid factor, anti-thyroid or anti-mitochondrial antibodies (AMA). The remaining 25% were seronegative for all of these autoantibodies, but were not tested for anti-LSP or anti-asialoglycoprotein receptor (anti-ASGP-R) (see below).

Although these findings have yet to be confirmed by other laboratories, some authorities have accepted anti-SLA positivity as defining a separate subgroup of AI-CAH. Nevertheless, there is no evidence that these patients differ in any significant respect from those with 'classical' AI-CAH. The female predominance, hypergammaglobulinaemia and steroid responsiveness were all similar to type 1 AI-CAH and indeed false-positive results with the Ortho anti-HCV test were seen as frequently as has been reported with type 1 disease (Manns, 1991). Furthermore, a later study showed that anti-SLA has no greater specificity for AI-CAH than any other autoantibody described, since it is found in other liver diseases as well as in normal subjects – albeit at lower titres (Wachter et al., 1990).

2.4. *Autoimmune chronic active hepatitis without ANA, SMA or anti-LKM*

Some patients with 'cryptogenic' CAH (i.e., no aetiologic factors and seronegative for ANA, SMA and LKM) are, in all respects (characteristic histology, high serum γ-globulin and IgG concentrations and, in particular, complete sensitivity to corticosteroids) other than their autoantibody status, similar to those classified as 'autoimmune' (Keating et al., 1987; Johnson et al., 1990). In these respects, the patients were indistinguishable from that small group of anti-SLA-positive patients who were seronegative for other autoantibodies described by Manns et al. (1987). Czaja et al. (1983) have also reported, in a review of the Mayo Clinic experience, that among patients with cryptogenic CAH, autoimmune features did not select a group which could be distinguished from those who did not. In particular, age, sex, frequency of progression to cirrhosis, response to treatment (Fig. 1) and prognosis were similar, irrespective of the presence or absence of immunological features.

Such patients may either never have had autoantibodies or lost them during a prolonged asymptomatic phase. In support of this latter contention, our cryptogenic patients were, on average, 10 years older and had a much higher frequency of cirrhosis at presentation, but still had anti-LSP and anti-ASGP-R

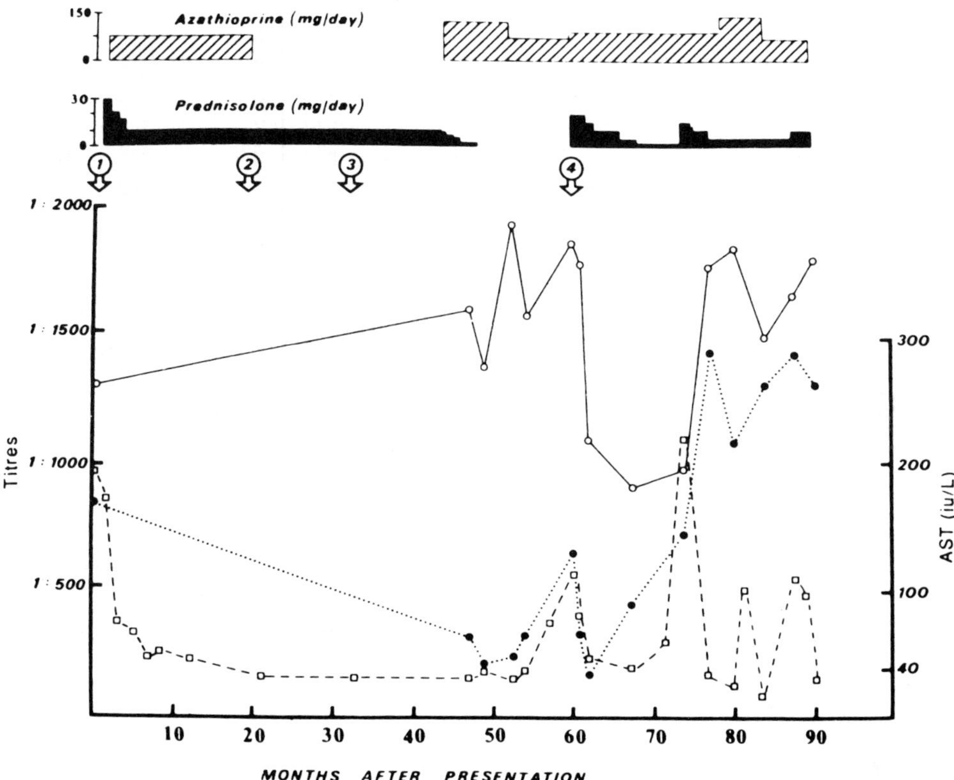

Fig. 1. Fluctuations in AST (□), and in anti-LSP (○) and anti-ASGP-R (●) titres, in relation to responses to alterations in immunosuppressive therapy in a patient with cryptogenic AI-CAH. This patient clearly illustrates the extreme sensitivity to immunosuppressive therapy which may be present even in the absence of any conventional, non-organ-specific antibodies. Numbered arrowheads indicate when liver biopsies were performed. Inflammatory activity in these biopsies, graded as defined in the text, was as follows: 1, severe; 2, mild; 3, inactive; and 4, moderate; and all 4 showed evidence of established cirrhosis. From Johnson et al. (1990).

antibodies at titres similar to those with classical AI-CAH (Johnson et al., 1990). The decision to classify such patients under the heading of autoimmune chronic active hepatitis is not entirely academic as there has been an increasing tendency to equate 'cryptogenic' CAH with chronic non-A, non-B (NANB) hepatitis. Nonetheless, it is clear that the composition of this cryptogenic group will vary from country to country and, whilst the conclusion drawn above may hold valid for the U.K. and the U.S.A., a significant number of cases from continental

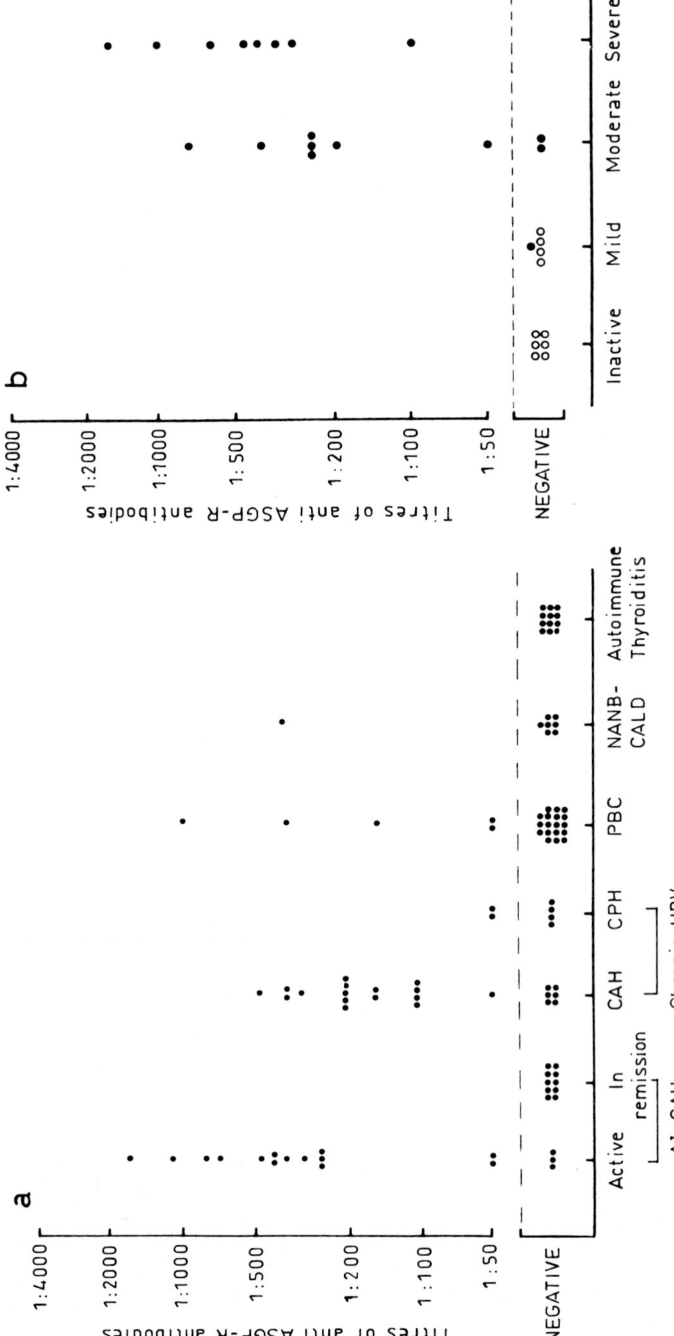

Fig. 2. a: Titres of anti-ASGP-R antibodies in sera from patients with AI-CAH and other conditions. b: relationship between titres of anti-ASGP-R and histologically assessed severity of portal tract inflammation and piecemeal necrosis in patients with AI-CAH with active disease (●) or in remission (○). From McFarlane, B.M. et al. (1986).

Europe will have genuine chronic HCV infection. Newly available assays for antibodies to HCV may help to clarify the situation (see below).

2.5. *Anti-LSP and anti-ASGP-R antibodies*

Anti-LSP represents a population of autoantibodies, some of which react with non-organ-specific liver cell determinants and others with liver-specific components (McFarlane, et al., 1984a; McFarlane and Williams, 1985). One of the latter is the galactose-specific hepatic ASGP-R (McFarlane et al., 1984b). Anti-LSP antibodies are found in a number of chronic liver disorders, primarily those with an underlying immunopathology and in which periportal inflammation is a feature, but is rare in chronic NANB. Titres of anti-LSP correlate with histologically assessed disease severity and fluctuate with response to immunosuppressive therapy (McFarlane et al., 1984a) (see Chapter 8). Anti-ASGP-R is more particularly associated with CAH (McFarlane B.M. et al., 1986; Treichel et al., 1990) and also correlates with one severity of periportal inflammation and piecemeal necrosis (Fig. 2a, b), occurring infrequently in other liver disorders and very rarely in acute or chronic NANB infections (McFarlane B.M. et al., 1986; Vento et al., 1988; Bedlow et al., 1989; Treichel et al., 1990). Neither antibody identifies a separate subgroup of AI-CAH. Indeed, virtually all AI-CAH patients including both type 1 and type 2 have high titres of both antibodies at presentation. The possible role of antibodies in the pathogenesis of AI-CAH is discussed below.

3. *Overlap with other conditions*

As Ludwig has pointed out, whilst it is true that all cases of AI-CAH have piecemeal necrosis and periportal inflammation, the reverse is not so (Ludwig, 1986). There are many other conditions which do not fall under the general heading of CAH in which the histological features of CAH may be seen. 'Overlap syndromes' are of 3 types.

(1) When a patient with another well-recognized cause of CAH has, in addition, all the features required to diagnose AI-CAH. For example, a patient with well-established Wilson's disease may have biopsy evidence of CAH, together with high titres of organ-non-specific autoantibodies and hypergammaglobulinaemia.

(2) When the histological features of CAH are present in a condition where they are not normally the prominent feature, for example in PBC or primary sclerosing cholangitis (PSC). Such cases are very poorly defined but unfortunately comprise a significant part of clinical practice.

(3) There may be temporal progression for classical AI-CAH to some other condition such as PBC or PSC.

3.1. Wilson's disease

Cirrhosis is a consistent feature of Wilson's disease, but a hepatic presentation occurs in only about 40% (Sternlieb and Scheinberg, 1987). Of these, a small number (less than 10%), present with a condition which bears histological and clinical similarities with CAH (Sternlieb and Scheinberg, 1972; Scott et al., 1978; Schilsky et al., 1991). Whether this represents a distinct pathological process or is part of a spectrum between the acute hepatitic picture which is sometimes seen in Wilson's disease and the characteristic inactive cirrhosis, is not clear; nor is it clear how this disease process relates to the well-recognized fulminant presentation. Although it has usually been stated that these patients do not have 'conventional' autoantibodies, we have detected both organ-non-specific, as well as anti-LSP and ASGP-R, in several cases.

Furthermore, it is now clear that the therapeutic effectiveness of penicillamine may be only partly related to its cupurietic effect – in 7 cases the liver copper concentration remained unchanged or continued to increase during treatment (Schilsky et al., 1991). It is also noteworthy that penicillamine is as effective as azathioprine or prednisolone in maintaining remission in autoimmune CAH (Stern et al., 1977) and there are anecdotal reports of CAH in Wilson's disease responding to corticosteroid therapy. The pathogenesis of CAH in Wilson's disease is, therefore, still obscure and detailed studies on the autoantibody and anti-HCV status at the time of presentation, and the tissue type of those presenting with CAH will be of considerable interest.

3.2. Alcoholic liver disease

Patients classified as suffering from alcoholic liver disease may have histological features of CAH (Crapper et al., 1983) and many of these will have detectable antibodies to LSP (Perperas et al., 1981). In some series, up to 70% of alcoholics with liver disease have titres of ANA of greater than 1:20 (Laskin et al., 1990) and in a population survey, 25% of patients with CAH were classified as being alcoholic (Hodges et al., 1982).

There are several interpretations of these observations. Firstly, it is conceivable that patients with AI-CAH who admit to taking some alcohol may be incorrectly classified as being alcoholic. Secondly, it is possible that alcohol may induce (trigger) the histological features of CAH and indeed there is considerable evidence for immunological mediation of alcoholic liver damage, not least of which is the increasingly strong evidence that immunosuppressive therapy may be effective in alcoholic hepatitis (Imperiale and McCullough, 1990; Hofer and McMahon, 1991). The extent to which immunosuppressive therapy might be effective when the histological picture is that of CAH, has received little attention. Finally, there is increasing evidence that, among the subgroup of alcoholic patients with CAH, HCV infection might be implicated (Brillanti et al., 1989).

3.3. Primary biliary cirrhosis

Overlap with PBC occurs in two ways. First, it is well accepted that about 20% of patients with classical type 1 AI-CAH have AMA. There is no doubt that in some earlier studies AMA were confused with anti-LKM antibodies, but even when these are recognized, a number remain positive and these appear to have characteristics of the M2 antigen. Secondly, at some stages in the development of PBC histological features of CAH can be seen, but taken with the other histological and clinical features the diagnosis is clear cut. There are, however, some true overlap cases in which the patient has florid clinical features of one condition with the histology of the other (Doniach and Walker, 1969; Kloppel et al., 1977; Okuno et al., 1987).

3.4. Primary sclerosing cholangitis

With the increasing use of endoscopic retrograde pancreatography (ERCP) this condition, characterized by chronic inflammation of the biliary tract, is being increasingly diagnosed (Chapman, 1991). The focus of the disease on the biliary tract, together with the strong association with ulcerative colitis and a marked male predominance, would seem to set it apart from AI-CAH. Furthermore, AMA and SMA are by most accounts unusual and only a small minority have antibodies to LSP or ASGP-R (Chapman et al., 1983; Lindor et al., 1986; Bedlow et al., 1987). Nonetheless, there is a high prevalence of HLA-B8 and -DR3 and it is well recognized that histological features akin to CAH may be seen at various stages in more than half the patients, and that hypergammaglobulinaemia is common (Chapman et al., 1983). These changes have been described in detail by Ludwig (1991).

The situation may, however, be much more complex than initially thought in view of recent studies in children. Mieli-Vergani et al. (1989) have recently reported a retrospective study of 13 children who fulfilled all the accepted criteria for the diagnosis of PSC, but who had presented with features of AI-CAH including high titres of autoantibodies and hypergammaglobulinaemia. When those with cholangiographic features of PSC were compared with those who appeared to have straight-forward AI-CAH, certain interesting immunological differences between the two groups became apparent. While in both groups K-cells appear to be implicated in mediation of cell damage, non-antigen-specific suppressor function was normal in patients with PSC, but significantly decreased in CAH (El-Shabrawi et al., 1987; Mieli-Vergani et al., 1989) (Fig. 3). These data add further support to the suggestion that abnormalities of immunomodulatory

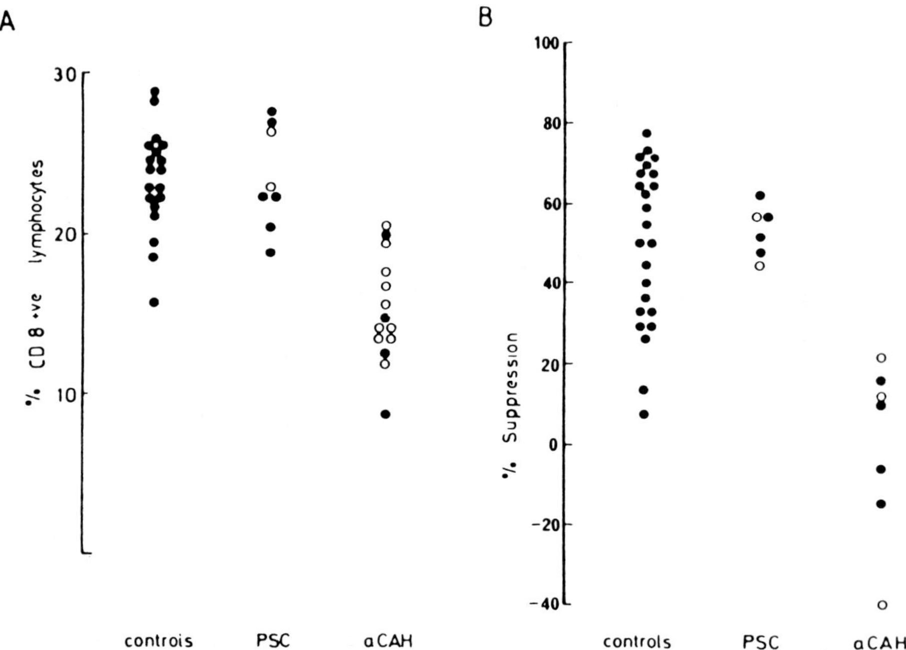

Fig. 3. Number and function of suppressor T-lymphocytes in normal controls, children with primary sclerosing cholangitis (PSC) and children with AI-CAH. A: percentage of circulating T-lymphocytes expressing suppressor/cytotoxic phenotype (CD8-positive cells). B: concanavalin A-induced suppression of immunoglobulin production by pokeweed mitogen-stimulated lymphocytes as measured by the haemolytic plaque assay. ●, untreated; ○, treated. From Mieli-Vergani et al. (1989).

cells, as originally hypothesized by Eddleston and Williams (1974), are of central importance in the pathogenesis of AI-CAH.

3.5. Chronic HCV infection

Chronic hepatitis NANB virus infection, particularly that following transfusion ('HCV'), is a recognized cause of chronic active hepatitis with both periportal inflammation and piecemeal necrosis (Koretz et al., 1976, 1985). Whilst the specific diagnosis cannot be established on histological grounds, certain additional features, including a prominent lobular component to the inflammation and cholangiolytic features are more frequently seen than in AI-CAH.

Before the development of serological tests for the HCV there was little to implicate this or any other NANB virus in liver autoreactivity. Mackay et al. (1985) used a panel of sera from patients with chronic hepatitis in 9 of whom the presence of a transmissible agent was confirmed by chimpanzee inoculation.

They tested for ANA, SMA, AMA, LMAg, and antibodies to actin and intermediate filaments and found only very low titres and at no higher frequency than that expected in the normal population. Among a group of 8 patients developing chronic liver disease after an outbreak of NANB hepatitis in a haemodialysis unit, none had autoantibody titres of greater than 1:10 (Galbraith et al., 1975). Similar findings were reported by Manns et al. (1989) and likewise others (Vento et al., 1988; McFarlane B.M. et al., 1986) could not detect antibodies to LSP or ASGP-R in any of 10 subjects with chronic NANB hepatitis. The findings were so clear cut that absence of autoantibodies in a patient with cryptogenic CAH was taken as an indication that a condition was most likely attributable to a NANB infection.

However, with the advent of serological tests for antibodies to the hepatitis C virus, large numbers of patients with various liver diseases were screened for infection with this virus and it was reported from Spain and Italy that up to 40% of AI-CAH patients were seropositive (Esteban et al., 1989; Lenzi et al., 1990). This appeared to be so, particularly among those with type 2 disease (Lenzi et al., 1990). The significance of these findings was questioned when there were several reports that the original (Ortho) assay used in these reports gave false-positive results in patients with high serum immunoglobulin levels (McFarlane et al., 1990) (Fig 4a).

Application of more specific tests supported this contention, particularly one based on the use of synthetic peptides from other HCV antigenic regions, which revealed that only 8% of U.K. patients were positive (and then only very weakly so) (Lenzi et al., 1991) (Fig. 4b). Subsequent testing by use of the polymerase chain reaction (PCR) has confirmed that these sera are invariably negative for HCV-RNA (Silva et al., 1993). Nonetheless, when the same test was applied to patients from Italy, a high percentage remained strongly positive, particularly those with type II disease (Lenzi et al., 1991) and these findings have been confirmed by other second-generation anti-HCV tests (Magrin et al., 1991; Todros et al., 1991) and, in some cases, by use of the PCR for HCV-RNA (Garson et al., 1991). (It is interesting to note that when anti-LKM was first described in association with the δ-virus, Rizzetto's group, speculated '…whether LKM (i.e. LKM-1) may also represent an epiphenomenon of infection with an unknown virus rather than reflect an autoimmune diathesis').

Very recently, the development of autoantibodies in patients with NANB hepatitis treated with interferon has been reported, suggesting that these were cases of autoantibody-negative AI-CAH whose disease was unmasked by this immunomodulatory therapy (Vento et al., 1990). Conversely, there has been a report of an autoantibody (anti-GOR) directed against a host peptide, which is detectable specifically in the patients with HCV infection (Mishiro et al., 1990).

The situation is clearly complicated, but at the time of writing it seems fair to conclude the following.

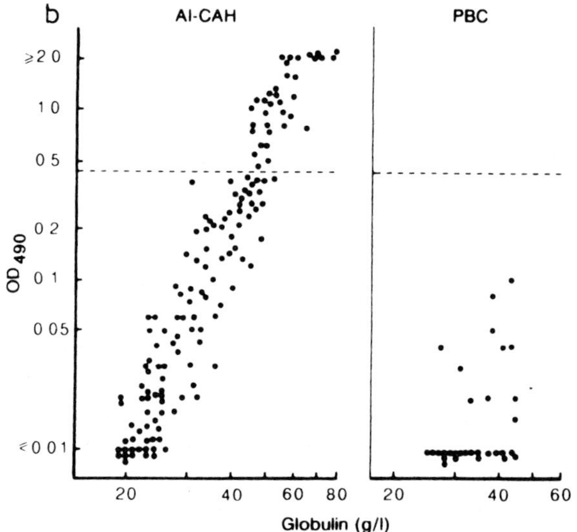

Fig. 4. a: frequency of antibodies to HCV using the original Ortho anti-HCV ELISA and a new assay based on synthetic HCV-peptides in U.K. and Italian patients with type 1 or type 2 AI-CAH. From Lenzi et al. (1991). b: correlation between serum globulin concentration and the optical density result in the original Ortho anti-HCV assay. From McFarlane, I.G. et al. (1990).

(1) Among Northern European caucasians with AI-CAH there is currently no evidence of infection with the HCV, or that HCV is in any way implicated in the pathogenesis of AI-CAH.

(2) Among patients from continental Europe, about 50% of those who are currently classified as suffering from type 1 and 80% of those with type 2 AI-CAH have evidence of active HCV infection. In the latter group, it is the older patients, (not the paediatric group) who are associated with HCV infection (Lunel et al., 1991).

How should we interpret the role of HCV when it is detected in patients who meet the criteria for a diagnosis of AI-CAH? The hypotheses that have been put forward include the following.

(a) HCV may, in susceptible individuals, trigger AI-CAH.
(b) HCV is the major aetiologic factor in CAH and the co-existing autoantibodies are but minor epiphenomena.
(c) HCV is superimposed on previously existing AI-CAH.

This latter suggestion would fit with the observation that HCV is detected mainly in areas of the world where sporadic HCV infection is common and that it can be detected in other non-liver conditions with immunological abnormalities such as essential mixed cryoglobulinaemia (Dammacco and Sansano, 1993). Whatever the correct interpretation, it must explain the basic enigma among the Italian patients as to why those patients primarily classified as suffering from chronic HCV infection do not have autoantibodies (see above), whereas those diagnosed as AI-CAH (on the basis of the *presence* of autoantibodies) are frequently anti-HCV-positive. These questions, which have major therapeutic implications pose one of the major problems for hepatology over the next decade.

4. Pathogenesis of liver damage

Major steps in understanding the pathogenesis of this condition have been made over the last 20 years. The most reasonable hypothesis is that AI-CAH arises in a genetically susceptible host who, by chance, comes in contact with the appropriate trigger. We therefore need to consider 4 closely interrelated areas of work: the genetic predisposition; the trigger; the effector mechanism; and the factors localizing the disease to the liver and more specifically to the periportal hepatocytes. Each of these aspects is considered in detail elsewhere in this book; the account given below is intended as a broad overview.

4.1. Immunogenetics

In common with a number of other autoimmune conditions, AI-CAH is strongly associated with the HLA-A1-B8-DR3 haplotype, at least among U.K., Australian and North American patients (Mackay and Morris, 1977; Opelz et al., 1977; Donaldson et al., 1991) and recent evidence suggests a secondary association with DR4 and a protective role for DR1. Since DR3/DR4 heterozygotes are relatively rare in this condition it would appear that the A1-B8-DR3 haplotype and DR4 are acting independently of each other and may identify two distinct subgroups of the disease. In support of this contention, those with DR4 presented at an older age than those without and relapsed on treatment less frequently. It should be stressed, however, that even amongst a rigorously selected caucasoid group, only about one-third of subjects have the HLA-A1-B8-DR3 haplotype (Donaldson et al., 1991).

4.2. The trigger

Although hepatotropic viruses have always been assumed to be the most likely triggers, it must be acknowledged from the outset that no trigger can be detected in most cases (McFarlane, 1991). It is perhaps unlikely that an initiating virus will be traceable, since triggering probably precedes clinical presentation by several months or years. For the same reason, it is also difficult to distinguish an initiating event, in a naive host, from a superimposed viral infection in patients with subclinical AI-CAH. Such problems arise in the case of AI-CAH apparently preceded by HBV infection (Laskus and Slusarczyk, 1989), but a recent study with hepatitis A is much more convincing.

Vento et al. (1991) have described a prospective study of first- and second-degree relatives of patients with AI-CAH. Three of these acquired well-documented acute hepatitis A virus (HAV) infection with development of anti-ASGP-R antibodies and T-cell sensitization to the ASGP-R. Subsequent investigation showed that two of these subjects who had inherited the antigen-specific (ASGP-R) suppressor T-cell defect (see below) both went on to develop classical type 1 AI-CAH. In contrast, the relative who did not inherit the defect made an uneventful recovery. It is worthy of note that both of those who developed AI-CAH lost antibodies to the HAV.

The rapidly expanding body of evidence implicating HCV infection has already been referred to in some detail. Some authors have taken this as evidence that HCV is a trigger for AI-CAH in many instances, particularly in Southern Europe, but this seems premature in view of the other possible interpretations of the data noted above.

4.2.1. Drugs as triggers

A syndrome identical to AI-CAH, including the presence of high titres of autoantibodies such as SMA and ANA (Homberg et al., 1987) has been recognized to follow ingestion of certain therapeutic drugs, notably oxyphenistan (Reynolds et al., 1971) and methyldopa (Tysell and Knauer, 1971). However, in most cases the disease resolves when the offending medication is withdrawn, but in others there is continuing activity (Schweitzer and Peters, 1974) suggesting that the drug has indeed acted as a trigger. The induction of a specific anti-LKM (anti-LKM-3) antibody by tienylic acid (ticrynafen) which causes chronic hepatitis in up to 10% of cases has already been mentioned. The value of immunosuppression in these cases is not well established.

4.3. Mechanism of hepatocyte damage

There is now compelling evidence that the, or at least a, specific target antigen for both humoral and cellular immune reactions is the ASGP-R (McFarlane et al., 1986, Lohr et al., 1990) which, in contrast to targets of the other autoantibodies so far described, is expressed on the hepatocyte membrane. As described above, more than 90% of patients with active disease will have high titres of circulating autoantibodies reacting with species cross-reactive determinants in ASGP-R.

Furthermore, most will also have T-cells sensitized to ASGP-R (as also happens in myasthenia gravis with respect to the acetyl-choline receptor (Newsom-Davis et al., 1989) which may assist B-cells in production of antibodies to this antigen. This has been suggested both by the use of an indirect agarose microdroplet assay for T-lymphocyte migratory inhibitory factor (T-LIF) production (Vento et al., 1986) and by the production of T-cell clones from AI-CAH patients which directed antigen-specific antibody production by autologous B-lymphocytes when exposed to LMA (Wen et al., 1990). Both these lines of investigation suggested that these circulating antigen-specific T-cells are predominantly of the CD4 (helper/inducer) subset, as are the T-cells isolated from the liver of AI-CAH patients. The most likely mechanism of tissue damage, based on the results of autologous cytotoxicity assays (Mieli-Vergani et al., 1979), is antibody-dependent cellular cytotoxicity in which ASGP-R antibodies and non-T-cells (K-cells) cooperate.

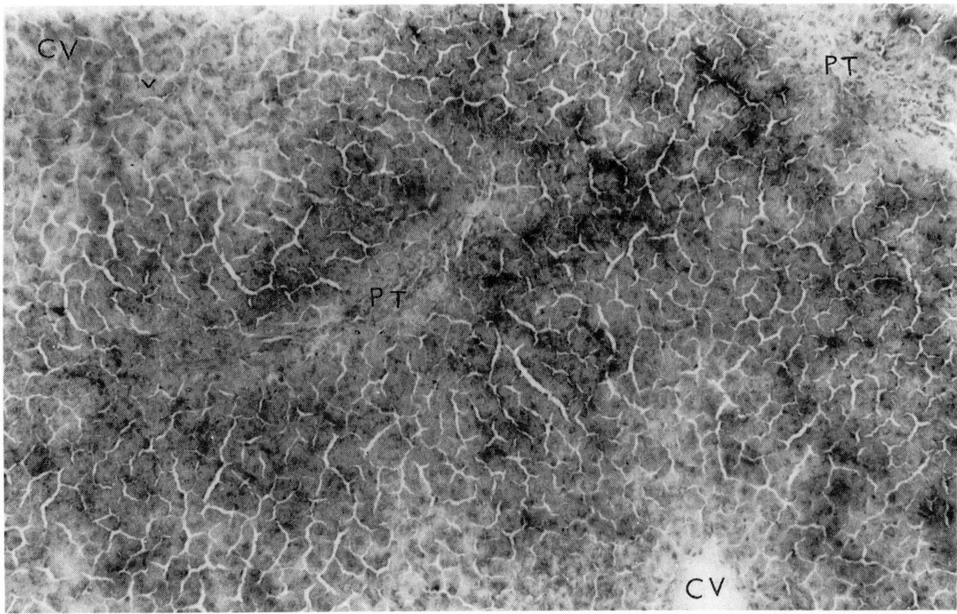

Fig. 5. Immunohistochemical localization of anti-ASGP-R antibodies in rat liver following in situ perfusion with guinea pig anti-ASGP-R in a retrograde direction. PT, portal tracts; CV central veins. From McFarlane, B.M. et al. (1990).

In common with other autoimmune diseases, there appears to be a non-antigen-specific suppressor cell defect, linked to the HLA-A1-B8-DR3 haplotype. It is this lesion which can be overcome by immunosuppressive therapy (Nouri-Aria et al., 1982; 1985) and also presumably explains the observation that subjects with this haplotype appear to have enhanced antibody responses to several common antigens (Galbraith et al., 1976). In addition, patients with AI-CAH may also have an antigen (ASGP-R) specific defect for control of autoimmune responsiveness, which is non-MHC-linked and not corrected by corticosteroid treatment (O'Brien et al., 1986). The possible pathogenetic relevance of this defect is clear from the report of HAV-triggered AI-CAH described above.

4.4. Organ and hepatocyte specificity

Any hypothesis relating to the pathogenesis of liver damage in AI-CAH must explain why the injury is confined to the liver and, in particular, to the periportal hepatocytes. The ASGP-R is specific to hepatocytes and preferentially expressed on the surfaces of periportal liver cells (Fig. 5) (Daniels et al., 1987; McFarlane B.M. et al., 1990) and as such provides an explanation for the focus of the disease.

5. Concluding remarks

Autoimmune chronic active hepatitis emerged from obscurity in the 1950s to reach maturity in the early 1970s when controlled trials confirmed the therapeutic efficacy of immunosuppression. Since then the diagnostic boundaries have become increasingly blurred, and the possible role of aberrant autoreactivity in several other areas of liver disease is an area of increasing research. Nonetheless, there does appear to be a group of patients with a true, primary autoimmune liver disease. Recognition of this group and dissection of the underlying immunological defects may permit the development of more specific therapy.

References

Bearn, A.G., Kunkel, H.G. and Slater, R.G. (1956) The problem of chronic liver disease in young women. Am. J. Med. 21, 3–15.

Beaune, P., Dansette P.M., Mansuy, D., Kiffel, L., Finck, M., Amar, C., Leroux, J.P. and Homberg, J.C. (1987) Human anti-endoplasmic reticulum autoantibodies appearing in a drug-induced hepatitis are directed against human liver cytochrome P-450 that hydroxylates the drug. Proc. Natl. Acad. Sci. U.S.A. 84, 551–555.

Bedlow, A.J., Donaldson, P.T., McFarlane, B.M., Lombard, M., McFarlane, I.G. and Williams, R. (1989) Autoreactivity to hepatocellular antigens in primary biliary cirrhosis and primary sclerosing cholangitis. J. Clin. Lab. Immunol. 30, 103–109.

Bianchi, L., De Groote, J., Desmet, V.J., Gedigk, P., Kork, G., Popper, H., Poulsen, H., Scheuer, P.J., Schmid, M., Thaler, H. and Wepler, W. (1977) Acute and chronic hepatitis revisited. Lancet 2, 914–919.

Brillanti, S., Barbara, L., Miglioli, M. and Bonino, F. (1989) Hepatitis C virus: a possible cause of chronic hepatitis in alcoholics. Lancet 2, 1390–1391.

Cattan, R., Vesin, P. and Bodin, H., (1957) Cirrhoses dysproteinemiques d'origine inconnue chez la femme. Bull. Soc. Med. Hop. Paris 73, 608–616.

Chapman, R.W. (1991) Aetiology and natural history of primary sclerosing cholangitis – a decade of progress? Gut 32, 1433–1435.

Chapman, R.W., Marburg, B.A., Rhodes, R.M., Summerfield, J.A., Dick, R., Scheuer, P.J. and Sherlock, S. (1983) Primary sclerosing cholangitis: a review of the clinical features, cholangiography, and hepatic histology. Gut 21, 870–877.

Cooksley, W.G.E., Bradbear, R.A., Robinson, W., Harrison, M., Halliday, J.W., Powell, L.W., Ng, H.-S., Seah, C.-S., Okuda, K., Scheuer, P.J. and Sherlock, S. (1986) The prognosis of chronic active hepatitis without cirrhosis in relation to bridging necrosis. Hepatology 6, 345–348.

Crapper, R.M., Bhathal, P.S. and Mackay, I.R. (1983) Chronic active hepatitis in alcoholic patients. Liver 3, 327–337.

Crivelli, O., Lavarini, C., Chiaberge, E., Amoroso, A., Farci, P., Negro, F. and Rizzetto M. (1983) Microsomal autoantibodies in chronic infection with the HBsAg associated delta (δ) agent. Clin. Exp. Immunol. 54, 232–238.

Czaja, A.J., Davis, G.L., Ludwig, J., Baggenstoss, A.H. and Taswell, H.F. (1983) Autoimmune features as determinants of prognosis in steroid-treated chronic active hepatitis of uncertain etiology. Gastroenterology 85, 713–717.

Dammacco, F. and Sansono, D. (1993) Antibodies to hepatitis C virus in essential mixed cryoglobulinaemia. Clin. Exp. Immunol., in press.

Daniels, C.K., Smith K.M. and Schmucker, D.L. (1987) Asialoorosomucoid hepato-biliary transport is unaltered by the loss of liver asialoglycoprotein receptors in aged rats. Proc. Soc. Exp. Biol. Med. 186, 246–250.

Diederichsen, H. and Riisom, K. (1980) Anti-actin antibodies revealed by counter-immunoelectrophoresis. J. Clin. Pathol. 33, 876–879.

Dighiero, G., Lymberi, P., Monot, C. and Abuaf, N. (1990) Sera with high levels of anti-smooth muscle and anti-mitochondrial antibodies frequently bind to cytoskeletal proteins. Clin. Exp. Immunol. 82, 52–56.

Donaldson, P.T., Doherty, D.G., Hayllar, K.M., McFarlane, I.G., Johnson, P.J. and Williams, R. (1991) Susceptibility to autoimmune chronic active hepatitis: HLA DR4 and A1-B8-DR-3 are independent risk factors. Hepatology 13, 701–706.

Doniach, D. and Walker, J.G. (1969) A unified concept of autoimmune chronic active hepatitis. Lancet i, 813–815.

Eddleston, A.L.W.F. and Williams, R. (1974) Inadequate antibody response to HBsAg or suppressor T cell defect in development of active chronic hepatitis. Lancet 2, 1543–1545.

El-Shabrawi, M., Wilkinson, M., Portmann, B., Mieli-Vergani, G., Chong, S.K.F., Williams, R. and Mowat, A.P. (1987) Primary sclerosing cholangitis in childhood, Gastroenterlogy 92, 1226–1235.

Esteban, J.I., Esteban, R., Viladomiu, L., Lopez-Talavera, J.C., Gonzalez, A., Hernandez, J.M., Roet, M., Vargas, V., Genesca, J., Buti, M., Guardia, J., Houghton, M., Choo, Q.L. and Kuo, G. (1989) Hepatitis C virus antibodies among risk groups in Spain. Lancet ii, 294–297.

Gabbiani, G., Ryan, G.B. and Lelein, J.P. (1973) Human smooth muscle autoantibody. Its identification as anti-actin antibody and a study of its binding to 'non-muscular' cells. Am. J. Pathol. 72, 473–488,

Galbraith, R.M., Eddleston, A.L.W.F., Portmann, B. and Williams, R. (1975) Chronic liver disease developing after outbreak of HBsAg negative hepatitis in haemodialysis unit. Lancet ii, 886–890.

Galbraith, R.M., Eddleston, A.L.W.F. and Williams, R. (1976) Enhanced antibody responses in active chronic hepatitis: relation to HLA-B8 and HLA-B12 and portosystemic shunting. Lancet, 1, 930–934.

Garson, J.A., Lenzi, M., Ring, C., Cassani, F., Ballardini, G., Briggs, M., Tedder, R. and Bianchi, F.B. (1991) Hepatitis C viraemia in adults with Type 2 autoimmune hepatitis. J. Med. Virol. 34, 223–226.

Gurian, L.E., Rogoff, T.M., Ware, A.J., Jordan, R.E., Combes, B. and Gilliam, J.N. (1985) The immunologic diagnosis of chronic active 'autoimmune' hepatitis: distinction from systemic lupus erythematosus. Hepatology 5, 397–402.

Hamlyn, A.N. and Berg, P.A. (1980) Haemagglutinating anti-actin antibodies in acute and chronic liver disease. Gut 21, 311–317.

Hay, J.E, Czaja, A.J., Rakela, J. and Ludwig, J. (1989) The nature of unexplained chronic aminotransferase elevations of a mild to moderate degree in asymptomatic patients. Hepatology 2, 193–197.

Hodges, J.R., Millward-Sadler, G.H. and Wright, R. (1982) Chronic active hepatitis: the spectrum of disease. Lancet i, 550–552.

Hofer, T. and McMahon, L. (1991) Corticosteroids and alcoholic hepatitis. Hepatology 13, 199–201.

Homberg, J.-C., Abuaf, N., Bernard, O., Islam, S., Alvarez, F., Khalil, S.H., Poupon, R., Darnis, F., Levy, V.-G., Grippon, P., Opolon, P., Bernuau, J., Benhamou, J.-P. and Alagille, D. et al. (1987) Chronic active hepatitis associated with antiliver/kidney microsome antibody Type 1: a second type of 'autoimmune' hepatitis. Hepatology 7, 1333–1339.

Imperiale, T.F. and McCullough, A.J. (1990) Do corticosteroids reduce mortality from alcoholic hepatitis? Ann. Int. Med. 11, 299–307.

Johnson, P.J., McFarlane, I.G., McFarlane, B.M. and Williams, R. (1990) Autoimmune features in patients with idiopathic chronic active hepatitis who are seronegative for conventional autoantibodies. J. Gastroenterol. Hepatol. 5, 244–251.

Joske, R.A. and King, W.E. (1955) The L.E.-cell phenomenon in active chronic viral hepatitis. Lancet ii, 477–480.

Keating, J.J., O'Brien, C.J., Stellon, A.J., Portmann, B.C., Johnson, R.D., Johnson, P.J. and Williams, R. (1987) Influence of aetiology, clinical and histological features on survival in chronic active hepatitis: an analysis of 204 patients. Q. J. Med. 62, 59–66.

Kloppel, G., Siefert, G. and Lindner, H. (1977) Histopathological features in mixed types of chronic aggressive hepatitis and primary biliary cirrhosis. Virchows Arch. Pathol. Anat. Pathol. 81, 143–160.

Konikoff, F., Isenberg, D.A. and Barrison, I. (1989) Antinuclear autoantibodies in chronic liver diseases. Hepatogastroenterlogy 36, 341–345.

Koretz, R.L., Suffin, S.C. and Gitnick, G.L. (1976) Post-transfusion chronic liver disease. Gastroenterology 71, 797–803.

Koretz, R.L., Stone, O., Moussa, M. and Gitnick, G.L. (1985) Non-A, non-B post-transfusion hepatitis – a decade later. Gastroenterology, 88, 1251–1254.

Kunkel, H.G., Ahrens, E.H. Jr, Eisenmenger, W.J., Bongiovanni, A.M. and Slater R.J. (1954) Extreme hypergammaglobulinemia in young women with liver disease of unknown etiology (abstract). J. Clin. Invest. 30, 654.

Kurki, P., Miettinen, A., Linder, E., Pikkarainen, P., Vuoristo, M. and Salaspuro, M.P. (1980) Different types of smooth muscle antibodies in chronic active hepatitis and primary biliary cirrhosis: their diagnostic and prognostic significance. Gut 21, 878–884.

Laskin, C.A., Vidins, E., Blendis, L.M. and Soloninka, C.A. (1990) Autoantibodies in alcoholic liver disease. Am. J. Med. 89, 129–133.

Laskus, T. and Slusarczyk, J. (1989) Autoimmune chronic active hepatitis developing after acute type B hepatitis. Dig. Dis. Sci. 34, 1294–1297.

Leevy, C.M., Popper, H. and Sherlock, S. (1976) Diseases of the Liver and Biliary Tract. Standardisation of Nomenclature, Diagnostic Criteria and Diagnostic Methodology. Fogarty International Centre Proceedings No. 22, U.S. Government Printing Office, Washington, DC.

Leggett, B.A., Collins, R.V., Cooksley, W.G.E., Prentice, D.I. and Powell, I.W. (1987) Evaluation of the Crithidia assay to distinguish between chronic active hepatitis and systemic lupus erythematosus. J. Gastroenterol. Hepatol. 21, 202–211.

Lenzi, M., Ballardini, G., Fusconi, M., Cassani, F., Seleri, L., Volta, U., Zauli, D. and Bianchi, F.B. (1990) Type 2 autoimmune hepatitis and hepatitis C virus infection. Lancet 335, 258–259.

Lenzi, M., Johnson, P.J., McFarlane, I.G., Ballardini, G., Smith, H.M., McFarlane, B.M., Bridger, C., Vergani, D., Bianchi, F.B. and Williams, R. (1991) Antibodies to hepatitis C virus and autoimmune liver disease: evidence for geographical heterogeneity. Lancet 338, 277–280.

Lindor, K.D., Wiesner, R.H., La Russo, N.F. and Dickson, E.R. (1986) Chronic active hepatitis: overlap with primary biliary cirrhosis and primary sclerosing cholangitis. In: A.J. Czaja and E.R. Dickson (Eds.) Chronic Active Hepatitis – The Mayo Clinic Experience, Marcel Dekker, New York, pp. 171–187.

Lohr, H., Treichel, U., Poralla, T., Manns, M., Meyer zum Büschenfelde, K.H. and Fleischer, B. (1990) The human asialoglycoprotein receptor is a target antigen for liver-infiltrating T cells in autoimmune chronic active hepatitis and primary biliary cirrhosis. Hepatology 12, 1314–1320.

Ludwig, J. (1986) Morphology of Chronic Active Hepatitis: Differential Diagnosis and Therapeutic Implication. In: A.J. Czaja and E.R. Dickson (Eds.) Chronic Active Hepatitis – The Mayo Clinic Experience, Marcel Dekker, New York, pp. 93–104.

Ludwig, J. (1991) Small-duct primary sclerosing cholangitis. Semin. Hepatol. 11, 11–17.

Lunel, E., Homberg, J.C., Grippon, P., Perrin, M., Blanc, C., Bernard, B., Cadranel, J.F., Abauf, N., Valla, D., Opolon, P. and Huraux, J.M. (1991) Type 2 autoimmune hepatitis and hepatitis C virus: a study of 83 patients. J. Hepatol. 13 (Suppl. 2), s47.

Mackay, I.R. and Morris, P. (1977) Association of autoimmune chronic hepatitis with HL-A1, 8. Lancet 2, 793–795.

Mackay, I.R., Taft, L.I. and Cowling, D.C. (1956) Lupoid hepatitis. Lancet 2, 1323–1326.

Mackay, I.R., Frazer, I.H., Toh, B.-H., Pederson, J.S. and Alter, H.J. (1985) Absence of autoimmune serological reactions in chronic non A, non B viral hepatitis. Clin. Exp. Immunol. 61, 39–43.

Mackworth-Young, C. and Schwartz, R.S. (1988) Autoantibodies to DNA. CRC Crit. Rev. Immunol. 8, 147–173.

Maddrey, W.C. (1987) Subdivisions of idiopathic autoimmune chronic active hepatitis. Hepatology 7, 1372–1376.

Magrin, S., Craxi, A., Fiorentino, G., Fabiano, C., Provenzano, G., Pinzello, G.B., Palazzo, U., Almasio, P. and Pagliaro, L. (1991) Is autoimmune chronic active hepatitis a HCV-related disease? J. Hepatol 13, 56–60.

Manns, M. (1989) Autoantibodies and antigens in liver diseases – updated. J. Hepatol. 9, 272–280.

Manns, M.P. (1991) Cytoplasmic autoantigens in autoimmune hepatitis: molecular analysis and clinical relevance. Semin. Liver Dis. 11, 205–214.

Manns, M., Gerken, G., Kyriatsoulis A., Staritz, M., Meyer Zum Büschenfelde, K.-H. (1987) Characterization of a new subgroup of autoimmune chronic active hepatitis by autoantibodies against a soluble liver antigen. Lancet i, 292–294.

Manns, M., Johnson, E.F., Griffen, K.J., Tan, E.M. and Sullivan, K.F. (1989) The major antigen target of liver kidney microsomal autoantibody in idiopathic autoimmune hepatitis is cytochrome P450db1. J. Clin. Invest. 83, 1066–1072.

McFarlane, B.M., McSorley, C.G., Vergani, D., McFarlane, E.G. and Williams, R. (1986) Serum autoantibodies reacting with the hepatic asialoglycoprotein receptor (hepatic lectin) in acute and chronic liver disorders. J. Hepatol. 3, 196–205.

McFarlane, B.M., Sipos, J., Gove, C.D., McFarlane, I.G. and Williams, R. (1990) Antibodies against the hepatic asialoglycoprotein receptor perfused in situ preferentially attached to periportal liver cells in the rat. Hepatology 11, 408–415.

McFarlane, I.G. (1984) Editorial review: Autoimmunity in liver disease. Clin., Sci. 67, 569–578.

McFarlane, I.G. (1991) Autoimmunity and hepatotropic viruses. Semin. Liver Dis. 11, 223–233.

McFarlane, I.G. and Williams, R. (1985) Review: Liver membrane antibodies. J. Hepatol. 1, 313–319.

McFarlane, I.G., Hegarty, J.E., McSorley, C.G., McFarlane, B.M. and Williams, R. (1984a) Antibodies to liver specific protein predict outcome of treatment withdrawal in autoimmune chronic active hepatitis. Lancet ii, 954–956.

McFarlane, I.G., McFarlane B.M., Major, G., Tolley, P. and Williams, R. (1984b) Identification of the hepatic asialoglycoprotein receptor (hepatic lectin) as a component of liver specific membrane lipoprotein (LSP). Clin. Exp. Immunol. 55, 347–354.

McFarlane, I.G., Smith, H.M., Johnson, P.J., Bray, G.P., Vergani, D. and Williams, R. (1990) Hepatitis C virus antibodies in chronic active hepatitis: pathogenetic factor of false-positive result? Lancet 335, 754–757.

Mieli-Vergani, G., Vergani, D., Jenkins, P.J. and Williams, R. (1979) Lymphocyte cytotoxicity to autologous hepatocytes in HBsAg-negative chronic active hepatitis. Clin. Exp. Immunol. 38, 16–21.

Mieli-Vergani, G., Lobo-Yeo, A., McFarlane, B.M., McFarlane, I.G., Mowat, A.P. and Vergani, D. (1989) Different immune mechanisms leading to autoimmunity in primary sclerosing cholangitis and autoimmune chronic active hepatitis of childhood. Hepatology 9, 198–203.

Mishiro, S., Hoshi, Y. and Takeda, K. (1990) Non-A, non-B hepatitis specific antibodies directed at host-derived epitope: implications for an autoimmune process. Lancet 336, 1400–1403.

Mistilis, S.P., Skyring, A.P. and Blackburn, R.B. (1968) Natural history of active chronic hepatitis. 1. Clinical features, course, diagnostic criteria, morbidity, mortality and survival. Aust. Ann. Med. 17, 214–223.

Newsom-Davis, J., Harcourt, G. and Sommer, N. (1989) T-cell reactivity in myasthenia gravis. J. Autoimmunity 2, 101–108.

Nouri-Aria, K.T., Hegarty, J.E., Alexander, G.J.M., Eddleston, A.L.W.F. and Williams, R. (1982) Effect of corticosteroids on suppressor-cell activity in 'autoimmune' and viral chronic active hepatitis. N. Engl. J. Med. 307, 1301–1304.

Nouri-Aria, K.T., Donaldson, P.T., Hegarty, J.E., Eddleston, A.L.W.F. and Williams, R. (1985) HLA A1-B8-DR3 and suppressor cell function in first-degree relatives of patients with autoimmune chronic active hepatitis. J. Hepatol. 1, 235–241.

O'Brien, C.J., Vento, S., Donaldson, T., McSorley, C.G., McFarlane, I.G., Williams, R. and Eddleston, A.L.W.F. (1986) Cell-mediated immunity and discrete suppressor T-cell defects to liver-derived antigens in families of patients with autoimmune chronic active hepatitis. Lancet i, 350–353.

Odievre, A.M., Maggiore, G., Homberg, J.C., Saadoun, F., Courouce, A.M, Yvart, J., Hadchouel, M. and Alagille, D. (1983) Seroimmunologic classification of chronic hepatitis in 57 children. Hepatology 3, 407–409.

Okuno, T., Seto, Y., Okanoue, T. and Takino, T. (1987) Chronic active hepatitis with features of primary biliary cirrhosis. Dig. Dis. Sci. 32, 775–779.

Opelz, G., Vogten, A.J.M., Summerskill, W.H.J., Schalm, S.W. and Terasaki, P.L. (1977) HLA determinants in chronic active liver disease: possible relation of HLA-Dw3 to prognosis. Tissue Antigens 1977 36–40.

Perperas, A., Tsantoulas, D., Portmann, B., Eddleston, A.L.W.F. and Williams, R. (1981) Autoimmuinity to a liver membrane lipoprotein and liver damage in alcoholic liver disease. Gut 22, 149–152.

Reynolds, T.B., Peters, R.L. and Yamada, S. (1971) Chronic active and lupoid hepatitis caused by a laxative, oxyphenisatin. N. Engl. J. Med. 285, 813–820.

Rizzetto, M., Swana, G. and Doniach, D. (1973) Microsomal antibodies in active chronic hepatitis and other disorders. Clin. Exp. Immunol. 15, 331–344.

Schilsky, M.L., Scheinberg, I.H. and Sternlieb, I. (1991) Prognosis of Wilsonian chronic active hepatitis. Gastroenterology 100, 762–767.

Schweitzer, I.L. and Peters, R.L. (1974) Acute submassive hepatic necrosis due to methyldopa. A case demonstrating possible initiation of chronic liver disease. Gastroenterology 66, 1203–1211.

Scott, J., Gollan, J.L., Samourian, S. and Sherlock, S. (1978) Wilson's disease presenting as chronic active hepatitis. Gastroenterology 74, 645–651.

Sherlock, S. (1964) Chronic hepatitis: the scope of the problem. Tijdschr. Gastro-Enterologie 7, 1–4.

Silva, A.E., Sallie, R., Tibbs, C., McFarlane, I.G., Johnson, P.J. and Williams, R. (1993) Absence of hepatitis C virus in U.K. patients with type 1 autoimmune chronic active hepatitis, in press.

Smeenk, R., van der Lelij, G. and Swaak, T. (1982) Specificity in systemic lupus erythematosus of antibodies to double-stranded DNA measured with the polyethylene glycol precipitation assay. Arthritis Rheum. 25, 631–638.

Smith, M.G.M., Williams, R., Walker, G., Rizzetto, M. and Doniach, D. (1974) Hepatic disorders associated with liver kidney microsomal antibodies. Br. Med. J. 2, 80–84.

Soloway, R.D., Summerskill, W.H.J., Baggenstoss, A.H. and Schoenfield, L.J. (1972) 'Lupoid hepatitis', a non-entity in the spectrum of chronic active liver disease. Gastroenterology 63, 358–365.

Stern, R.B., Wilkinson, S.P., Howorth, P.J.N. and Williams, R. (1977) Controlled trial of synthetic D-penicillamine in maintenance therapy for active chronic hepatitis. Gut 18, 19–22.

Sternlieb, I. and Scheinberg, H. (1972) Chronic hepatitis as a first manifestation of Wilson's disease. Ann. Int. Med, 76. 59–64.

Sternlieb, I. and Scheinberg, I.H. (1987) Wilson's disease. In: R. Wright, G.H. Millward-Sadler, A. Alberti and S. Karran (Eds.) Liver and Biliary Disease, Baillière Tindall, London, pp. 949–962.

Tan, E.M. (1989) Antinuclear antibodies: diagnostic markers for autoimmune diseases and probes for cell biology. Adv. Immunol. 44, 93–151.

Tan, E.M. Feltkamp, T.E.W. and Alarcon-Segovia, D. (1988) Reference reagents for antinuclear antibodies. Arthritis Rheum. 31, 1331.

Todros, L., Touscoz, G., D'Urso, N., Durazzo, M., Albano, E., Poli, G., Baldi, M. and Rizzetto, M. (1991) Hepatitis C virus-related chronic liver disease with autoantibodies to liver–kidney microsomes (LKM). J. Hepatol. 13, 128–131.

Toh, B. (1973) Smooth muscle autoantibodies and autoantigens. Clin. Exp. Immunol. 15, 331–344.

Treichel, U., Poralla, T., Hess, G., Manns, M. and Meyer zum Büschenfelde, K.H. (1990) Autoantibodies to human asialoglycoprotein receptor (ASGP-R) in autoimmune-type chronic hepatitis. Hepatology 11, 606–612.

Tysell, J.E. and Knauer, C.M. (1971) Hepatitis induced by methyldopa (Aldomet): a case report and review of the literature. Am. J. Dig. Dis. 16, 849–855.

Vento, S., O'Brien, C.J., McFarlane, B.M., McFarlane, I.G., Eddleston, A.L.W.F. and Williams, R. (1986) T-lymphocyte sensitisation to hepatocyte antigens in autoimmune chronic active hepatitis and primary biliary cirrhosis: evidence for different underlying mechanisms and different antigenic determinants as targets. Gastroenterology 91, 810–817.

Vento, S., McFarlane, B.M., McSorley, C.G., Ranieri, S., Giuliani-Piccari, G., Dal Monte, P.R., Verucchi, G., Williams, R., Chiodo, F. and McFarlane, I.G. (1988) Liver autoreactivity in acute virus A, B and non-A, non-B hepatitis. J. Clin. Lab. Immunol. 25, 1–7.

Vento, S., Di Perri, G., Garofano, T., Cosco, L., Concia, E., Ferraro, T. and Bassetti, D. (1990) Hazards of interferon therapy for HBV-seronegative chronic hepatitis. Lancet ii, 926 (letter).

Vento, S., Garofano, T., Di Perri, G., Dolci, L., Concia, E. and Bassetti, D. (1991) Identification of hepatitis A virus as a trigger for autoimmune chronic active hepatitis type 1 in susceptible individuals. Lancet 337, 1183–1187.

Wachter, B., Kyriatsoulis, A., Lohse, A.W., Gerken, G., Meyer zum Büschenfelde, K.-H. and Manns, M. (1990) Characterisation of liver cytokeratin as a major target antigen of anti-SLA antibodies. J. Hepatol. 11, 232–239.

Waldenstrom, J. (1950) Leber, Blutproteine und Nahrungseiweiss: Dtsch Ges. Verdau. Stoffwechselkr. 15, 113–119.

Wen, L., Peakman, M., Lobo-Yeo, A., McFarlane, B.M., Mowat, A.P., Mieli-Vergani, G. and Vergani, D. (1990) T-cell-directed hepatocyte damage in autoimmune chronic active hepatitis. Lancet 336, 1527–1530.

Whittingham, S.F., Irwin, J., Mackay, I.R. and Smalley, M. (1966) Smooth muscle autoantibody in 'auto-immune' hepatitis. Gastroenterology 51, 499–505.

Wood, J.R., Czaja, A.J., Beaver, S.J., Hall, S., Ginsburg, W.W., Kaufman, D.K. and Markowitz, H. (1986) Frequency and significance of antibody to double-stranded DNA in chronic active hepatitis. Hepatology 6, 976–980.

Yadin, O., Sarov, B., Naggan, L., Slor, H. and Schoenfeld, Y. (1989) Natural antibodies in the serum of healthy women – a five year follow-up. Clin. Exp. Immunol. 75, 402–406.

Autoimmune Hepatitis
Edited by M. Nishioka, G. Toda and M. Zeniya
© 1994, Elsevier Science B.V. All rights reserved

Chapter 13

Immunological aspects of autoimmune hepatitis: lymphocyte responses

Shinichi Kakumu

Department of Internal Medicine (III), Nagoya Univerisity,
School of Medicine, Turumai-Cyo 65, Syowa-ku, Nagoya 466 (Japan)

1. Introduction

Autoimmune chronic active hepatitis (CAH) is characterized histologically by hepatocellular necrosis, and a dense portal tract mononuclear cell infiltrate mainly composed of T-lymphocytes. In normal subjects, the regulatory apparatus of the immune system suppresses responses directed to self-components. Autoimmune disease may occur as a defect of this immunoregulatory system including a failure to differentiate self from non-self either due to a primary lack of the immunoregulatory system or because of the changes in the antigenicity of the tissue and in the secondary immune response. When autoimmune reactions target membrane-associated antigens, they may be of importance in the hepatocyte damage. Alternatively, those directed to cytoplasmic components may be diagnostically useful, although the pathogenic significances are frequently difficult to define. The defect of the immune system may be generalized or limited to certain autoantigens. Thus autoimmune disease may be either multi- or unisystemic. The recent development of experimental techniques allowing the continuous growth of antigen-specific and/or autoreactive T-cells of peripheral blood and liver tissue have contributed to a better understanding of the immunological mechanisms involved in autoimmune CAH. However, precise antigen-specific immunoregulatory function is still not clear.

                    S. Kakumu

2. *Lymphocyte subsets in peripheral blood and liver*

Kung and his colleagues (1979) produced a series of antibodies that identified surface markers on mononuclear cells which were related to maturity or function. Frequently used monoclonal antibodies are described in Table 1. More precise analysis of function and activity of mononuclear cells is now available using two-color flow cytometry. Some examples are shown in Table 2.

Thomas et al. (1982) found that the CD4/CD8 ratio was increased in patients with autoimmune CAH and returned to normal with successful therapy of prednisolone. In contrast, others demonstrated normal populations of T-cell subsets, but some patients had lymphocytes positive for both CD4 and CD8 and when this group was excluded from analysis, the CD4/CD8 ratio was noted to be

Table 1
A guide to the monoclonal antibodies used to identify lymphocytes
PMN, polymorphonuclear.

Monoclonal antibodies	Lymphocytes
CD3 (Leu-4, OKT-3)	T-cells
CD4 (Leu-3a, OKT-4)	T-cell subset (helper/inducer)
CD5 (Leu-1)	T-cells, B-cell subset
CD8 (Leu-2a, Leu-2b, OKT-8)	T-cell subset (suppressor/cytotoxic)
CD11b (Leu-15, OKM-1)	CR3; suppressor T-cells, NK-cells, monocytes, PMN
CD11c (Leu-M5, OKM-5)	Monocytes, PMN
CD16 (Leu-11a, Leu-11b, Leu-11c, OK-NK	IgG Fc receptors on NK cells and PMN
CD19 (Leu-12, B4, OKB-7)	B-cells
CD20 (Leu-16, B1, OKB-16)	B-cells
CD21 (CR2, B2, OKB-7)	B-cells (matured)
CD22 (Leu-14, B3, OKB-22)	B-cells
CD25 (IL-2R, IL-1R1)	IL-2 receptor on activated T-cells
CD45 (HLe-1)	Pan leukocytes
CD45RA (Leu-18, 2H4)	T-cell subset (suppressor/inducer), NK-cells, B-cells
CD57 (Leu-7)	Subset of NK-cells and T-cells

Table 2
Discrimination of lymphocyte subset by two-color flow cytometry.

Combination	Significance
CD8 and CD11	Discrimination between suppressor and cytotoxic T-cells
CD4 and Leu-8	Discrimination between helper and suppressor/inducer T-cells
CD57 and CD16	Evaluation of NK-cell activity
CD3 and HLA-DR	Simultaneous measurement of T-cells, B-cells and activated T-cells
CD4 and HLA-DR	Discrimination between rest and activated helper/inducer T-cells
CD8 and HLA-DR	Discrimination between rest and activated suppressor/cytotoxic T-cells

increased in the remainder (Back and Back, 1981; Carella et al., 1982; Frazer and Mackay, 1982; Raedler et al.,1986).

Nouri-Aria et al. (1982) observed the presence of a marked impairment of suppressor cell function in autoimmune CAH, which was corrected by in vitro incubation of their lymphocytes with prednisolone. This finding is inconsistent with the alteration in T-cell subsets and suggests a maturation process that may be related to the presence of immature double-staining lymphocytes in patients with active disease (Carella et al., 1982). Recently, Wen et al. (1990) demonstrated the presence of T-cell clones specific for liver-membrane antigen. Six of 7 clones reacted with liver-specific lipoprotein complex, one clone responded to the asialoglycoprotein receptor (ASGP-R), both known targets of immune attack in autoimmune CAH. Most of them were CD4-positive. Thus, they suggested that liver-membrane-specific activated T-lymphocytes in peripheral blood may be important in the autoimmune attack of CAH.

Lymphocyte subsets at the sites of inflammation may differ from those in peripheral blood in patients with acute and chronic liver diseases (Pape et al., 1983). Alternatively, there is a report that in the mononuclear cell infiltrate in the liver, the ratio of inducer to cytotoxic/suppressor cells was greater in patients with autoimmune CAH, primary biliary cirrhosis (PBC) and anti-HBe-positive hepatitis B virus (HBV)-induced chronic active liver disease than in HBeAg-positive HBV-induced chronic hepatitis (Montano et al., 1983). This finding shows a relative deficiency of the cytotoxic/suppressor population of T-cells even in liver tissue in autoimmune liver diseases.

Eggink et al. (1982) studied the inflammatory infiltrate in liver biopsies of patients with chronic active liver disease, with specific reference to areas of piecemeal necrosis. In those with autoimmune CAH, areas with piecemeal necrosis CD8+ and OKM+ lymphocytes and IgG plasma cells were present, whereas in chronic active hepatitis B, almost exclusively CD8+ T-cells were found. They concluded that T-cell cytotoxicity and antibody-dependent cell-mediated cytotoxicity (ADCC) might be responsible for liver cell damage in autoimmune CAH. Franco et al. (1990) obtained 16 CD4+ T-cell clones and 14 CD8+ T-cell clones. Among them, 5 CD4+ and 4 CD8+ T-clones proliferated in response to autologous hepatocytes. The hepatocyte recognition was major histocompatibility complex (MHC)-restricted because only class II MHC-matched hepatocytes were able to stimulate the CD4+ T-clones, while only class I-matched hepatocytes stimulated CD8+ clones. These findings, together with the observation that autologous irradiated peripheral blood mononuclear cells were unable to stimulate the clones, indicated that the response of these clones was directed to a liver membrane antigen in association with class II or class I MHC molecule on the surface of the hepatocytes. The class II antigen expression on hepatocytes may be regulated by γ-interferon (γ-IFN) released by infiltrating T-lymphocytes, thus, the activated liver cells could present autoantigens to autoreactive T-cell clones (Barnaba and Balsano, 1989).

3. Immunoregulatory T-cell function

The mechanisms allowing continuous liver-damaging autoimmune reactions in autoimmune CAH appear to be closely relevant to the pathogenesis. In particular, defects in immunoregulation have been implicated. Early studies evaluated non-organ-specific suppressor T-cell function using the system of concanavalin A-stimulated lymphocyte proliferation and pokeweed mitogen-induced immunoglobulin synthesis. These studies showed that suppressor T-cell function was clearly decreased in patients with chronic active liver disease (Kakumu et al., 1980; Kashio et al., 1981; Nouri-Aria et al., 1982). In vivo administration of prednisolone significantly improved decreased suppressor activity of T-cells in these patients, suggesting that impaired suppressor cell activity was secondary to intra-hepatic inflammation.

However, it is also likely that this is a primary event, because defective suppressor cell function has been found in healthy first-degree relatives of patients with autoimmune CAH (Nouri-Aria et al., 1985). We also demonstrated that concanavalin A-induced suppressor activity of spleen cells was substantially decreased in mice with autoimmune hepatitis immunized with syngeneic liver proteins (Kuriki et al., 1983).

Defective non-organ and non-antigen specific suppressor cell function may result in the appearance of non-organ-specific autoantibodies and hypergammaglobulinemia. In addition, it is unlikely that this non-specific defect itself induces highly organ-specific disease. Therefore, additional antigen- and/or organ-specific defects are likely to be more deeply associated and crucially important for the development and persistence of this illness.

Vento et al. (1984, 1986) demonstrated the presence of T-lymphocytes specific for liver-specific lipoprotein complex (LSP) in most of patients with autoimmune CAH using an indirect migration inhibition assay. In contrast, such T-lymphocyte migration inhibitory factors (T-LIF) were generated in only one of 21 patients with HBsAg-positive chronic liver disease and none of 19 controls. Furthermore, the generation of T-LIF activity by T-cells from autoimmune CAH patients was suppressed when these cells were co-cultured with T-cells from normal subjects, and patients with type 2 chronic liver disease and PBC, but was unaffected if co-cultured with T-cells from other patients with autoimmune CAH. Thus they hypothesized that there exists a defect in the specific suppressor T-cell population controlling the immune response to LSP in autoimmune CAH which is unaffected by disease activity and treatment and which may be of fundamental importance in the pathogenesis of the disease.

In addition to LSP, T-cell sensitization to the ASGP-R, a liver-specific protein on the surface of hepatocytes and contained in LSP preparation, was also invariably found in those with autoimmune CAH by means of a T-LIF assay, but not in healthy relatives or spouses (O'Brien et al., 1986; Vento et al., 1986). In contrast to the findings with the purified ASGP-R, there was a functional defect in the suppressor T-lymphocytes specific for LSP complex in 50% of first-degree relatives and 43% of second-degree relatives, but in only 9% of spouses, suggesting that the abnormality of immunoregulation may be genetically determined and crucial to the development of the disease. Thus cumulatively it appears that the ASGP-R is a target for cellular immune reactions and is associated with a suppressor T-cell defect for liver cell antigens.

Vento et al. (1987) also implied that CD4+ T-cell inducers of suppressor T-lymphocytes specific for liver cell surface antigens exits in the peripheral blood of healthy people, while such T-cells are defective in patients with autoimmune CAH. These suppressor T-cell-inducer cells seem to be activated in vivo in healthy subjects and may form part of an immunoregulatory network which actively prevents autoimmunity. Alternatively, a generalized increase in immunoglobulin secretion, which is a prominent feature of autoimmune disease, may be due to intrinsic abnormality of B-lymphocytes as suggested in mouse models (Bocchieri, 1989; Aldo-Benson et al., 1989).

In addition to the abnormalities of lymphocyte function, some cytokines are implicated in autoimmune phenomena. For example, initial studies on the role of interleukin-2 (IL-2) in autoimmunity indicated a deficiency in the production of this lymphokine in autoimmune disease. However, recent data support the notion that an excess endogenous or exogenous IL-2 may aggravate autoaggression by triggering autoreactive effector cells, and that IL-2 may favor the de novo development of autoimmunity by breaking autotolerance (Kroemer and Wick, 1989).

According to the results of these recent findings, an initial event in autoimmune CAH may occur due to the loss of T-cell tolerance to the hepatic antigens or receptors such as the LSP complex or ASPG-R. Alternatively, different mechanisms by T-cell circuits involved in idiotype/anti-idiotype interactions could play a role in the control of immune reactions against hepatocytes as suggested by Tsubouchi et al. (1985).

4. Lymphocyte-mediated liver cell damage

The initial study demonstrated that lymphocytes from patients with autoimmune CAH were directly cytotoxic to isolated rabbit hepatocytes, and the addition of either human or rabbit LSP preparation reduced the cytotoxicity, indicating this cytotoxicity was a consequence of specific sensitization to LSP (Thomson et al., 1974). Subsequently, the cytotoxicity was observed in a non-T-cell population of peripheral blood lymphocytes bearing Fc receptors (Cochrane et al., 1976) However, these test systems are not suitable for disclosing T-cell-mediated cytotoxicity, because it depends on histocompatibility antigen between target and effector cells (Zinkelnagel and Doherty, 1979). Mieli-Vergani et al. (1979) investigated the cytotoxic activity using autologous hepatocytes in microcytotoxicity assay system. The results with T- and non-T-lymphocytes and the blocking study with LSP complex showed ADCC (anti-LSP) is the major cytotoxic mechanism in autoimmune CAH.

Some studies disclosed different mechanisms responsible for in vitro cell-mediated cytotoxicity to autologous hepatocytes between autoimmune and HBsAg-positive chronic liver disease (Mondelli et al., 1985; Barnaba et al., 1986). In autoimmune CAH and HBsAg-positive CAH without HBcAg in liver tissue, cytotoxicity was sustained by non-T-lymphocytes and was confined to M1-positive cells bearing Fc receptors; M1 cytotoxicity inhibition by adding agregated IgG suggested that these cells were responsible for an ADCC. T-cell (CD8 + subset) cytotoxicity was exclusively found in patients with HBcAg in the liver. Moreover, the inhibition of T-cell cytotoxicity by preincubating liver cells with monoclonal antibody (MoAb) anti-HLA-ABC and not with MoAb anti-HLA-DR or aggregated IgG, supported the involvement of class I MHC expressed on the hepatocyte surface.

Although a number of observations suggest that ADCC may be a major mechanism for liver cell damage in patients with autoimmune CAH, it remains unknown whether a similar mechanism operates in vivo. Furthermore, CD8 + cytotoxic T-cells are major elements of infiltrating lymphocytes at portal tracts in these patients. Thus definitive cytotoxic studies will clarify the mechanism of hepatocellular lysis by using cloned cell lines including T-cell clones isolated from liver tissue, specific for liver cell membrane antigens, with autologous hepatocytes or HLA-class I-matched cell lines expressing liver cell membrane antigens as target cells.

References

Aldo-Benson, M., Brooks, M.S. and Scheiderer-Pratt, L. (1989) B cell hyperactivity in autoimmune continuous B cell lines. Immunol. Res. 8, 271–280.

Bach, M.A. and Bach, J.F. (1981) The use of monoclonal anti-T cell antibodies to study T-cell imbalances in human diseases. Clin. Exp. Immunol. 45, 449–456.

Barnaba, V., Levrero, M., Franco, A., Ruberti, G., Musca, A., Bonavita, M.S. and Balsano, F. (1986) Characterization of effector cells in lymphocytotoxicity to autologous hepatocytes in HBsAg-positive and autoimmune chronic active hepatitis (CAH). Liver 6, 45–52.

Barnaba, V., Franco, A. and Balsano, F. (1989) Autoimmune chronic liver disease as a model of human autoimmunity. Clin. Exp. Rheum. 7, 47–50.

Bocchieri, M.H. (1989) Immunoregulatory effects of cloned T-cells on B-cell responses: comparison of autoimmune and non-autoimmune derived clones. Immunology 66, 526–531.

Carella, G., Chatenoud, L., Degos, F. and Bach, M.A. (1982) Regulatory T-cell subset imbalance in chronic active hepatitis. J. Clin. Immunol. 2, 93.

Cochrane, A.M.G., Moussouros, A., Thomson, A.D., Eddleston, A.L.W.F. and Williams, R. (1976) Antibody-dependent cell-mediated (K cell) cytotoxicity against isolated hepatocytes in chronic active hepatitis. Lancet 1, 441–444.

Eggink, H.F., Houthoff, H.J., Huitema, S., Gips, C.H. and Poppema, S. (1982) Cellular and humoral immune reactions in chronic active liver disease. I. Lymphocyte subsets in liver biopsies of patients with untreated idiopathic autoimmune hepatitis, chronic active hepatitis B and primary biliary cirrhosis. Clin. Exp. Immunol. 50, 17–24.

Franco, A., Barnaba, V., Ruberti, G., Benvenuto, R., Balsano, C. and Musca, A. (1990) Liver-derived T cell clones in autoimmune chronic active hepatitis: accessory cell function of hepatocytes expressing class II major histocompatibility complex molecules. Clin. Immunol. Immunopathol. 54, 382–394.

Frazer, I.H. and Mackay, I.R. (1982) T-lymphocyte subpopulations defined by two sets of monoclonal antibodies in chronic active hepatitis and systemic lupus erythematosus. Clin. Exp. Immunol. 50, 107–114.

Kakumu, S., Yata, K. and Kashio, T. (1980) Immunoregulatory T-cell function in acute and chronic liver disease. Gastroenterology 79, 613–619.

Kashio, T., Hotta, R. and Kakumu, S. (1981) Lymphocyte suppressor cell activity in acute and chronic liver disease. Clin. Exp. Immunol. 44, 459–466.

Kroemer, G. and Wick, G. (1989) The role of interleukin 2 in autoimmunity. Immunol. Today 10, 246–251.

Kung, P.C., Goldstein, G., Reinherz, E.L. and Schlossman, S.F. (1979) Monoclonal antibodies defining distinctive human T-cell surface antigens. Science 206, 347–349.

Kuriki, J., Murakami, H., Kakumu, S., Sakamoto, N., Yokochi, T., Nakashima, I. and Kato, N. (1983) Experimental autoimmune hepatitis in mice after immunization with syngeneic liver proteins together with the polysaccharide of *Klebsiella pneumoniae*. Gastroenterology 84, 596–603.

Mieli-Vergani, G., Vergani, D., Jenkins, P.J., Portmann, B., Mowat, A.P., Eddleston, A.L.W.F. and Williams, R. (1979) Lymphocyte cytotoxicity to autologous hepatocytes in HBsAg-negative chronic active hepatitis. Clin. Exp. Immunol. 38, 16–21.

Mondelli, M., Mieli-Vergani, G., Bortolotti, F., Cadrobbi, P., Portmann, B., Alberti, A., Realdi, G., Eddleston, A.L.W.F. and Mowat, A.P. (1985) Different mechanisms responsible for in vitro cell-mediated cytotoxicity to autologous hepatocytes in children with autoimmune and HBsAg-positive chronic liver disease. J. Pediatr. 106, 899–906.

Montano, L., Aranguibel, F., Boffill, M., Goodall, A.H., Janossy, G. and Thomas, H.C. (1983) An analysis of the composition of the inflammatory infiltrate in autoimmune and hepatitis B virus-induced chronic liver disease. Hepatology 3, 292–296.

Nouri-Aria, K.T., Hegarty, J.E., Alexander, G.J.M., Eddleston, A.L.W.F. and Williams, R. (1982) Effect of corticosteroids on suppressor-cell activity in 'autoimmune' and viral chronic active hepatitis. N. Engl. J. Med. 307, 130–1304.

Nouri-Aria, K.T., Donaldson, P.T., Hegarty, J.E., Eddleston, A.L.W.F. and Williams, R. (1985) HLA A1–B8-DR3 and suppressor cell function in first-degree relatives of patients with autoimmune chronic active hepatitis. J. Hepatol. 1, 235–241.

O'Brien, C.J., Vento, S., Donaldson, P.T., McSorley, C.G., McFarlane, I.G., Williams, R. and Eddleston, A.L.W.F. (1986) Cell-mediated immunity and suppressor-T-cell defects to liver-derived antigens in families of patients with autoimmune chronic active hepatitis. Lancet 1, 350–353.

Pape, G.R., Rieber, E.P., Eisenburg, J., Hoffmann, R., Balch, C.M., Paumgartner, G. and Riethmuller, G. (1983) Involvement of the cytotoxic/suppressor T-cell subset in liver tissue injury of patients with acute and chronic liver diseases. Gastroenterology 85, 657–662.

Raedler, A., Bredow, G., Kirch, W., Thiele, H.G. and Greten, H. (1986) In vivo activated peripheral T cells in autoimmune disease. J. Clin. Lab. Immunol. 19, 181–186.

Thomas, H.C., Brown, D., Carbrody, J. and Epstein, D. (1982) T-cell subsets in autoimmune and HBV induced chronic liver disease: a review of the abnormalities and effects of treatment. Liver 2, 266–269.

Thomson, A.D., Cochrane, M.A.G., McFarlane, I.G., Eddleston, A.L.W.F. and Williams, R. (1974) Lymphocyte cytotoxicity to isolated hepatocytes in chronic active hepatitis. Nature 252, 721–722.

Tsubouchi, A., Yoshioka, K. and Kakumu S. (1985) Naturally occurring serum antiidiotypic antibody against antiliver-specific membrane lipoprotein in patients with hepatitis. Hepatology 5, 752–757.

Vento, S., Hegarty, J.E., Bottazzo, G., Macchia, E., Williams, R. and Eddleston, A.L.W.F. (1984) Antigen specific suppressor cell function in autoimmune chronic active hepatitis. Lancet 1, 1200–1204.

Vento, S., O'Brien, J., McFarlane, B.M., McFarlane, I.G., Eddleston, A.L.W.F. and Williams, R. (1986) T-Lymphocyte sensitization to hepatocyte antigens in autoimmune chronic active hepatitis and primary biliary cirrhosis. Gastroenterology 91, 810–817.

Vento, S., O'Brien, C.J., McFarlane, I.G., Williams, R. and Eddleston, A.L.W.F. (1987) T-cell inducers of suppressor lymphocytes control liver-directed autoreactivity. Lancet 1, 886–888.

Wen, L., Peakman, M., Lobo-Yeo, A., McFarlane, B.M., Mowat, A.P., Mieli-Vergani, G. and Vergani, D. (1990) T-cell-directed hepatocyte damage in autoimmune chronic active hepatitis. Lancet 336, 1527–1530.

Zinkernagel, R.M. and Doherty, P.C. (1979) MHC-restricted cytotoxic T-cells: Studies on the biological role of polymorphic major transplantation antigens determining T-cell restriction-specificity, function and responsiveness. Adv. Immunol. 27, 109–141.

Autoimmune Hepatitis
Edited by M. Nishioka, G. Toda and M. Zeniya
© *1994, Elsevier Science B.V. All rights reserved*

Chapter 14

Idiotype network and autoimmune hepatitis

Toshio Morizane

Department of Internal Medicine, Kanagawa Dental College,
82 Inaoka-chou, Yokosuka, Kanagawa 238 (Japan)

1. Introduction

Most immunological theories up to now have attempted to explain the phenomena of immune responsiveness by emphasizing the lack of autoreactivity to be the major underlying factor, and immune reactivity to self components has always been related to autoimmune diseases. The phenomenon of autoimmunity or autoreactivity is now considered not 'horror autotoxicus' but a normal inherent property of a functionally autonomous immune system (Kaushik, 1992). Autoimmune reactions are 'self-to-self interactions' between the molecules of the body and cells comprising the immune system. It seems evident that there are natural autoantibodies (Bussard, 1966; Avrameas et al., 1981; Dighiero et al., 1986, 1987; Tomer and Shoenfeld, 1988), autoreactive B-cells (Shoenfeld et al., 1982; Cairns et al., 1984) and autoreactive T-cells (Wekster et al., 1981; Zauderer 1989) in normal individuals or non-immunized animals (Pages and Bussard, 1978; Dighiero et al., 1983; Prabhakar et al., 1984; Underwood et al., 1985; Box and Meenuwsen, 1989) as well as in patients or animals with 'autoimmune diseases'. The physiologic role of autoantibodies is unclear, as is their relationship with pathogenic autoantibodies (Van Es et al., 1992). Although it has now become possible to investigate the antibody-variable regions of pathogenic autoantibodies derived from patients with autoimmune disease, the difference between natural autoantibodies and pathogenic autoantibodies is still unknown. In autoimmune hepatitis (AIH) it is naturally expected that autoreactive lymphocytes and auto-antibodies recognizing autoantigens expressed in liver cells will be detectable.

However, clonal deletion of autoreactive B-cells and T-cells (Burnet, 1959) or clonal anergy (Nossal, 1983) are definitely operating to insure tolerance to autoantigens, although the normal presence of autoreactive B-cells, T-cells and autoantibodies seems to contradict these mechanisms which account for immunological tolerace (Hasek et al., 1986). Two studies on the fate of autoreactive B-cells in transgenic mice provided for both clonal deletion (Nemazee and Burki, 1989) and clonal anergy (Goodnow et al., 1988, 1989). For T-cells, the thymus plays an important role in the development of tolerogenesis during intra-thymic differentiation. It was shown, using transgenic mice in which anti-self T-cell receptors (TCR) were expressed in the developing T-cells, that clonal deletion of autoreactive T-cells occurs during intra-thymic differentiation (Kisielow et al., 1988; Sha et al., 1988). Several in vitro experimental approaches also suggest clonal anergy of autoreactive T-cells (Nossal, 1989). It seems that autoimmunity and immunological tolerance co-exist and constitute the underlying framework of immunophysiological processes critical to homeostasis, tolerance, and the development of immune responses.

Autoimmune diseases are of multifactorial origin involving genetic, environmental and hormonal factors. Several hypotheses have been put forward in an attempt to explain the etiopathogenesis of autoimmune diseases. They include: (1) dysregulation of the immune system; and (2) molecular mimicry of autoantigens by foreign antigenic determinants. Although autoantibodies and autoreactive lymphocytes are found in normal subjects, they are linked with disease in some patients, and the contribution of certain kinds of these autoantibodies (Datta et al., 1992) and autoreactive lymphocytes (Heber-Katz, 1992) in the development of autoimmune diseases is now well established. Several investigators have found that the serum levels of autoantibodies reactive with liver cell components are elevated in patients with AIH and chronic hepatitis of viral origin (Jensen et al., 1978; McFarlane et al., 1984, 1986; Swanson et al., 1989), although it is unknown which antibodies are really pathognomonic in these liver diseases. There are also several reports of autoreactive lymphocytes (Vergani et al., 1979; Wen et al., 1991) which respond to liver cell components in AIH or chronic hepatitis.

The idiotype (Id) of an immunoglobulin (Ig) molecule is defined as the total set of antigenic determinants on the variable region of the Ig molecule (idiotopes) which are recognized by anti-idiotypic antibodies. This concept can also be extended to TCR consisting of a heterodimer of α and β or δ and γ. By virtue of the very large diversity of idiotypic structures it is postulated that any external antigen is potentially represented within the antibodies or lymphocyte antigen receptors as an idiotypic determinant. A theory proposed by Jerne (1973) is that interaction between idiotypes of both antibody molecules and lymphocyte antigen receptors may form a network in which a series of idiotypic–anti-idiotypic interactions regulate the immune response and in which a state of dynamic equilibrium exists. Jerne's concept is based on the dual character of Ig molecules, i.e., as antigen and antigen receptor (Jerne, 1984). The administration of antigen changes this equilibrium and evokes an immune response. Antibody (Ab-1) will be produced in response to this antigenic stimulus. Because of immunogenic idiotopes located on Ab-1 and the diversity and completeness of the antibody repertoire, anti-idiotypic antibody (Ab-2) will be formed. Much evidence has accumulated supporting the concept that anti-idiotypic antibodies work as regulatory signals (Zanetti, 1986a).

Anti-idiotypic antibodies have been shown to emerge spontaneously in humans with such diseases as myasthenia gravis (Lefvert, 1981; Dwyer et al., 1983), systemic lupus erythematosus (SLE) (Abdou et al., 1981; Nasu et al., 1982, 1983; Zouali and Eyquem, 1983, Silvestris et al., 1984; Taniguchi et al., 1984), rheumatoid arthritis (Heimer et al., 1982; Birdsall et al., 1983), autoimmune thyroiditis (Teuber and Helmke, 1981; Islam et al., 1983), hepatitis (Troisi and Hollinger, 1985; Tsubouchi et al., 1985), and other diseases in which hypergammaglobulinemia is a symptom. In this chapter, the significance of idiotype network in the pathogenesis of AIH will be discussed.

2. Principles of idiotypy

The heterogeneity of Ig can be defined at 3 levels of variation: isotypic; allotypic; and idiotypic. Most of the isotypic and allotypic antigenic determinants are located in the constant region of the Ig molecule. Isotypes define the class and subclass of an immunoglobulin. In humans, 5 classes (IgG, IgA, IgM, IgD and IgE) and 6 subclasses (IgG-1, IgG-2, IgG-3, IgG-4, IgA-1 and IgA-2) are recognized. Isotypes are present in all individuals of a species, while allotypes represent the variations between groups of individuals of a species.

Idiotypes are antigenic determinants located in the hypervariable region of the Ig, in the antigen-binding site (paratope), or near the paratope. Each antigenic determinant expressed on the surface of the V-region of an individual antibody molecule is called an idiotope. Each idiotope has a single determinant, and the unique collection of idiotopes present on an antibody forms the Id of that antibody.

Idiotypes can be classified into two large categories, private Id and public Id. Private Id, also called IdI, consists of determinants that are found only in that individual person or animal in which the Ab-1 was generated against a specific antigen. Alternatively, public Id, also called cross-reactive, shared Id or IdX, includes determinants present on Ab-1 produced in different individuals of a species in response to an antigen. Public Id can cross species boundaries as well. It should be noted that a particular idiotope may also be expressed on antibodies which have different antigenic specificities, while another idiotope may be directly related to the antigenic specificity of that antibody.

Jerne and co-workers classified anti-idiotypic antibodies (Ab-2) into two categories, Ab-2α and Ab-2β. The Ab-2α binding to its Ab-1 may or may not be inhibited by the antigen inducing the Ab-1. Anti-Id of this group recognize determinants distinct from the antigen-binding site of the Ab-1 and may actually be bound to the Ab-1 at the same time the antigen is. The Ab-2β mimics the antigen used to generate the Ab-1 and can substitute for the nominal antigen, and it is, therefore, called internal image anti-Id. However, Bona and Köhler modified the classification by splitting Ab-2α into two groups (Ab-2α and Ab-2γ) and adding a fourth category, Ab-2ε. According to them, anti-idiotypic antibodies are classified into 4 major categories.

(1) Ab-2α: antibodies directed against an antigen-non-inhibitable idiotope or against an individual idiotope, i.e., antibodies recognizing non-antigen combining site idiotopes, which are usually private idiotopes.
(2) Ab-2β: antibodies carrying the internal image of the antigen (homobody).
(3) Ab-2γ: antibodies recognizing an antigen-inhibitable idiotope, i.e., antibodies recognizing an antigen-combining site idiotope, but having neither an internal image nor biological mimicry of the antigen (because they may only sterically hinder antigen-binding), which may be representative of recurrent intra-strain or intra-species idiotopes.
(4) Ab-2ε: antibodies recognizing an idiotope and an epitope on the antigens recognized by the Ab-1 (epibody).

Anti-idiotypes can not only mimic the antigenic structure of pathogenic organisms, but also substitute for certain hormones by binding s-specific cell receptors. The Ab-1 is generated against a hormone and the Ab-2 mimicry is demonstrated by its functional binding to the hormone receptor of the cell. In this system, the Ab-2 can behave as an agonist or antagonist (Shechter et al., 1982; Wasserman et al., 1983).

The antibody-combining region of Ig molecules is located in the variable regions of the heavy (H) and light (L) chains. Each H- or L-chain variable region is subdivided into 4 framework regions separated by 3 hypervariable regions or complementarity-determining regions (CDR) (Fig. 1). Recombination of gene segments allows for the formation of the variable region of an antibody and accounts, in part, for antibody diversity. In humans, V_H-genes have been assigned to 6 families (I–VI) based on homology in DNA sequence (Kodaira et al., 1986; Schroeder et al., 1987; Shen et al., 1987; Berman et al., 1988). Within H-chains, any one of a few hundred variable (V) region segments may recombine with one of several diversity (D) region segments and one of several joining (J) region segments making a single variable region (Taub and Greene, 1992; Van Es et al., 1992).

With regard to human autoantibodies, it has been argued that natural autoantibodies, mostly derived from CD5+ B-cells (Casali and Notkins, 1989), preferentially use the small human V_H-gene families (IV–VI) of germ-line genes (Sanz et al., 1989a). Capra's group has recently shown that these small human V_H-families display remarkably little polymorphism (Makar et al., 1988; Sanz

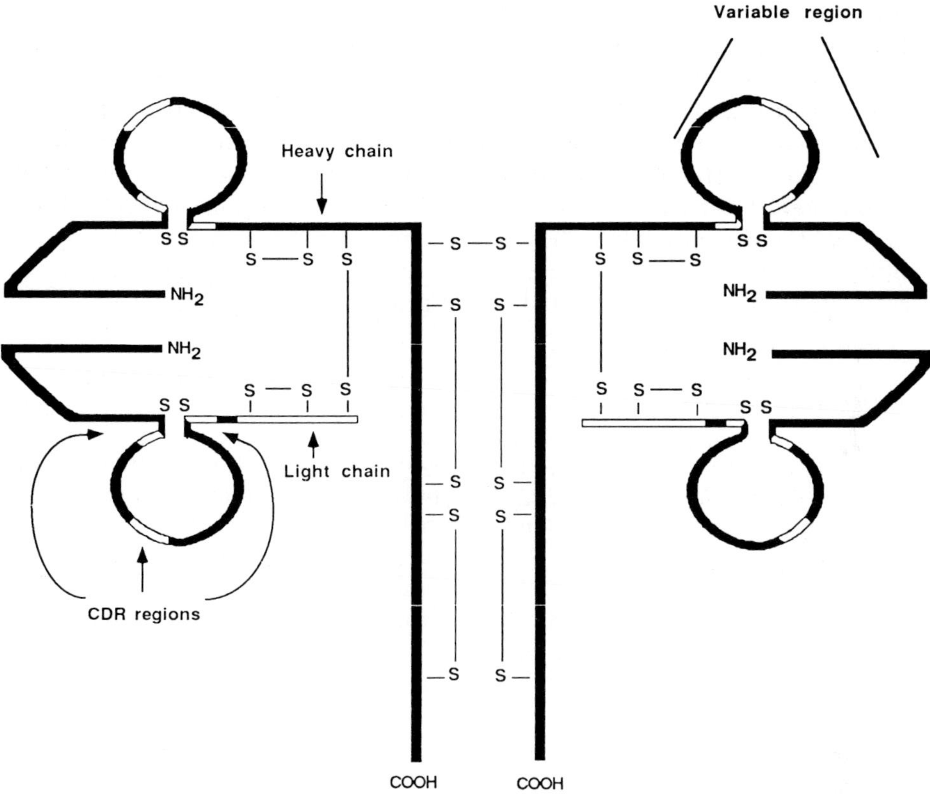

Fig. 1. Structure of an antibody molecule and complementarity-determining regions (CDR). Modified from Taub and Greene (1979).

et al., 1989b). They analyzed the nucleotide sequence of a human monoclonal Ab-2 which naturally arose in an individual during the course of a routine rabies immunization protocol and which was derived from a CD5 + EBV-transformed human B-cell clone (Van der Heijden et al., 1990). They found that the H-chain of this antibody derives from the small V_H-V-family of human V-region gene segments and that the germ-line V_H-V-gene isolated from the same individual reveals that the expressed molecule contains 19 nucleotide differences in the V_H-gene segment. However, an exhaustive computer comparison between the amino acid sequence of this V_H and the rabies virus glycoprotein failed to reveal any significant homology. Bruck et al. determined the nucleic acid sequence of an internal image-bearing monoclonal anti-idiotype and compared it with the sequence of the external antigen, the virus-neutralizing epitope on the mammalian reovirus type 3 hemagglutinin. The sequence analysis reveals that the same V_H and J_H are used by this Ab-2 and two other unrelated antibodies. However, amino acid sequence comparison between the viral hemagglutinin and this monoclonal Ab-2 L-chain internal image, reveals an area of significant homology (Bruck et al., 1986). Taub and Greene found such a similarity in other systems including: (1) platelet fibrinogen receptor and its internal image Ab-2; and (2) thyroxin-stimulating hormone and its internal image Ab-2 (Taub and Greene, 1992). The similarity was found in the CDR region of the L-chain. However, the sequence similarities between antigen or ligand and anti-idiotypic antibody seem very limited. Alternatively, similarity may be based solely on secondary or tertiary structure and not on primary amino acid sequence.

3. Idiotype cascade

Anti-idiotypic antibodies (Ab-2) can be generated not only by exposure to Ab-1, but also by exposure to the antigen. Exposure to the antigen induces Ab-1 production and Ab-2 is produced in response to the rising level of Ab-1 and Ab-3 is produced in response to Ab-2. Thus, a series of immune responses may continue. Within the framework of Jerne's initial network theory, Ab-3 can be produced with the specificity to bind the original antigen by mimicking the Ab-1.

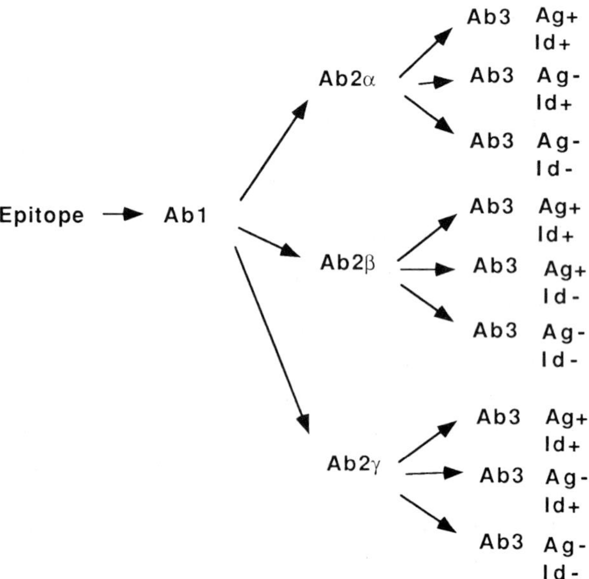

Fig. 2. Idiotype cascade.

Thus, the Ab-3 has the structure or conformation which allows it to bind the Id expressed on the surface of the Ab-2. The Id of the Ab-1 also has the structural conformation which confers to the Ab-2 favorable attractive forces for binding to the Ab-1 preparation. Therefore, the conformation of the Ab-3 represents the Id of the Ab-1 and therefore has the capacity to bind antigen.

The antibody response induced by Ab-2, i.e., Ab-3 response, depends on the kind of Ab-2 used for immunization (Schick and Kennedy, 1989) (Fig. 2). Immunization with Ab-2α can result in 3 types of Ab-3 antibodies: (1) Ab-3 antibodies which neither share idiotopes with Ab-1 nor bind to the same epitope as Ab-1 (Id–, Ag–); (2) Ab-3 antibodies which share idiotopes with Ab-1 but differ in antigen epitope specificity (Id +, Ag–); and (3) Ab-3 antibodies which are idiotypically similar to Ab-1 and which bind the same antigen epitope as Ab-1 (Id +, Ag +). Ab-2β can also induce 3 types of Ab-3, i.e., Id +/Ag + Ab-3, Id–/ Ag + Ab-3 and Id–/Ag–Ab-3. Thus, theoretically, Ab-2α and Ab-2β can induce antigen-binding antibodies and are able to substitute for antigen in the induction of antigen-specific immune responses. This phenomenon has been demonstrated with regard to various antigen systems including infectious agents, tumor antigens, hormones and complement factors.

4. Immunoregulatory function of anti-idiotype

Anti-idiotypic antibodies with the internal image of an antigen (Ab-2β) can induce immune reactions against the corresponding antigen. This is also possible with the autoantigen–autoantibody system (Essani et al., 1986). It was also reported that Ab-2 can activate T-cells in the mycobacterial antigen system (Rees et al., 1987). However, there are many studies showing that anti-idiotypic antibodies function as a substitute for antigens as well as functioning as an immunoregulatory molecule (Bona et al., 1984; Rimmelzwaan et al., 1989; Zanetti et al., 1992).

A number of studies have demonstrated directly or indirectly that anti-idiotypic antibodies are powerful agents for the suppression of antibodies possessing the appropriate idiotype. This suppressive activity of anti-idiotypic antibodies is observed in autoantibodies as well (Eichmann and Rajewsky, 1974; Binz and Wigzell, 1976; Bona and Paul, 1979; Weinberger et al., 1980; Geha and Cmunale, 1983; Takeuchi et al., 1985). The immune response to autoantigens in vivo can be suppressed by anti-idiotypic antibodies administered before immunization with autoantigen (Zanetti, 1986b) and the humoral response can be suppressed in vivo by active immunization with the idiotype on autoantibodies to the same autoantigen (Zouali et al., 1985). In NZB/NZW F1 female mice which spontaneously develop lupus nephritis associated with anti-DNA antibodies, repeated inoculation of the mice with monoclonal anti-idiotypic antibody which is directed against a major cross-reactive Id on IgG antibody to DNA can suppress the production of anti-DNA and delay the onset of nephritis so that survival is prolonged (Hahn and Ebling, 1983, 1984). It was shown in patients with SLE that a monoclonal anti-idiotypic antibody that recognizes a cross-reactive determinant on anti-DNA antibodies specifically suppressed anti-DNA production by peripheral blood mononuclear cells in vitro (Epstein et al., 1987). A similar suppression induced by anti-idiotypic antibody was reported with anti-U1-ribonucleoprotein antibody in patients with mixed connective tissue disease or SLE (Koide et al., 1988). In a mouse model it was shown that an antigen present in a mouse at birth is able to generate a T-cell-dependent suppressive mechanism that controls expression of antigen-specific antibodies through the recognition of antibody idiotypes (Tokuhisa and Rajewsky, 1985). The association of the suppression of disease activity with an anti-idiotypic antibody is observed in patients with SLE (Abdou et al., 1981) as well as in experimental autoimmune uveoretinitis (De Kozak and Mirshahi, 1990).

It has been shown that T-cell idiotypes can also suppress immune responses to the corresponding antigen. It was reported that humoral and cellular autoresponses can be suppressed in vivo by active immunization with antigen-reactive, idiotype-positive T-cells (Neilson and Phillips, 1982; Lider et al., 1988). It has also been revealed that the humoral autoresponse can be suppressed in vivo by passive transfer of idiotype-primed T-cells (Neilson et al., 1984; Zanetti et al., 1986). Furthermore, a segment of TCR peptides was tested to see whether it affected the autoimmune reactions and it was discovered that active immunization with a synthetic peptide of the TCR common idiotype leads to prevention of T-cell-mediated autoimmune disease. Therefore, idiotypes expressed by TCR also seem to operate as immunoregulators suppressing immune responses (Howell et al., 1989; Vandenbark et al., 1989).

5. Liver-specific idiotype-bearing antibody in chronic hepatitis

Autoantigens expressed in human liver cells which would be the targets of autoantibodies or autoreactive T-cells have been extensively searched for in several laboratories (Fletcher et al., 1970; Espinosa, 1973; Mihas et al., 1977; Behrens and Paronetto, 1978; McFarlane et al., 1980; Nerenberg et al., 1980). Liver-specific protein (LSP), first reported by Meyer zum Büschenfelde and Miescher in 1972, is one which has attracted many investigators (Hopf et al., 1974; McFarlane et al., 1977; Jensen et al., 1983). However, LSP has not yet been successfully purified as a single molecule. Therefore, studies using LSP preparation always have a limitation that the target antigens are unclear, because this preparation is a supernatant of liver homogenate spun at 100,000 g and contains many different components. Sodium dodecyl sulfate–polyacrylamide gel electrophoresis reveals more than 20 bands (Shelton et al., 1983) indicating that this preparation is a mixture of various components (Riisom and Diederichsen, 1983;

Murakami et al., 1984) of which some should be liver-specific antigens (Frazer and Mackay, 1984).

In our laboratory, we have produced a murine monoclonal antibody designated H2. This monoclonal antibody recognizes an epitope which is expressed solely on human liver cells (Morizane et al., 1986). We thought that if this H2 mAb possesses an interspecies, cross-reactive Id, it would be a useful tool for studying the workings of the antigen–idiotype–anti-idiotype network in cases of liver disease. We produced rabbit antiserum raised against H2 mAb. After extensive absorption with normal mouse serum and IgG, this anti-H2 rabbit antibody showed a fine specificity to H2 Id. The specificity for H2 Id was demonstrated by a solid-phase enzyme-linked immunosorbent assay (ELISA) against an assortment of murine mAbs and mouse IgGs. A competitive ELISA also revealed that this anti-H2 Id rabbit antibody is exclusive, that is, it reacts with H2 mAb but not with other mAb of the same subclass having different specificity. A competitive ELISA also showed that this anti-H2 Id prevents the binding of H2 mAb to the antigen. Therefore, it is thought that this anti-H2 rabbit antibody recognizes the paratope or idiotope which is near the paratope of H2 mAb since it blocks the binding of Ab-1 to the antigen. Using this anti-H2 Id, it became possible to detect antibodies possessing the same cross-reactive Id as the H2 mAb. We named these antibodies with the cross-reactive Id 'liver-specific idiotype-bearing antibodies' (LSIA), since their Id is shared by an mAb which is specific for human liver-specific antigen. The serum level of LSIA was revealed to be elevated in AIH, chronic hepatitis B and chronic hepatitis C, but not in acute viral hepatitis or SLE (Saito et al., 1990) (Fig. 3).

Although we do not have direct evidence showing that LSIA causes liver cell damage in AIH, chronic hepatitis B and C, it was shown that LSIA can mediate antibody-dependent cell-mediated cytotoxicity (ADCC) against Chang liver cells in vitro. This result suggests that LSIA is a pathogenic antibody. Another piece of information suggesting that LSIA is causing liver cell damage in vivo is that there is a significant correlation between the serum level of alanine aminotransferase

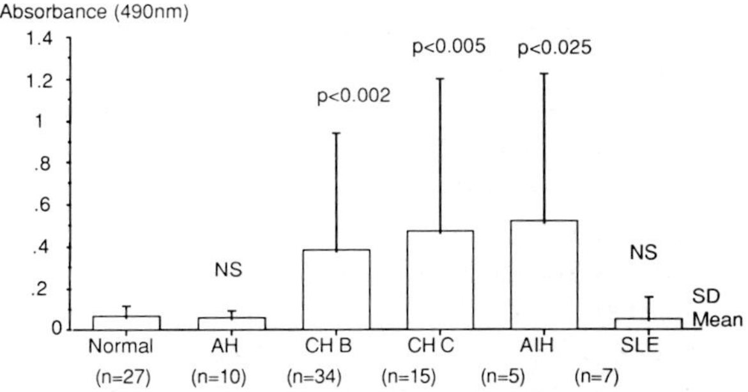

Fig. 3. Serum level of liver-specific idiotype-bearing antibody (LSIA). Statistical analysis was made by Student's *t*-test between the normal group and each of the patient groups. NS, not significant.

(ALT) and the serum level of LSIA in chronic hepatitis B. However, this might merely reflect the fact that LSIA is produced in response to the antigen released into the circulation as a result of liver cell damage. It is not surprising that LSIA is not only found in AIH, but also in chronic hepatitis caused by hepatitis viruses, because, as described in the first part of this chapter, liver cells damaged by T-cells which are directed against virus-associated antigens or by any other mechanisms release various liver cell components and may give antigenic stimulation with autoantigens, and, as a result, autoantibodies directed against liver cell components may be produced. In other antigen systems, it is known that chronic infection of a pathogen or a chemical can induce autoimmune responses (Abu-Shakra and Shoenfeld, 1992; Pelletier et al., 1992).

From the data on LSIA, it seems difficult to explain the difference between AIH and chronic hepatitis associated with hepatitis B virus or hepatitis C virus infection. However, we might speculate that autoantibodies as well as autoreactive T-cells towards liver cells play a central role in AIH and that they play only a cosmetic or a marginal role in chronic hepatitis of viral origin. In this view, in other words, autoantibodies towards liver cell antigens are solely pathogenic in AIH, but are part of a liver cell destruction mechanism in chronic hepatitis B and C.

6. Idiotype network in AIH and chronic hepatitis

In order to further pursue the nature of the idiotype network in AIH and other liver diseases, we need purified target antigens for which the amino acid sequence has been defined and for which some information on conformational structure has been made available. Because immune reactions, both humoral and T-cell-mediated, are directed to an epitope expressed in a very narrow segment of a molecule, we can garner little insight into the idiotype network if we use crude antigen preparations. These putative target antigens should be derived from liver cells, since only liver cells are damaged in AIH and other types of chronic liver diseases. However, antigens shared by other types of cells in the body may also be involved in the induction of autoantibodies and autoreactive T-cells. These autoimmune reactions, however, should not have pathogenic implications, but should only be marginal epiphenomena. Even epiphenomena may have clinical implications, however. Since gene cloning is now available as a routine technique, it seems possible to produce target antigens with defined primary structure.

We also need monoclonal antibodies (Ab-1) and T-cell clones that are reactive with liver-associated antigens derived from patients. For screening these autoreactive antibodies and T-cells we need an antigen. Although human monoclonal antibodies have been produced using the Epstein–Barr virus or by using a hybridoma technique, they have yielded only limited success. If we can obtain Ab-1 clones, it will then enable us to search for Ab-2 clones.

Currently favored hypothetical mechanisms relating to the idiotype network which might operate in AIH or chronic hepatitis are suggested in Fig. 4. As described above, anti-idiotypic antibodies tend to suppress immune responses against antigens. It is reasonable to think that in normal subjects sufficient Ab-2 is produced to suppress excessive production of Ab-1. Therefore, I am inclined to believe that in patients with AIH (excluding other types of chronic hepatitis) Ab-2 response is weak enough to allow excessive production of Ab-1 against liver cell antigens and that if the Ab-1 level reaches a certain threshold, liver cell destruction will begin by means of ADCC and complement-dependent antibody-dependent cytotoxicity.

On the other hand, in patients with chronic hepatitis of viral origin, I believe that the Ab-2 response is fairly good, although not up to the normal level, but being exposed to liver cell antigens provided by liver cells which have been destroyed in interactions between cytotoxic T-cells and viral antigens expressed on liver cell surfaces in conjunction with HLA-class I gives a constant stimulation to the production of Ab-1. This should result in a high level of Ab-1 and also a high level of Ab-2 and Ab-1 may participate in liver cell destruction through ADCC and complement cytotoxicity. We have found that serum level of Ab-2 against LSIA is low in patients with AIH, but at the same level in chronic hepatitis B or C as in normal subjects (unpublished data).

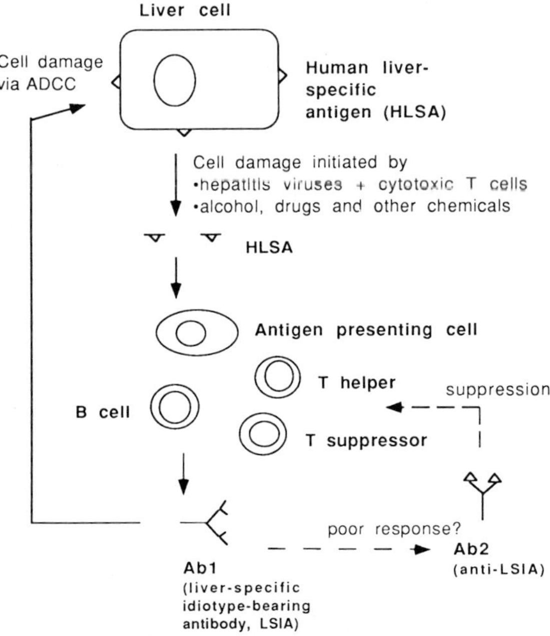

Fig. 4. Hypothesis on the role of LSIA and anti-idiotypic antibody.

    T. Morizane

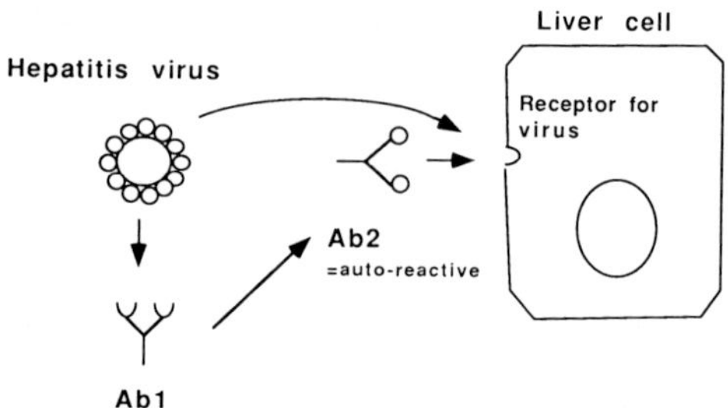

Fig. 5. Hypothesis on autoantibody production induced by hepatitis virus infection.

Another possible mechanism to account for the induction of autoantibodies towards liver cells in viral hepatitis can be derived from the idiotype network theory. Hepatitis viruses, both type B and type C, must bind to a liver cell plasma membrane in order to gain access to the intra-cellular space for proliferation. A receptor or a receptor-like structure on the liver cell surface is thought to be an access point, one that should only be expressed on liver cells, since hepatitis viruses can infect and proliferate only in liver cells. Conversely, the hepatitis viruses should have a structure on their surfaces which has a high affinity for the receptor or receptor-like structure on the liver cell surface, i.e., an acceptor structure of the virus surface proteins. If this acceptor structure evokes immune responses so that antibodies are produced in the virus-infected host, these antibodies (Ab-1) can induce Ab-2 production and the Ab-2 can then react with the virus receptors on the liver cells. Thus, Ab-2 against Ab-1 which was in its turn raised against hepatitis virus surface structure can behave as an autoantibody towards liver cells. A schematic of this hypothesis is shown in Fig. 5.

7. Conclusions

The investigation of the functioning of the idiotype network in AIH and chronic hepatitis of other types is still in its infancy. However, the ever-expanding frontiers of biotechnology continue to put ever better tools in our hands, so that in the near future it might be possible for researchers to use idiotypic structures for suppressing immune responses or enhancing immune responses in a specific manner.

Acknowledgements

I thank Mr. Martin Peters for his rapid English corrections and Ms. Misao Imasaki for help with preparation of the manuscript. This work was supported in part by a Grant-in-Aid for 'Intractable Liver Disease' from the Ministry of Health and Welfare of Japan.

References

Abdou, N.I., Wall, H., Lindsley, H.B. et al. (1981) Network theory in autoimmunity. In vitro suppression of serum anti-DNA antibody binding to DNA by anti-idiotypic antibody in systemic lupus erythematosus. J. Clin. Invest. 67, 1297–1304.

Abu-Shakra, M. and Shoenfeld, Y. (1992) Chronic infections and autoimmunity. In: C.A. Bona and A.K. Kaushik (Eds.), Molecular Immunobiology of Self-Reactivity, Marcel Dekker, New York, pp. 285–314.

Avrameas, S., Guilbert, B. and Dighiero, G. (1981) Natural antibodies against tubulin, actin, myoglobulin, fetuin, albumin and transferrin are present in normal human sera and monoclonal immunoglobulins from multiple myeloma and Waldenström's macroglobulinaemia may express similar antibody specificities. Ann. Immunol. (Inst. Pasteur) 132C 231–236.

Behrens, U.J. and Paronetto, F. (1978) Liver-specific and shared cell membrane antigens: studies by light- and electron microscopy. Immunology 35, 289–298.

Berman, J.E., Millis, S.J., Pollock, R. et al. (1988) Content and organization of the human IgV$_H$ locus: definition of three new V$_H$ families and linkage to the Ig C$_H$ locus. EMBO J. 7, 727–738.

Binz, H. and Wigzell, H. (1976) Shared idiotype determinants on B and T lymphocytes reactive against the same antigenic determinants. V. Biochemical and serological characteristics of naturally occurring, soluble antigen-binding T-lymphocyte-derived molecules. Scand. J. Immunol. 5, 559–571.

Birdsall, H.H., Lidsky, M.D. and Rossen, R.D. (1983) Anti-Fab' antibodies in rheumatoid arthritis. Measurement of the relative quantities incorporated in soluble immune complexes in sera and supernatants from cultured peripheral blood lymphocytes. Arthritis Rheum. 26, 1482–1492.

Bona, C. and Paul, W.E. (1979) Cellular basis of regulation of expression of idiotype. I. T-suppressor cells specific for MOPC-460 idiotype regulate the expression of cells secreting anti-TNP antibodies bearing 460 idiotype. J. Exp. Med. 149, 592–600.

Bona, C.A., Victor-Kobrin, C., Manheimer, A.J. et al. (1984) Regulatory arms of the immune network. Immunol. Rev. 79, 25–44.

Box, N.A. and Meenuwsen, C.G. (1989) B cell repertoire in adult antigen free and conventional neonatal mice. I. Preferential utilization of the CH-proximal V$_H$ gene family 7183. Eur. J. Immunol. 19, 1811–1815.

Bruck, C., Co, M.S., Slaoui, M. et al. (1986) Nucleic acid sequence of an internal image-bearing monoclonal anti-idiotype and its comparison to the sequence of the external antigen. Proc. Natl. Acad. Sci. U.S.A. 83, 6578–6582.

Burnet, F.M. (1959) The Clonal Selection Theory of Acquired Immunity. Cambridge University Press, Cambridge.

Bussard, A.E. (1966) Antibody formation in non-immune peritoneal cells after incubation in gum containing antigen. Science 153, 887–888.

Cairns, E., Block, J. and Bell, D.A. (1984) Anti-DNA autoantibody producing hydridomas of normal human lymphoid cell origin. J. Clin. Invest. 74, 880–887.

Casali, P. and Notkins, A.L. (1989). Probing the human B-cell repertoire with EBV: polyreactive antibodies and CD5$^+$ B lymphocytes. Annu. Rev. Immunol 7, 513–535.

Datta, S.K., Rajagopalan, S., O'Keefe, T.L. et al. (1992) Pathogenic anti-DNA autoantibodies and pathogenic autoantibody-inducing T cells. In: C.A. Bona and A.K. Kaushik (Eds.) Molecular Immunobiology of Self-Reactivity. Marcel Dekker, New York, pp. 133–153.

De Kozak, Y. and Mirshahi, M. (1990) Experimental autoimmune uveoretinits: idiotypic regulation and disease suppression. Int. Ophthalmol. 14, 43–56.

Dighiero, G., Lymberi, P., Mazie, J.C. et al. (1983) Murine hybridomas secreting natural monoclonal antibodies reacting with self antigens. J. Immunol 131, 2267–2272.

Dighiero, G., Lymberi, P., Guilbert, B. et al. (1986) Natural autoantibodies constitute a substantial part of normal circulating immunoglobulins. Ann. N.Y. Acad. Sci. 475, 135–145.

Dighiero, G., Kaushik, A., Poncet, P. et al. (1987) Origin and significance of autoantibodies. Concepts Immunopathol. 4, 42–76.

Dwyer, D.S., Bradley, R.J. Urquhart, C.K. et al. (1983) Naturally occurring anti-idiotypic antibodies in myasthenia gravis patients. Nature 301, 611–614.

Eichmann, K. and Rajewsky, K. (1974) Induction of T and B cell immunity by anti-idiotypic antibody. Eur. J. Immunol. 5, 661–669.

Epstein, A., Greenberg, M., Diamond, B. et al. (1987) Suppression of anti-DNA antibody synthesis in vitro by a cross-reactive antiidiotypic antibody. J. Clin. Invest. 79, 997–1000.

Espinosa, E. (1973) Circulating tissue antigens. II. Studies on an organ-specific antigen of human liver. Lab. Invest. 29, 556–561.

Essani, K., Srinivasappa, J., McClintok, R. et al. (1986) Multiorgan reactive IgG antibody induced by antiidiotypic antibody to a human monoclonal IgM autoantibody. J. Exp. Med. 163, 1355–1360.

Fletcher, A.P., Neuberger, A., Ratcliffe, W.A. et al. (1970) Tamm-Horsfall urinary glycoprotein: the subunit structure. Biochem. J. 120, 425–432.

Frazer, I.H. and Mackay, I.R. (1984) Immune responses to liver-specific lipoprotein and liver membrane antigen: a tabular interpretative review. J. Clin. Lab. Immunol. 14, 165–167.

Geha, R.S. and Cmunale, M. (1983) Regulation of immunoglobulin E. Antibody synthesis in man by anti-idiotypic antibodies. J. Clin. Invest. 71, 46–55.

Goodnow, C.C., Crosbie, J., Adelstein, S. et al. (1988) Altered immunoglobulin expression and functional silencing of self-reactive B lymphocytes in transgenic mice. Nature 334, 676–682.

Goodnow, C.C., Crosbie, J., Jorgensen, M. et al. (1989) Induction of self-tolerance in mature peripheral B lymphocytes. Nature 342, 340–341.

Hahn, B.H. and Ebling, F.M. (1983) Suppression of NZB/NZW murine nephritis by administration of syngeneic monoclonal antibodies to DNA. Possible role of anti-idiotypic antibodies. J. Clin. Invest. 71, 1728–1736.

Hahn, B.H. and Ebling, F.M. (1984) Suppression of murine lupus nephritis by administration of an anti-idiotypic antibody to anti-DNA. J. Immunol. 132, 187–190.

Hasek, M., Holan, V. and Hraba, T. (1986) From immunological tolerance to immunoregulation. Cellular and molecular aspects. Concepts Immunopathol. 3, 158–175.

Heber-Katz, E. (1992) The autoimmune T-cell receptor in experimental disease. In: C.A. Bona and A.K. Kaushik (Eds.) Molecular Immunobiology of Self-Reactivity. Marcel Dekker, New York, pp. 155–169.

Heimer, R., Wolfe, L.D. and Abruzzo, J.L. (1982) IgM and IgG anti-F(ab′)2 antibodies in rheumatoid arthritis and systemic lupus erythematosus. Arthritis Rheum. 25, 1298–1306.

Holmes, C.H., Hawkey, C.J., Gunn, B. et al. (1983) A monoclonal antibody reactive with human hepatocytes. Liver 3, 295–301.

Hopf, U., Meyer zum Büschenfelde, K.H., Freudenberg, J. et al. (1974) Liver-specific antigens of different species. II. Localization of a membrane antigen at surface of isolated hepatocytes.. Clin. Exp. Immunol. 16, 117–123.

Howell, M.D., Winters, S.T., Olee, T. et al. (1989) Vaccination against experimental allergic encephalomyelitis with T cell receptor peptides. Science 246, 668–670.

Islam, M.N., Pepper, B.M., Briones-Urbina, R. et al. (1983) Biological activity of anti-thyrotropin anti-idiotypic antibody. Eur. J. Immunol. 13, 57–63.

Jensen, D.M., McFarlane, I.G., Portmann, B. et al. (1978) Detection of antibodies directed against a liver-specific membrane lipoprotein in patients with acute and chronic active hepatitis. N. Engl. J. Med. 299, 1–7.

Jensen, D.M., Hall, C. and Majewski, T. (1983) The plasma membrane origin of liver-specific protein (LSP). Liver 3, 213–219.

Jerne, N.K. (1973) Towards a network theory of the immune system. Ann. Immunol. (Inst. Pasteur) 125C, 373–389.

Jerne, N.K. (1984) Idiotypic networks and other preconceived ideas. Immunol. Rev. 79, 5–24.

Kaushik, A.K. (1992) A synopsis of self-reactivity. In: C.A. Bona and A.K. Kaushik (Eds.) Molecular Immunobiology of Self-Reactivity. Marcel Dekker, New York, pp. 1–24.

Kisielow, P., Bluthmann, H., Staerz, V.D. et al. (1988) Tolerance in T cell receptor transgenic mice involves deletion of non-mature $CD4^+ 8^+$ thymocytes. Nature 333, 742–746.

Kodaira, M., Kinashi, T., Umemura, I. et al. (1986) Organization and evolution of variable region genes of the human immunoglobulin heavy chain. J. Mol. Biol. 190, 529–541.

Koide, J., Takeuchi T., Hosono, O. et al. (1988) Suppression of in vitro production of anti-U1-ribonucleoprotein antibody by monoclonal anti-idiotypic antibody to anti-U1-ribonucleoprotein antibody. Scand. J. Immunol. 28, 687–696.

Lambert, K.J., Major, G.N., Welsh C.J.R. et al. (1984) Production and preliminary characterization of monoclonal antibodies to human liver-specific lipoprotein (LSP). Liver 4, 122–127.

Lefvert, A.K. (1981) Anti-idiotypic antibodies against the receptor antibodies in myasthenia gravis. Scand. J. Immunol. 13, 493–497.

Lider, O., Reshef, T., Beraud, E. et al. (1988) Anti-idiotypic network induced by T-cell vaccination against experimental autoimmune encephalomyelitis. Science 239, 181–183.

Makar, R., Sanz, I., Thomas, J.W. et al. (1988) A structural basis for human cross-reacting idiotypes. Ann. Immunol. (Inst. Pasteur) 139, 651–657.

McFarlane, B.M., McSorley, C.G., Vergani, D. et al. (1986) Serum autoantibodies reacting with the hepatic asialoglycoprotein receptor protein (hepatic lectin) in acute and chronic liver disorders. J. Hepatol. 3, 196–205.

McFarlane, I.G., Wojcicka, B.M., Zucker, G.M. et al. (1977) Purification and characterization of human liver-specific lipoprotein (LSP). Clin. Exp. Lmmunol. 27, 381–390.

McFarlane, I.G., Wojcicka, B.M. and Williams, R. (1980) Antigens of the human liver. Clin. Exp. Immunol. 40, 1–7.

McFarlane, I.G., Hegarty, J.E., McSorley, C.G., et al. (1984) Antibodies to liver-specific protein predict outcome of treatment withdrawal in autoimmune chronic active hepatitis. Lancet ii: 954–956.

Meyer zum Büschenfelde, K.H. and Miescher, P.A. (1972) Liver-specific antigens. Purification and characterization. Clin. Exp. Immunol. 10, 89–102.

Mihas, A.A., Saccomani, G., Tomana, M. et al. (1977) Isolation and characterization of liver-specific antigen (F-Ag) from human liver. Immunochemistry 14, 727–731.

Morizane, T., Tsuchimoto, K., Iino, A. et al. (1986) Two different murine monoclonal antibodies B2 and H2 which are specific for human hepatocytes. Acta Hepatol. Jap. 27, 726–735 (in Japanese).

Murakami, H., Kuriki, J., Kakumu, S. et al. (1984) The specificity of human liver membrane lipoprotein: studies with monoclonal antibodies. Hepatology 4, 192–198.

Nasu, H., Chia, D.S., Taniguchi, O. et al. (1982) Characterization of anti-F(ab′)2 antibodies in SLE patients. Evidence for cross-reacting of autoanti-idiotypic antibodies. Clin. Immunol. Immunopathol. 25, 80–90.

Nasu, H., Chia, D.S., Taniguchi, O. et al. (1983) Characterization of anti-F(ab′)2 antibodies in SLE patients. Evidence for cross-reacting of autoanti-idiotypic activity in a single patient. Ann. Immunol. (Inst. Pasteur) 134C, 377–382.

Neilson, E.G. and Phillips, M.S. (1982) Suppression of interstitial nephritis by auto-anti-idiotypic immunity. J. Exp. Med. 155, 179–189.

Neilson, E.G., McCafferty, E., Phillips, S.M., et al. (1984) Anti-idiotypic immunity in interstitial nephritis. II. Rats developing anti-tubular basement membrane disease fail to make an anti-idiotypic regulatory response: the modulatory role of a TR7.1$^+$, OX8$^-$ suppressor T cell mechanism. J. Exp. Med. 159, 1009–1026.

Nemazee, D.A. and Burki, K. (1989) Clonal deletion of B lymphocytes in a transgenic mouse bearing anti-MHC class-I antibody genes. Nature 337, 562–566.

Nerenberg, S.T., Prasad, R. Inboriboon, P. et al. (1980) Isolation and characterization of a human liver and kidney-specific protein: the hepato-renal (H-R) antigen. Clin. Exp. Immunol. 39, 626–634.

Nossal, G.J.V. (1983) Cellular mechanisms of immunologic tolerance. Annu. Rev. Immunol 1, 33–62.

Nossal, G.J.V. (1989) Immunologic tolerance: collaboration between antigen and lymphokines. Science 245, 147–153.

Pages, J.M. and Bussard, A.E. (1978) Establishment and characterization of permanent murine hybridoma secreting monoclonal autoantibodies. Cell. Immunol. 41, 188–194.

Pelletier, L., Bellon, B., Tournade, H. et al. (1992) Chemical-induced autoimmunity. In: C.A. Bona and A.K. Kaushik (Eds.) Molecular Immunobiology of Self-Reactivity. Marcel Dekker, New York, pp. 315–354.

Prabhakar, B.S., Saegusa, J., Onodera, T. et al. (1984) Lymphocytes capable of making monoclonal autoantibodies that react with multiple organs are a common feature of the normal B cell repertoire. J. Immunol. 133, 2815–2817.

Rees, A.D.M., Scoging, A., Dobson, N. et al. (1987) T cell activation by anti-idiotypic antibody: mechanism of interaction with antigen reactive T cells. Eur. J. Immunol. 17, 197–201.

Riisom, K. and Diederichsen, H. (1983) Demonstration of organ-nonspecific antigens in liver-specific antigens in liver-specific protein. Gastroenterology 85, 1271–1276.

Rimmelzwaan, G.F., Bunschoten, E.J., UytdeHaag, F.G.C.M. et al. (1989) Monoclonal anti-idiotypic antibody vaccines against poliovirus, canine parvovirus, and rabies virus. Methods Enzymol. 178, 375–390.

Saito, H., Morizane T., Tsuchimoto, K. et al. (1990) Liver-specific idiotype-bearing antibody in autoimmune hepatitis. In: M. Tsuchiya, H. Nagura, T. Hibi and I. More (Eds.) Frontiers of Mucosal Immunology, Vol. 2, Elsevier Science Publisher, Amsterdam, pp. 65–68.

Sanz, I., Casali P., Thomas, J.W. et al. (1989a) Nucleotide sequences of eight human natural auto-antibody V_H gene regions reveals apparent restricted use of V_H families. J. Immunol. 142, 4054–4061.

Sanz, I., Kelly P., Williams, C. et al. (1989b) The smaller human V_H gene families display remarkably little polymorphism. EMBO J. 8, 3471–3478.

Schick, M.R. and Kennedy, R.C. (1989) Production and characterization of anti-idiotypic antibody reagents. Methods Enzymol. 178, 36–48.

Schroeder, H.W., Hillson, J.L. and Perlmutter R.M. (1987) Early restriction of the human antibody repertoire. Science 238, 791–793.

Sha, W.C., Nelson, C.A., Newberry, R.D. et al. (1988) Positive and negative selection of an antigen receptor on T cells in transgenic mice. Nature 336, 73–76.

Shechter, Y., Maron, R., Elias, D. et al. (1982) Autoantibodies to insulin receptor spontaneously develop as anti-idiotypes in mice immunized with insulin. Science 216, 542–545.

Shelton, L.L., Lee, W.M., Curtis, G.M. et al. (1983) Membrane antigens in chronic active hepatitis: physicochemical and immunological studies of soluble liver homogenate fractions. Clin. Immunol. Immunopathol. 28, 135–141.

Shen, A., Humphries, C., Tucker, P. et al. (1987) Human heavy chain variable region gene family nonrandomly rearranged in familial chronic lymphocytic leukemia. Proc. Natl. Acad. Sci. U.S.A. 84, 8563–8567.

Shoenfeld, Y., Hsu-Lin, S.C., Gabriels, J.E. et al. (1982) Production of autoantibodies by human–human hybridomas. J. Clin Invest. 70, 205–208.

Silvestris, F., Bankhurst, A.D., Searles, R.P. et al. (1984) Studies on anti-F(ab′)2 antibodies and possible immunologic control mechanisms in systemic lupus erythematosus. Arthritis Rheum. 27, 1387–1396.

Swanson, N.R., Reed, W.D., Yarred, L.J. et al. (1989) Autoantibodies to isolated human hepatocyte plasma membrane in liver disease. I. Specificity for chronic active hepatitis. Clin. Immunol. Immunopathol. 52, 291–304.

Takeuchi, T., Hosono, O., Koide, J. et al. (1985) Suppression of rheumatoid factor synthesis by anti-idiotypic antibody in rheumatoid arthritis patients with cross-reactive idiotypes. Arthritis Rheum. 28, 873–881.

Taniguchi, O., Chia, D.S. and Barnett, E. (1984) Auto-anti-DNA antibodies from SLE patients and normals. J. Rheumatol. 11, 291–297.

Taub, R. and Greene, M.I. (1992) Functional validation of ligand mimicry by anti-receptor antibodies: structural and therapeutic implications. Biochemistry 31, 7431–7435.

Teuber, J. and Helmke, K. (1981) Immunoregulation by anti-idiotypic antibodies during the course of autoimmune disorders of the thyroid. Immunobiology 160, 120–127.

Tokuhisa, T. and Rajewsky, K. (1985) Antigen induces chronic idiotype suppression. Proc. Natl. Acad. Sci. U.S.A. 82, 4217–4220.

Tomer, Y. and Shoenfeld, Y. (1988) The significance of natural autoantibodies. Immunol. Invest. 17, 389–424.

Troisi, C.L. and Hollinger, F.B. (1985) Detection of an IgM antiidiotype directed against anti-HBs in hepatitis B patients. Hepatology 5, 758–762.

Tsubouchi, A., Yoshioka, K. and Kakumu, S. (1985) Naturally occurring serum antiidiotypic antibody against antiliver-specific membrane lipoprotein in patients with hepatitis. Hepatology 5, 752–757.

Underwood, J.R., Pedersen, J.S., Chalmers, P.J. et al. (1985) Hybrids from normal germfree nude and neonatal mice produce monoclonal autoantibodies to eight different intracellular structures. Clin. Exp. Immunol., 60, 417–426.

Vandenbark, A.A., Hashim, G. and Offner, H. (1989) Immunization with a synthetic T-cell receptor V-region peptide protects against experimental autoimmune encephalomyelitis. Nature 341, 541–544.

Van der Heijden, R.W.J., Bunschoten, H., Pascual, V. et al. (1990) Nucleotide sequence of a human monoclonal anti-idiotypic antibody specific for a rabies virus-neutralizing monoclonal idiotypic antibody reveals extensive somatic variability suggestive of an antigen-driven immune response. J. Immunol. 144, 2835–2839.

Van Es, J.H., Schutte M.E.M., Ebeling, S.B. et al. (1992) Immunoglobulin variable gene expression in human autoantibodies In: C.A. Bona and A.K. Kaushik (Eds.) Molecular Immunobiology of Self-Reactivity. Marcel Dekker, New York, pp. 119–131.

Vergani, G.M., Vergani, D., Jenkins, P.J. et al. (1979) Lymphocyte cytotoxicity to autologous hepatocytes in HBsAg-negative chronic active hepatitis. Clin. Exp. Immunol. 38, 16–21.

Wasserman, N.H., Penn, A.S., Freimuth, P.I. et al. (1983) Anti-idiotypic route to anti-acetylcholine receptor antibodies and experimental myasthenia gravis. Proc. Natl. Acad. Sci. U.S.A. 79, 4810–4814.

Weinberger, J.Z., Germain, R.N., Benacerraf, B. et al. (1980) Hapten-specific T cell responses to 4-hydroxy-3-nitrophenyl acetyl. V. Role of idiotypes in the suppressor pathway. J. Exp. Med. 152, 161–169.

Weksler M.E., Moody, C.E. and Kozak, R.W. (1981) The autologous mixed lymphocyte reaction. Adv. Immunol., 31, 271–312.

Wen, L., Peakman, M., Lobo-Yeo, A. et al. (1991) T-cell-directed hepatocyte damage in autoimmune chronic active hepatitis. Lancet i, 9–15.

Zanetti, M. (1986a) Idiotype network and its relevance to autoimmune diseases. Functional considerations. Concepts Immunopathol. 3, 253–284.

Zanetti, M. (1986b) Idiotypic regulation of autoantibody production. Crit. Rev. Immunol. 6, 151–183.

Zanetti, M., Glotz, R. and Rogers, J. (1986) Pertubation of the autoimmune network. II. Immunization with isologous idiotype induces auto-anti-idiotypic antibodies and suppresses the immune response elicited by antigen. J. Immunol. 137, 3140–3146.

Zanetti, M., Sollazzo, M. and Billetta, R. (1992) Functions and structures in a regulatory network for self-reactivity. In: C.A. Bona, and A.K. Kaushik (Eds.) Molecular Immunobiology of Self-Reactivity. Marcel Dekker, New York, pp. 221–238.
Zauderer, M. (1989) Origin and significance of autoreactive T cells. Adv. Immunol. 45, 417–437.
Zouali, M. and Eyquem, A. (1983) Idiotypic-anti-idiotypic interactions in SLE: demonstration of oscillatory levels of anti-DNA autoantibodies and reciprocal anti-idiotypic activity in a single patient. Ann. Immunol. (Inst. Pasteur) 134C, 377–391.
Zouali, M., Jolivet, M., LeClerc, C. et al. (1985) Suppression of murine lupus autoantibodies to DNA by administration of muramyl dipeptide and syngenetic anti-DNA IgG. J. Immunol. 135, 1091–1096.

Section VI

Genetic Aspects of Autoimmune Hepatitis

Autoimmune Hepatitis
Edited by M. Nishioka, G. Toda and M. Zeniya
© 1994, Elsevier Science B.V. All rights reserved

Chapter 15

Immunogenetic background of autoimmune hepatitis

Brian D. Tait[1] and Ian R. Mackay[2]

[1]*Tissue Typing Laboratory, Centre for Medical Research, Royal Melbourne Hospital, Parkville 3050, Victoria (Australia) and* [2]*Centre for Molecular Biology and Medicine, Monash University, Clayton 3168, Victoria (Australia)*

1. Background

Chronic active hepatitis (CAH) was first recognized as a disease entity in the early 1950s (Mackay, 1975). Most of the early cases described were young females from populations of European origin. Subsequently, such cases were found to have serological markers of autoimmune disease. This type of CAH was soon to become the prototype for the disease and provided the basis for definition by the Fogarty-IASL nomenclature group (Fogarty International Centre and International Association for Study of the Liver Standardization Conference, 1976). Subsequent experience, however, established CAH as an heterogeneous entity (see Chapter 1) with 4 major types being identified.

(1) The autoimmune prototype found predominantly in females (AI-CAH).
(2) The type associated with seropositivity for the hepatitis B surface antigen (HBsAg) and occurring more commonly in males (CAH-B).
(3) A cryptogenic form of the disease with no evident cause or associated serological markers, but now mainly accountable for by infection with hepatitis C virus (CAH-C).
(4) A drug-induced type of CAH (DI-CAH).

There appears to be further clinical and serological heterogeneity within the AI-CAH category. First, there are two distinct peaks of incidence, one in adolescent females (disease onset 10–30 years) and one in older women (50–70 years) (Mackay, 1978), and among the latter, there appears to be co-occurrence of other autoimmune diseases including thyroiditis and Sjögren's syndrome. Second, there is serological heterogeneity with two types, 1 and 2, specified according to reactivity with either nuclei/actin or with liver and kidney microsomes (see Chapter 1).

Despite this apparent disease heterogeneity, the histopathology of AI-CAH and in fact most types of CAH, appears relatively uniform. There are characteristic alterations revealed on liver biopsy, including lymphocyte–plasma cell infiltration into portal tracts and piecemeal necrosis of liver cells extending outward into the parenchyma from the limiting plate, with eventual development of macronodular cirrhosis. The concomitant clinical and genetic subgrouping has permitted the validation of the autoimmune type of CAH as a distinct entity by virtue of its strong HLA associations, which are absent in the virus-associated forms of the disease. This chapter re-examines the HLA association with AI-CAH in the light of advances in our understanding of the structure of HLA gene products and discusses possible mechanisms that may explain the observed associations.

2. *Immunological features of AI-CAH*

One of the major features of CAH is hypergammaglobulinaemia, which in AI-CAH is associated with the presence of autoantibodies of multiple specificities. Unlike various other autoimmune diseases, e.g., myasthenia gravis in which the acetylcholine receptor antibody is clearly organ/tissue specific and can be interpreted as responsible for the disease pathogenesis, the autoantibodies of AI-CAH are non-organ-specific and generally lack disease specificity, although anti-actin is a strong marker for AI-CAH. It is still not clear whether autoantibodies present in AI-CAH are implicated in the disease process, or whether they are simply an end result of cell destruction and the exposure of the immune system to cryptic antigenic epitopes. The autoantibodies observed in AI-CAH include the following.

(1) Anti-nuclear antibody (ANA) which is a common feature of AI-CAH and is detected by immunofluorescence on various substrates. The pattern of nuclear immunofluorescence observed can be homogeneous (usually) or speckled, the former being associated with more severe disease at a young age of onset (Terada et al., 1991). The reactivity is believed to be due to nuclear histones, although ANA with undefined specificities are found in some cases of AI-CAH. Antibodies to double-stranded DNA occur in about 20% of cases of AI-CAH, particularly in the acute phase of the disease (Smeenk et al., 1982).

(2) Smooth muscle antibody (SMA) which is detected by immunofluorescence using a rodent stomach wall substrate and is present in approximately 70% of CAH patients with AI-CAH (Czaja et al., 1983). Using special preparations of substrate (cultured cells or phalloidin-treated rat liver), SMA can be shown to consist of antibodies to components of the cellular cytoskeleton, more

particularly actin in AI-CAH and intermediate filaments in viral types of CAH (Pedersen et al., 1982).

(3) Antibodies to liver and kidney microsomal antigen (LKM-1) are markers for type 2 AI-CAH (Homberg et al., 1987) which is associated with a seemingly different set of extra-hepatic autoimmune diseases from that associated with type 1 AI-CAH. The LKM-1 autoantigen has been shown to be cytochrome P-450 (Manns, 1991).

3. Major histocompatibility complex (MHC) associations with CAH

Most reports on HLA associations with AI-CAH have dealt with Caucasoid populations since the disease is mostly represented among these groups. However, reference is made below to recent results obtained in the Japanese population.

3.1. MHC associations in Caucasoids

In 1971, an association was described between two HLA class I antigens, A1 and B8, and autoimmune chronic active hepatitis (Mackay and Morris, 1972). This finding was confirmed in a larger group of patients where the frequency of B8 was found to be 69% compared with 24% in controls with a relative risk of 7 (Morris et al., 1977). An independent study from Germany (Freudenberg et al., 1977) reported B8 occurring in 82% of patients and 19% of controls with a relative risk of 25. Opelz et al. (1977) first reported an association of CAH with a class II specificity (Dw3) defined by mixed lymphocyte reactivity. The increase in Dw3 appeared to be greater than that seen for B8 which suggested that the primary association was with the class II region and the increase in B8 was merely a result of linkage disequilibrium. The first study of AI-CAH with the serologically defined DR specificities was undertaken as part of the Seventh International Histocompatibility Workshop (Joint Report-Active Chronic Hepatitis, 1977). As expected, DR3 was significantly increased in frequency in a group of 50 Caucasian patients with a particularly strong association in those with a high titre of anti-SMA, and to a lesser extent in those with high titre ANA. The class I specificity B12 and the class II specificity DR5 were decreased in frequency.

Mackay and Tait (1980) studied 43 cases of AI-CAH, confirming the increase in frequency of DR3, and demonstrating a decrease in frequency of both DR2 and DR5. The previously observed decrease in B12 was also observed, which cannot be explained by linkage disequilibrium with either DR2 or DR5, since the two DR alleles in linkage disequilibrium with B12 in Caucasoids are DR4 and DR7, neither being decreased significantly in this study. Associations of HLA alleles with CAH were studied in patients from France, former Yugoslavia and Australia as part of the 8th International Workshop (Tait et al., 1980). In Caucasoid patients, the A1-B8-DR3 association appeared strongest in those patients with high levels of SMA and ANA. Subgrouping of female patients with high-titre autoantibodies, according to age at clinical onset of the disease revealed the A1-B8-DR3 association was most prominent in those patients less than 30 years of age, corresponding to the 'archetypal' cases of AI-CAH reported on in the 1950s and 1960s. Differences in HLA frequencies in female patients included in the 8th International Workshop based on age of disease onset, were also observed in the 2nd Asian and Oceania Workshop (Tait et al., 1981). In addition, the decrease previously seen in B12 (B44) appeared confined to patients with an older age of onset (> 30 years), and was accompanied by a decrease in DR7 suggestive of a haplotype effect. A1-B8-DR3 in the older female group was present in approximately normal frequency, and the increase seen in younger patients was replaced by a significant increase in the B27-Cw1 haplotype.

In the families of 14 probands studied by Mackay and Tait (1980) B8 and DR3 were formally shown to be coded for by genes on the same chromosome, i.e., the same HLA haplotype. In 10 of these cases, the entire A1-B8-DR3 was present. These data suggested that the susceptibility gene(s) were most likely to be located in the B/DR region of the MHC. Subsequently, a study was undertaken in which other markers on the A1-B8-DR3 haplotype were measured to determine whether a subset of this haplotype conferred an increased risk for AI-CAH (Tait et al., 1989). Of particular interest was the diallelic glyoxylase locus which is located at the centromeric end of the MHC, approximately 15 μm from HLA-DP. Both alleles GLO1 and GLO2 occurred in CAH. This was in contrast with data reported for insulin-dependent diabetes mellitus (IDDM or type 1 diabetes), for which a previous report indicated that B8-DR3-GLO1 was not a risk haplotype for disease development (Raum et al., 1984). The reported association of GLO2 with IDDM has not been confirmed, but if true, may indicate that the extended haplotypes in the two diseases are different, suggesting the possibility that influence of the B8-DR3 haplotype in the two diseases is acting by a different mechanism(s).

Eckardt et al. (1989) searched for informative heterogeneity in the A1-B8-DR3 haplotype in AI-CAH by using a representative set of DNA restriction enzymes selected to maximize the number of restriction sites screened, and probed for restriction fragment length polymorphisms (RFLP) with DRB and DQB probes. None of the fragments obtained was informative for AI-CAH when compared with HLA-matched controls. Although no disease related polymorphism was detected, the possibility could not be excluded that a polymorphism existed but was not detected due to an insufficient number of enzymes being used.

There is an absence of studies to date on type 2 LKM-positive AI-CAH. It would be interesting to establish whether there is an A1-B8-DR3 association in this group, since the autoantibody profile is clearly different from that seen in type 1 AI-CAH.

3.2. MHC associations in Japanese

A non-significant increase in DR4 was observed in a group of Japanese patients with CAH-B studied as part of the 8th International Workshop (Tait et al., 1980). More recently, female patients with AI-CAH were studied by Seki et al. (1992). Amplification of the second exon of the DR, DQ, DP genes by the polymerase chain reaction technique was performed and the resultant product digested with restriction enzymes to generate allele-specific fragments. Although DR4 was increased in frequency, no increase in any DR4 subtype was found, suggesting that the association was primarily with the broad DR4 specificity. An observed increase of DQA1*0301 and DQB1*0401 appeared to be due to linkage disequilibrium with DR4. No DP allelic associations were observed in this group of patients. The association with DR4 in Japanese is clearly different from the DR3 association observed in Caucasians. However, it is consistent with the report of Williams et al. (1978) and Donaldson et al. (1991) that DR4 in Caucasians represents a weaker secondary association with AI-CAH. The DR4 association may be more readily observed in Japanese by virtue of the fact that DR3 is absent from this population.

4. Immunoglobulin gene (Gm allotype) association with CAH

Genes coding for immunoglobulin (Gm) allotypes which are found on the heavy chain of IgG exist as haplotypes, some of which have been shown to be increased in frequency in certain diseases, and in some cases Gm alleles have been shown to interact with HLA class II alleles (Farid et al., 1977; Nakao et al., 1980; Whittingham et al., 1983; Tait et al., 1986). A study of Gm allotypes in Caucasoid patients with AI-CAH (Whittingham et al., 1981) revealed interactive effects of allotype Gm a+ x+ b+ with B8 (and presumably DR3 although class II antigens were not tested for) in conferring susceptibility.

5. What genes are responsible for disease susceptibility on the A1-B8-DR3 haplotype?

A1-B8-DR3 represents one of approximately 20 conserved ancestral haplotypes (Tokunaga et al., 1988). It is unique to Caucasoid groups and is the most frequent haplotype, displaying the strongest degree of linkage disequilibrium from HLA-A to HLA-DQ. The alleles which are currently defined and known to comprise this haplotype are shown in Table 1. The A1-B8-DR3 haplotype is often referred to as the autoimmune haplotype because of its association with many diseases of an autoimmune nature, but with differing immunopathology. These

    B.D. Tait and I.R. Mackay

Table 1
Alleles comprising the A1-B8-DR3 autoimmune haplotype

Locus	Allele	Serological specificity
Class 1		
A	A*0101	A1
B	B*0801	B8
C	Cw*0701	Cw7
Class II		
DRB1	DRB1*0301	DR3
DRB3	DRB3*0101	DR52
DQA1	DQA1*0501	
DQB1	DQB1*0201	DQ2
Class III		
Bf	S	
C4A	QO (null)	
C4B	1	
TNF[a]	Ncol 5.5 kb[b]	
HSP 70[a]	Pst-1 8.5 kb[c]	
BAT 2[a]	Rsa-1 2.7 kb[d]	

[a] Defined by RFLP (restriction fragment length polymorphism).
[b] Dawkins et al. (1989a). The 5.5- and 10.5-kb fragments were defined using the Ncol enzyme. The 5.5-kb fragment is associated with the A1-B8-DR3 haplotype.
[c] Caplen et al. (1990). The 8.5- and 9.0-kb fragments were defined using the Pst1 enzyme. The 8.5-kb fragment always occurs in association with C4A null, i.e., the A1-B8-DR3 haplotype.
[d] Fugger et al. (1991). The 3.3-, 2.7- 2.3- and 0.9-kb fragments were defined using the Rsal enzyme. The 2.3-kb fragment is negatively associated with the A1-B8-DR3 haplotype (Williams et al., 1978).

include IDDM, myasthenia gravis, coeliac disease, dermatitis herpetiformis, autoimmune Addison's disease, primary Sjögren's syndrome and AI-CAH. The association of diseases with such widely differing immunopathology and tissue distribution suggests a non-specific effect of this haplotype on disease development, possibly involving a general defect in immune regulation. This is supported by the observation that individuals with the A1-B8-DR3 haplotype may be deficient in antigen degradation (Legrand et al., 1982) and have impaired T-cell responses (Kallenberg et al., 1981).

The critical issue is whether the pathogenic effects are attributable to a single allele at one locus or to a combination of alleles at several loci which combine to cause a 'multiple hit' effect resulting in disease susceptibility. Focussing on the disease-causing gene is made difficult by the extreme linkage disequilibrium of the A1-B8-DR3 haplotype. One approach to overcome this problem is to examine the presence or absence of individual alleles at each of the polymorphic loci on other haplotypes, and determine whether these haplotypes are associated with any increase in susceptibility to the disease in question.

6. Class II loci

6.1. General molecular structure

There are 3 major class II subregions, DR, DQ and DP, each containing several genes. In each region, the product expressed on the cell surface is a dimer, consisting of the product of an A-gene (α-chain) and the product of a B-gene (β-chain). In the DR subregion, there is a non-polymorphic DRA gene, the product of which can form a dimer with the product of each of the 4 expressed DRB genes (DRB1, DRB3, DRB4 and DRB5). The DRB1 gene is highly polymorphic and codes for the serologically defined series of DR epitopes. The DRB3 gene has limited polymorphism with 4 identified alleles and is located on DR3, DR5 and DR6 haplotypes. The DRB4 gene is non-polymorphic, and the DRA/DRB4 dimer is present on DR4, DR7 and DR9 haplotypes. The DRB5 gene has 4 identified alleles occurring on different DR2 haplotypes. All haplotypes, therefore, code for an expressed DRA/DRB1 dimer and either DRA/DRB3, DRA/DRB4 or DRA/DRB5, depending on the haplotype involved. In the DQ and DP subregions there is one set of expressed genes DQA1, DQB1 and DPA1, DPB1 and one set of non-expressed genes DQA2, DQB2 and DPA2, DPB2. Unlike the DRA gene both DQA1 and DPA1 are polymorphic. The A1-B8-DR3 haplotype, therefore, expresses the following class II dimeric molecules: DRA1/DRB1, DRA1/DRB3, DQA1/DQB1 and DPA1/DPB1.

The majority of sequence differences in the class II genes resulting in amino acid substitutions are found in the second exon coding for the first domain of the molecule which forms an integral part of the peptide binding groove of the MHC class II molecule. The sequences coding for the serologically defined specificities are mainly found in the first hypervariable region which is located in the floor of the groove. Alleles that share common sequences in this region differ at other hypervariable regions, and hence serologically defined epitopes can be shared by several allelic products. The nomenclature discriminates between alleles and serologically defined epitopes (antigens). For example, the sequence that specifies DR3 is found on two alleles, DRB1*0301 and DRB1*0302. The first 4 letters refer to the locus DRB1, the first two numbers to the serological epitope coded for by the allele 03 (DR3) and the last two numbers indicate the subtype. The reader is referred to the most recent WHO nomenclature report for a detailed listing (Bodmer et al., 1992).

6.2. Individual class II genes conferring susceptibility

The selective presentation of either viral or self-peptide to cytotoxic and helper T-cells by both class I and class II molecules, respectively, is the most likely mechanism to explain many HLA and disease associations. Amino acid substitutions at critical hypervariable sites on the class II MHC molecule appear to influence the interaction of peptide with the class II binding site and the ensuing recognition of the complex by the T-cell receptor (Falk et al., 1991; Geluk et al., 1992). Experiments in mice involving site-directed mutagenesis have demonstrated that one or two amino acid substitutions within the class II molecule can result in failure of T-cell recognition (Ronchese et al., 1987). It follows, therefore, that allelic sequences resulting in amino acid substitutions may confer either susceptibility or resistance to particular molecules by virtue of their ability to bind disease-related peptides, i.e., virally-derived peptide or endogenous protein-derived autopeptide.

6.3. DRB1 and DRB3 loci

In vitro experiments that measure T-cell responsiveness have demonstrated that some peptides are able to bind to only one, or a limited range of class II molecules. For example, a peptide derived from the heat shock protein (HSP) 65 of mycobacteria binds only to the DR3 molecule which is coded for by DRB1*0301 (Geluk et al., 1992). This finding is particularly relevant to many DR3-associated autoimmune diseases. The generation of cytotoxic T-cells with specificity for a bacterial HSP-derived peptide may result in the destruction of cells, with release of self peptides and precipitation of an autoimmune response in genetically susceptible individuals. The conservation of HSP sequences during evolution (Hunt and Morimoto, 1985) suggests this observed DRB1*0301 association may have wider implications with respect to other organisms which may initiate autoimmune disease. The DRB1*0301 allele, however, exists as part of other haplotypes, e.g., A30-B18-DR3 which is not associated with autoimmunity in general. Hence an involvement of the DRB1*0301 product in presentation of disease-related peptide cannot be the sole explanation for the association of the A1-B8-DR3 haplotype with autoimmune disease. The product of the DRB3 locus expressed on DR3, DR5 and DR6 haplotypes has been shown to bind peptides and act as a restriction element (O'Sullivan et al., 1990). The DRB3 allele on the B8-DR3 haplotype (DRB3*0101) is unique and distinct from the DRB3 allele on the B18-DR3 haplotype (DRB3*0201) (Bontrop et al., 1987) with substitutions of amino acid residues at positions 11, 26, 28, 30, 37, 38, 51, 57, 60, 74 and 86 (Gregersen et al., 1987). These changes are sufficient to alter the peptide-binding property of the molecule. The possibility exists, therefore, that the DRB3 product on the A1-B8-DR3 haplotype can act as a unique restriction element for a relevant disease-related peptide.

6.4. DQ loci

Both α- and β-chains contribute to DQ polymorphism in contrast to the DR molecules in which the α-chain is invariant. The DQ alleles associated with the A1-B8-DR3 haplotype are DQA1*0501 and DQB1*0201. These DQ α- and

β-alleles occur in linkage disequilibrium with other DR alleles; for example, DQB1*0201 is present on some DR7 haplotypes but this particular α, β combination is unique to DR3 haplotypes. The same combination, however, is also present on the B18-DR3 haplotype and so does not readily explain the autoimmune nature of the A1-B8-DR3 haplotype.

6.5. DP loci

There are reports indicating HLA-DP associations with some autoimmune diseases (Hoffman et al., 1986; Bugawan et al., 1989; Easteal et al., 1990) suggesting that this locus may also confer degrees of susceptibility. In the normal Caucasian population, DRB1*0301 is in linkage disequilibrium with DPB1*0101 (Tait et al., 1992a). In IDDM, the majority of DR3 haplotypes appear to be DPB1*0401 or DPB1*0301 (Tait et al., 1992b) suggesting DP or a closely linked gene makes an additional contribution to susceptibility. It would be of interest to examine the DP status of DR3-positive patients with AI-CAH, but this study has not been performed to date.

7. Class I loci

The class I alleles HLA-A1 and HLA-B8 found on the A1-B8-DR3 haplotype are also located on other haplotypes which do not confer susceptibility and there is no evidence that these serologically identical specificities on the various haplotypes differ in amino acid sequence.

The conclusion to be drawn from these data, therefore, is that with the exception of the DRB3 gene, there is little evidence that susceptibility is conferred by a single allele or locus of any of the known HLA class I and class II loci on the A1-B8-DR3 haplotype. Hence the question remains whether there are individual polymorphisms at other loci on this haplotype that are responsible for susceptibility, or whether there is a 'haplotype effect', i.e., a synergistic effect of several susceptibility loci acting in concert at various stages of immune responsiveness. This synergistic effect could include molecules responsible for antigen presentation to helper and cytotoxic T-cells (class II and class I molecules), cytokines (tumour necrosis factor (TNF)-α and -β), complement factors (C2, C4, BF (properdin factor)) and possibly other molecules of unknown function including the products of the B-associated transcripts' (BAT) genes (see below).

8. Other MHC loci

There are other candidate gene loci within the MHC responsible for autoimmunity including genes for TNF-α and -β, HSP 70, serum complement (C4A,

C4B, Bf) and the BAT proteins. Limited polymorphism of the TNF genes has been demonstrated including a polymorphism found on the B8-DR3 haplotype (Dawkins et al., 1989a). There is some evidence that this polymorphism may be translated into functional differences, since individuals with this haplotype have been reported to secrete high levels of TNF-α and -β on stimulation (Jacob et al., 1990). Also, polymorphism of the HSP 70 genes has been described, but in the absence of any functional correlation (Caplen et al., 1990).

Polymorphisms of the BAT genes exist in association with the B8-DR3 haplotype (Fugger et al., 1991), but the function of these genes has not been elucidated.

The B8-DR3 haplotype includes a deletion of the complement C4A gene (i.e., C4A null), but with an expressed gene on the second haplotype, the level of serum complement detected in individuals with this haplotype is associated at most with only marginal complement deficiency. It is possible, however, that a marginal deficiency may result in impaired viral clearance which in turn could act as a trigger for autoimmune disease.

Genes have recently been mapped in the class II region between DQ and DP (Spies et al., 1990; Glynne et al., 1991; Robertson, 1991) which encode products that appear to exert a central role in both proteolysis of exogenous and endogenous proteins, and the transport of resultant peptides into the endoplasmic reticulum for presentation on class I molecules (Robertson, 1991).

The genes coding for the proteolytic enzymes are referred to as LMP-7 (or Ring 10) and LMP-2 (or Ring 12) and the transporter molecules are termed TAP-1 (Ring 4) and TAP-2 (Ring 11) (Bodmer et al., 1992). Polymorphisms of the Tap-1 and Tap-2 genes have been described, (Powis et al., 1992) including one which appears to be associated with IDDM (Colonna et al., 1992), but no associated functional correlations have been found to date. The number of proteolytic and transporter genes, and the uniqueness of any polymorphisms on the A1-B8-DR3 haplotype have not been described.

9. *Haplotype effects*

The autoimmune properties of the A1-B8-DR3 haplotype according to available evidence must depend on either a single as yet unidentified allele at a single gene locus within the A1-B8-DR3 haplotype or a combination of alleles at several loci. One intriguing aspect of the A1-B8-DR3 haplotype is that it is the haplotype with the strongest degree of linkage disequilibrium between the A and DQ loci. This extreme linkage disequilibrium infers that the maintenance of a number of alleles operating in tandem has resulted in a survival advantage. This advantage at a functional level is likely to be related to optimal immune responsiveness to the point of 'overbalance' in the direction of autoimmunity. The combination of alleles which confer this hyper-responsiveness, or the mechanisms by which it is achieved, have not yet been identified. It is interesting to speculate that the A1-B8-DR3 haplotype which in evolutionary terms is the most recent, with extensive gene duplications and deletions (Dawkins et al., 1989b) may have lost critical regulatory genes (perhaps immune-suppressor genes) during this formative process, shifting the balance of immune regulation towards hyper-responsiveness and susceptibility to autoimmune disease. It is important to stress, however, in the context of autoimmune disease, in general, and CAH, in particular, that the development of clinical disease may also be dependent on a number of non-MHC genes such as those encoding the T-cell receptor, immunoglobulins and various cytokines. Whether it is possible to dissect the influence of these genes in terms of disease-related polymorphisms or demonstrate their interaction with MHC genes, remains to be determined.

10. Future directions

The improved identification of autoantibody specificities with cloning and sequencing of autopeptides and resultant clinical subgrouping, in parallel with an expanding knowledge of MHC genes and their function, is required for an unravelling of the genetic and environmental interactions which result in CAH. With the sequencing of autoantigens, such as actin and LKM-1, and the recognition of immunodominant epitopes, it should be possible to examine in vitro, T-cell responsiveness to peptides derived from these antigens presented on various class I and class II HLA molecules. The eluting and sequencing of peptides (Rudensky et al., 1991) from antigen-presenting cells of normals and patients with CAH at different stages of the disease could indicate which peptides are likely to be relevant to the disease process, and their likely origin.

The complete mapping of the A1-B8-DR3 haplotype and its comparison with non-autoimmune haplotypes will indicate where deletions or change in gene number have occurred. The elucidation of the precise function of many of the non-HLA MHC genes will be required before their contribution to the autoimmune disease process can be fully appreciated. Finally, an understanding of the mechanism of interaction of MHC genes with non-MHC genes in conferring susceptibility will complete the picture.

References

Bodmer, J.G., Marsh, S.G.E., Albert, E.D., Bodmer, W.F., Dupont, B., Erlich, H.A., Mach, B., Mayr, W.R., Parham, P., Sasazuki, T., Schreuder, G.M.T., Strominger, J.L., Svejgaard., A. and Terasaki, P.I. (1992) Nomenclature for factors of the HLA system 1991. Tissue Antigens 39, 161–173.
Bontrop, R., Ballas, M., Madrigal, A., Hermans, P., Fuggle, S., Otting, N., Carter, C., Sacks, S., Kaplan, C., Morel, M.-C., Radka, S.F., Nepom, B., Bow, L., DuToit, E., Crawford, S., Knitter-Jack, N.,

Nepom, G., Mazzilli, M.C., Brahmi, Z. and Charron, D. (1987) DRW52: 2-D gel patterns. In: B. Dupont (Ed.), Immunobiology of HLA, Vol. 1, Springer, New York, pp. 401–404.

Bugawan, T.L., Angelini, G., Larrick, J., Auricchio, S., Ferrara, G.B. and Erlich, H.A. (1989) A combination of a particular HLA-DP beta allele and an HLA-DQ heterodimer confers susceptibility to coeliac disease. Nature 339, 470–473.

Caplen, N.J., Patel, A., Millward, A., Campbell, R.D., Ratanachaiyavong, S., Wong, F.S. and Demaine, A.G. (1990) Complement C4 and heat shock protein 70 (hsp) genotypes and type 1 diabetes. Immunogenetics 32, 427–430.

Collona, M., Bresnahan, M., Bahram, S., Strominger, J.L. and Spies, T. (1992) Allelic variants of the human putative peptide transporter involved in antigen processing. Proc. Natl. Acad. Sci. U.S.A. 89, 3932–3936.

Czaja, A.J., Davis, G.L., Ludwig, J., Baggenstoss, A.H. and Taswell, H.F. (1983) Autoimmune features as determinants of prognosis in steroid treated chronic active hepatitis of uncertain etiology. Gastroenterology 85, 713–717.

Dawkins, R.L., Leaver, A., Cameron, P.U., Martin, E., Kay, P.H. and Christiansen, F.T. (1989a) Some disease-associated ancestral haplotypes carry a polymorphism of TNF. Human Immunol. 26, 91–97.

Dawkins, R.L., Kay, P.H., Martin, E., and Christiansen, F.T. (1989b) The genomic structure of ancestral haplotypes revealed by pulsed field gel electrophoresis (PFGE). In: B. Dupont, (Ed.) Immunobiology of HLA. Histocompatibility Testing 1987. Springer, New York, pp. 893–895.

Donaldson, P.T., Doherty, D.G., Hayllar, K.M., McFarlane, I.G., Johnson, P.J. and Williams, R. (1991) Susceptibility to autoimmune chronic active hepatitis: human leukocyte antigens DR4 and A1-B8-DR3 are independent risk factors. Hepatology 13, 701–706.

Easteal, S., Kohonen-Corish, M.R.J., Zimmet, P. and Serjeantson, S.W. (1990) HLA-DP variation as additional risk factor in IDDM. Diabetes 39, 855–857.

Eckardt, G.S., O'Brien, R.M., Mackay, I.R., DeMartinis, L. and Tait, B.D. (1989) Lack of informative HLA restriction fragment length polymorphisms in autoimmune chronic active hepatitis. Tissue Antigens 34, 270–278.

Falk, K., Rotzschke, O., Stevanovic, S., Jung, G. and Rammensee, H.-G. (1991) Allele specific motifs revealed by sequencing of self peptides eluted from MHC molecules. Nature 351, 290–296.

Farid, N.R., Newton, R.M., Noel, E.P. and Marshall, W.H. (1977) Gm phenotypes in autoimmune thyroid disease. J. Immunogenet. 4, 429–432.

Fogarty International Centre and International Association for Study of the Liver Standardization Conference (1976) Fogarty International Centre Proceedings No. 22 Dhew Publications No (NIH) 76-725, Bethesda, MD, 1–212.

Freudenberg, J., Baumann, H., Arnold, W., Berger, J. and Meyer zum Buschenfelde, K.-H. (1977) HLA in different forms of chronic active hepatitis. A comparison between adult patients and children. Digestion 15, 260–270.

Fugger, L., Morling, N., Ryder, L.P., Jakobsen, B.K., Anderson, V., Oxholm, P., Dalhoff, K., Heilmann, C., Pedersen, F.K., Friis, J., Halberg, P., Spies, T., Strominger, J.L. and Svejgaard, A. (1991) Restriction fragment length polymorphism of two HLA-B associated transcript genes in five autoimmune diseases. Human Immunol. 30, 27–31.

Geluk, A., Bloemhoff, W., De Vries, R.R.P. and Ottenhoff, T.H.M. (1992) Binding of a major T cell epitope of mycobacteria to a specific pocket within HLA-DRW17 (DR3) molecules. Eur. J. Immunol. 22, 107–113.

Glynne, R., Powis, S.H., Beck, S., Kelly, A., Kerr, L.-A. and Trowsdale, J. (1991) A proteasome related gene between the two ABC transporter loci in the class II region of the human MHC. Nature 353, 357–360.

Gregersen, P.K., Todd, J.A., Erlich, H.A., Long, E., Servenius, B., Choi, E., Hung, T.K., and Lee, J.S. (1987) First domain sequence diversity of DR and DQ subregion alleles. In: B. Dupont (Ed.) Immunobiology of HLA, Vol. 1, Springer, New York, pp. 1027–1031.

Hoffman, R.W., Shaw, S., Francis, L.C., Larsen, M.G., Petersen, R.A., Chylack, L.T. and Glass, D.N. (1986) HLA-DP antigens in patients with pauciarticular juvenile rheumatoid arthritis. Arthritis Rheum. 29, 1057–1062.

Homberg, J.C., Abraf, N., Bernard, O., Islam, S., Alvarez, F., Khalil, S.M., Poupon, R., Darnis, F., Levy, V.G., Grippon, P., Opolon, P., Bernuau, J., Benhamou, J.-P. and Alagille, D. (1987) Chronic active hepatitis associated with antiliver/kidney microsome antibody type 1: a second type of autoimmune hepatitis. Hepatology 7, 1333–1339.

Hunt, C. and Morimoto, R.I. (1985) Conserved features of eukaryotic hsp 70 genes revealed by comparison with the nucleotide sequence of human hsp70. Proc. Natl. Acad. Sci. U.S.A. 82, 6455–6459.

Jacob, C.O., Fronek, Z., Lewis, G.D., Koo, M., Hansen, J.A. and McDevitt, H.O. (1990) Heritable major histocompatibility complex class 2 associated differences in production of tumour necrosis factor alpha: relevance to genetic pre-disposition to systemic lupus erythematosus. Proc. Natl. Acad. Sci. U.S.A. 87, 1233–1237.

Joint Report-Active Chronic Hepatitis (1977) In: Bodmer, W.F., Batchelor, J.R., Bodmer, J.G., Festenstein, H., Morris, P.J. (Eds.) Histocompatibility Testing 1977. Munksgaard, Copenhagen, pp. 214–217.

Kallenberg, C.G.M., Van Der Voort-Beelen, J.M., D'Amaro, J. and The, T.H. (1981) Increased frequency of B8/DR3 in scleroderma and association of the haplotype with impaired cellular immune response. Clin. Exp. Immunol. 43, 478–485.

Legrand, L., Rivat-Perran, L., Huttin, C. and Dausset, J. (1982) HLA and Gm-linked genes affecting the degradation rate of antigens (sheep red blood cells) endocytized by macrophages. Hum. Immunol. 4, 1–13.

Mackay, I.R. (1975) Chronic active hepatitis. In: L. Van Der Reis (Ed.) Frontiers of Gastrointestinal Research, Vol. 1, Karger, Basel, pp. 142–187.

Mackay, I.R. (1978) Chronic active hepatitis, cirrhosis and other diseases of the liver. In: M. Samter (Ed.) Immunological Disease, 3rd edn., Little Brown, Boston, pp. 1454–1477.

Mackay, I.R. and Morris, P.J. (1972) Association of autoimmune active chronic hepatitis with HLA-A1, 8. Lancet 2, 793–795.

Mackay, I.R. and Tait, B.D. (1980) HLA associations with autoimmune type chronic active hepatitis: identification of B8-DRw3 haplotype by family studies. Gastroenterology 79, 95–98.

Manns, M.P. (1991) Liver kidney microsomal autoantibodies and their antigens in chronic hepatitis. In: M. Tsuchiwa et al. (Eds.) Frontiers of Mucosal Immunology, Vol. 2, Elsevier, Amsterdam, pp. 47–51.

Morris, P.J., Vaughan, H., Tait, B.D. and Mackay, I.R., (1977) Histocompatibility antigens (HLA): association with immunopathic diseases and with response to microbial antigens. Aust. N.Z. J. Med. 7, 616–624.

Nakao, Y., Matsumoto, H., Miyazaki, T., Nishitani, H., Ota, K., Fujita, T. and Tsuji, K. (1980) Gm allotypes in myasthenia gravis. Lancet 1, 677–680.

Opelz, G., Vogten, A.J.M., Summerskill, W.H.J., Schalm, S.W. and Terasaki, P.I. (1977) HLA determinants in chronic active liver disease: possible relation of HLA-DW3 to prognosis. Tissue Antigens 9, 36–40.

O'Sullivan, D., Sidney, J., Appella, E., Walker, L., Phillips, L., Colon, S.M., Miles, C., Chesnut, R.W. and Sette, A. (1990) Characterization of the specificity of peptide binding to four DR haplotypes. J. Immunol. 145, 1799–1808.

Pedersen, J.S., Toh, B.H., Mackay, I.R., Tait, B.D., Gust, I.D., Kastelan, A. and Hadzic, N. (1982) Segregation of autoantibody to cytoskeletal filaments, actin, and intermediate filaments with two types of chronic active hepatitis. Clin. Exp. Immunol. 48, 527–532.

Powis, S.H., Mockridge, I., Kelly, A., Kerr, L.-A., Glynne, R., Gileadi, U., Beck, S. and Trowsdale, J. (1992) Polymorphism in a second ABC transporter gene located within the class II region of the human major histocompatibility complex. Proc. Natl. Acad. Sci. U.S.A. 89, 1463–1467.

Raum, D., Awdeh, Z., Yunis, E.J., Alper, C.A. and Gabbay, K.H. (1984) Extended major histocompatibility complex haplotypes in type I diabetes mellitus. J. Clin. Invest. 74, 449–454.

Robertson, M. (1991) Proteosomes in the pathway. Nature 353, 300–301.

Ronchese, F., Brown, M.A. and Germain, R.N. (1987) Structure–function analysis of the A mutation using site-directed mutagensis and DNA mediated gene transfer. J. Immunol. 139, 629–638.

Rudensky, A.Y., Preston-Hurlburt, P., Hong, S.-C., Barlow, A. and Janeway, C.A. (1991) Sequence analysis of peptides bound to MHC class II molecules. Nature 353, 622–627.

Seki, T., Ota, M., Furuta, S., Fukushima, H., Kondo, T., Hino, K., Mizuki, N., Ando, A., Tsuji, K., Inoko, H. and Kiyosawa, K. (1992) HLA class II molecules and autoimmune hepatitis susceptibility in Japanese patients. Gastroenterology 103, 1041–1047.

Smeenk, R., Van der Lelij, G., Swaak, T., Groenwold, J. and Aarden, L. (1982) Specificity in systemic lupus erythematosus of antibodies to double-stranded DNA measured with polyethylene glycol precipitation assay. Arthritis Rheum. 25, 631–638.

Spies, T., Bresnahan, M., Barham, S., Arnold, D., Blanck, G., Mellins, E., Pious, D. and DeMars, R. (1990) A gene in the human major histocompatibility complex class II region controlling the class I antigen presentation pathway. Nature 348, 744–747.

Tait, B.D., Mackay, I.R., Kastelan, A., Dausset, J., Mayer, S. and Okochi, K. (1980) Chronic liver disease including chronic active hepatitis. In: P.I. Terasaki (Ed.) Histocompatibility Testing 1980. UCLA Tissue Typing Laboratory, pp. 657–661.

Tait, B.D., Mackay, I.R., Whittingham, S., Gust, I., Kirk, R., Hirota, M., Naito, S., Takata, H., Chandanayingyong, D. and Lingao, A. (1981) In: M.J. Simons., B.D. Tait (Eds.) Proceedings of the Second Asian and Oceania Histocompatibility Workshop Conference. Immunopublishing, Melbourne, pp. 316–331.

Tait, B.D., Propert, D.N., Harrison, L.C., Mandel, T. and Martin, F.I.R. (1986) Interaction between HLA antigens and immunoglobulin (Gm) allotypes in susceptibility to type I diabetes. Tissue Antigens 27, 249–255.

Tait, B.D., Mackay I.R., Board, P., Coggan, M., Emery, P. and Eckardt, G. (1989) HLA A1 B8 DR3 extended haplotypes in autoimmune chronic hepatitis. Gastroenterology 97, 479–481.

Tait, B.D., Bodmer, J.G., Erlich, H.A., Ferrara, G.B., Albert, E., Begovich, A., Kimura, A., Varney, M.D. and Klitz, W. (1992a) DNA typing: DPA and DPB analysis. In: HLA 1991. Proceedings of the 11th International Histocompatibility Workshop, Yokohama, 1991.

Tait, B.D., Harrison, L.C., Drummond, B.P., Stewart, V., Varney, M.D. and Honeyman, M.C. (1992b) HLA heterogeneity associated with age at diagnosis of insulin dependent diabetes, submitted.

Terada, S., Hong, S.H., Watanabe, Y., Morshed, S.A. and Nishioka, M. (1991) Analysis of antinuclear antibodies (ANA) in autoimmune hepatitis. In: M. Tsuchiya et al. (Eds.) Frontiers of Mucosal Immunology, Vol. 2, Elsevier, Amsterdam, pp. 39–42.

Tokunaga, K., Saueracker, G., Kay, P.H., Christiansen, F.T., Anand, R. and Dawkins, R.L. (1988) Extensive deletions and insertions in different MHC supratypes detected by pulsed gel electrophoresis. J. Exp. Med. 168, 933–940.

Whittingham, S., Mathews, J.D., Schanfield, M.S., Tait, B.D. and Mackay, I.R. (1981) Interaction of HLA and Gm in autoimmune chronic active hepatitis. Clin. Exp. Immunol. 43, 80–86.

Whittingham, S., Mathews, J.D., Schanfield, M.S., Tait, B.D. and Mackay, I.R. (1983) HLA and Gm genes in systemic lupus erythematosus. Tissue Antigens 21, 50–57.

Williams, R.M., Martin, S., Falchuk, K.R., Trey, C., Dubey, D.P., Cannady, W.G., Fitzpatrick, D., Noreen, H., Dupont, B. and Yunis, E.J. (1978) Increased frequency of DRW4 in chronic active hepatitis. Vox Sang. 35, 366–369.

Autoimmune Hepatitis
Edited by M. Nishioka, G. Toda and M. Zeniya
© *1994, Elsevier Science B.V. All rights reserved*

Chapter 16

Genetic background of autoimmune hepatitis in Japan

Mikio Zeniya, Fumitoki Watanabe, Yoshio Aizawa,

and Gotaro Toda

Department of Internal Medicine I, The Jikei University School of Medicine, Tokyo (Japan)

1. Introduction

Autoimmune-type chronic active hepatitis (AI-CAH) is a specific form of liver disease in which immune reactions against autoantigens are believed to be the major pathogenesis. This particular disease was first described by Waldenström (Waldenström, 1950), followed by the report by Kunkel (Kunkel et al., 1951) as an immune-associated disease featured by lupus erythematosus (LE) cell phenomenon. Later, Mackay et al. (Mackay et al., 1956) advocated the term 'lupoid hepatitis' to this disease, i.e., CAH with immune system disorders characterized by LE cell phenomenon. Though the vicissitude of the clinical entity of this disease was fully described in Mackay et al.'s report, with the description of anti-smooth muscle antibodies (anti-SMA) (Whittingham et al., 1966) and a distinct difference between lupoid hepatitis and systemic lupus erythematosus, this disease was defined and named 'autoimmune hepatitis' (AIH).

Nowadays, AIH is regarded as a clinical syndrome distinguished by features such as a predominant occurrence in women, familial occurrence, frequent association with other autoimmune disorders and the appearance of various serum autoantibodies, It has been well documented that genetic factors might play an important role in the pathogenesis of AIH.

During the last decade, analytical methods at the molecular level have greatly progressed. It was shown that by using clones that can recognize autoantigen(s) the immunopathogenesis of autoimmune disorders could be identified. Furthermore, the genes responsible for altered immune functions such as autoimmune processes are postulated to be closely linked to HLA genes and these HLA phenotypes may restrict the disease susceptibility of autoimmune diseases including AIH.

In this chapter, renewal analysis of HLA phenotype and molecular analysis of susceptible genes for AIH in Japan are discussed.

2. Geographic differences of HLA haplotypes

Interestingly, there are marked geographic differences in the frequency of AIH between Western and Asian countries. In Southeast Asia, the carrier rate of the hepatitis B virus (HBV) is clearly high compared to Western countries, and AIH is less common, whereas in the U.K., AIH is one of the major causes of liver cirrhosis. The environmental and socioeconomic state can partly explain such geographic variation. However, genetic background expressed by HLA is also one of the candidates to induce such different susceptibility for AIH and viral hepatitis (Zeniya et al., 1993). Table 1 shows the different HLA frequencies between Caucasians and Japanese. There are marked differences of HLA phenotypes between Caucasians and Japanese in both class I and class II HLA. HLA-A1, -A28, -B8, -Cw3, -Cw4, -Cw5 and -DR3 are more frequent in Caucasians. On the other hand, the frequency of HLA-A9, -A24, -A11 -A31, -Bw52, -Bw22, -Bw54, -Cw1, -DR4, -DRw8, and -DRw9 is higher in the Japanese population. Furthermore, there was different HLA phenotypic linkage between Japanese and Caucasians (Table 2).

In 1976, Mackay and Morris reported (Mackay and Morris, 1976) a strong association between HLA-A1 and -B8, the association rate was 60 and 68%, respectively, among the patients, most of whom were diagnosed as autoimmune-type chronic hepatitis. Later, the HLA-A1 excess was attributed to the linkage disequilibrium of the gene for A1 with that for HLA-B8. This observation further extended to all definitely diagnosed AIH, and 69% were typed as HLA-B8. With reference to the HLA-C locus, Lepage (Lepage et al., 1981) reported there was an association between Cw7 and AIH. In 1977, it was reported in the Seventh International Histocompatibility Workshop (Bodmer et al., 1978) that the frequency of DR3 had significantly increased and HLA-DR2 and -DR5 had decreased in AIH (Opelz et al., 1977). Moreover, it was confirmed that most of the cases carried both HLA-DR3 and -B8, indicating that a much stronger linkage disequilibrium between HLA-DR3 and -B8 existed (Mackay et al., 1956). In Europe, especially in Germany, the frequency of HLA-B8 was 82% in patients who satisfied the criteria for AIH (Freudenberg et al., 1977). Furthermore, in the U.K., it was reported there was corroboration of the increase in HLA-B8 and -DR3 in AIH (Eddleston et al., 1978). These reports confirmed that there may be major histocompatibility-linked gene effects in AIH associated with both susceptibility to and outcome of the disease and HLA-B8/DR3 may identify a 'core' group within the general category of AIH. In Japan, however, these HLA

Table 1
Racial difference of HLA frequencies

HLA	Japanese ($n=472$)	North Am. Caucasoid ($n=236$)	Australian Caucasoid ($n=144$)	HLA	Japanese ($n=472$)	North Am. Caucasoid ($n=236$)	Australian Caucasoid ($n=144$)
A1	1.3	28.2	32.4	B27	0.4	11	4.9
A2	40.7	49.3	48.6	B35	15.5	15	17.6
A3	1.5	23.3	26.1	B37	1.4	3.5	2.8
A9	69	24.7	19	B40	33.7	11	15.5
A23	0	7.9	4.9	Bw60	10.6	7.5	8.5
A24	68.4	14.1	14.1	Bw61	23.8	3.1	5.7
A10	21.4	11.9	9.1	Bw41	0.3	0.9	0.7
A25	0	3.5	3.5	Bw42	0.3	0	0
A26	21.2	7.6	5.6	Bw46	10.1	0	0
Aw34	0	0.9	0	Bw47	0	1.3	0
Aw66	0	0	0	Bw48	4.6	0.9	0
A11	17.1	9.2	10.6	Bw53	0	0	0
Aw19	21.6	25.1	27.5	Bw59	7	1.3	0
A29	0	6.1	5.6	Bw67	1.2	0	0
A30	0.5	4.4	8.5	Bw70	1.8	0.5	1.4
A31	12.5	4.8	3.5	Bw71	0	1	1.4
A32	0	7.5	9.2	Bw72	0	0	0
Aw33	9.5	2.6	2.1	Bw73	0	0	0
A28	0.2	10.8	5.6	Bw4	55.9	65	62.3
Aw68	0.6	0.9	3.5	Bw6	89.8	86.4	84.3
Aw69	0.6	0.9	2.1	Cw1	27.6	9.4	4.7
Aw36	0	0	0	Cw2	0	11.1	3.9
Aw43	0	0	0	Cw3	49.3	23.7	29.7
B5	36.2	15.8	9.2	Cw4	7.2	21.6	21.1
B51	14.2	11.4	6.3	Cw5	0.5	13.7	18.8
Bw52	23.5	3.9	1.4	Cw6	1.9	13.9	16.4
B7	12.9	16.7	19	Cw7	22.8	33	33.1
B8	0	18.9	26.1	Cw8	0.2	3.6	0.8
B12	10.8	20.6	31.7	DR1	12.4	16.9	18.9
B44	10.8	18	29.6	DR2	34.3	27.4	26.8
B45	0	1.8	2.1	DR3	0	21.9	21.2
B13	3.8	5.3	5.6	DR4	41.6	29.9	26.8
B14	0	7	6.3	DR5	18.7	27.9	22.8
Bw64	0	0	2.6	DRw11	6.1	7.8	7.3
Bw65	0	3.9	2.6	DRw12	7.6	9.7	5.5
B15	17.2	11.8	7	DRw6	16.1	20.4	22.8
Bw62	15.5	9.2	6.3	DRw13	6.2	7.3	7.3
Bw63	0.4	2.2	0.7	DRw14	5.5	4.7	8.7
B16	7.4	12.7	5.6	DR7	0.9	22.9	31.5
B38	0	7.5	1.4	DRw8	24.8	7.5	5.5
B39	7.2	4.8	4.2	DRw9	26.1	4.5	3.2
B17	0.6	10.1	10.6	DRw10	0.9	4	0
Bw57	0.2	7	8.5	DRw52	52.3	64.7	59.2
Bw58	0.5	1.8	2.8	DRw53	64.9	51.7	60.8
B18	0	8.3	8.5	DQw1	64.4	57.2	61.6
B21	0	7.5	4.2	DQw2	0.7	35.8	42.9
B49	0	3.1	2.1	DQw3	54.7	57.7	60
Bw50	0	4.4	2.1	TA10	18.6	13.8	70.6
Bw22	19.1	3.9	5.6	DQwA	10.2	8.3	0
Bw54	14	0	0				
Bw55	3.8	3.5	4.2				
Bw56	1.3	0.4	0.7				

Table 2
Haplotype frequencies with significant linkage disequilibria

Japanese ($n=472$)			North American Caucasoid ($n=236$)			Australian Caucasoid ($n=144$)		
HLA-A	HLA-B	$\chi^{2\,a}$	HLA-A	HLA-B	$\chi^{2\,a}$	HLA-A	HLA-B	$\chi^{2\,a}$
A1	B37	191.7	A1	B8	67.8	A1	B8	60.3
A1	Bw57	71.7	A23	Bw50	25.4	A31	Bw56	27.6
A3	B44	27.1	A25	B18	31.7			
A24	Bw52	42.9	Aw34	B45	27.1			
A11	Bw67	25.2	Aw33	Bw58	35.5			
Aw33	B44	279.9	Aw69	Bw65	24.7			
HLA-B	HLA-DR	$\chi^{2\,a}$	HLA-B	HLA-DR	$\chi^{2\,a}$	HLA-B	HLA-DR	$\chi^{2\,a}$
B7	DR1	255	B8	DR3	72.7	B7	DR2	21.4
Bw52	DR2	147.8	B13	DR7	23.9	B8	DR3	64.2
Bw54	DR4	38.7	Bw57	DR7	21.1	Bw63	DRw9	30.5
Bw59	DR4	31.1	Bw48	DRw9	20.6			
B44	DRw11	24.3	B57	DRw10	27.4			
B44	DRw13	122.2						
Bw57	DR7	140.7						
Bw46	DRw8	58						
Bw61	DRw9	21.1						
B37	DRw10	159.7						
HLA-B	HLA-C	$\chi^{2\,a}$	HLA-B	HLA-C	$\chi^{2\,a}$	HLA-B	HLA-C	$\chi^{2\,a}$
Bw54	Cw1	201.3	B27	Cw1	46.9	B27	Cw1	73.8
Bw59	Cw1	71	B27	Cw3	27	Bw61	Cw2	29.7
Bw61	Cw3	39.9	Bw62	Cw3	22.8	Bw62	Cw3	25.2
B35	Cw3	43.7	Bw60	Cw3	33.2	Bw35	Cw4	63.7
Bw62	Cw4	52.7	B35	Cw4	79.4	B44	Cw5	50.2
Bw56	Cw4	32.1	B44	Cw5	47.3	B8	Cw7	34
B37	Cw6	138.3	B8	Cw7	24.1			
B7	Cw7	160.3	Bw65	Cw8	24.7			
B39	Cw7	66.3						

$^a\chi^2 > 20.$

haplotypes are less common compared to Europe and Australia. Indeed, the frequency of AIH in the general population of Japan is apparently lower than that of Western countries, indicating there are ony a few people in Japan who have disease-susceptible HLA. This different genetic background may be one of the major causes of the different frequency of diseases, including AIH.

3. HLA analysis in Japan

3.1. Diagnostic criteria and clinical manifestations of AIH using HLA analysis

The diagnosis of AIH was made according to the following criteria advocated by the Japanese Hepatitis Research Group in 1980 and revised in 1992 (Ohta, 1993).

(1) Seronegativity for HBsAg and/or low titer of anti-HBc antibody, and negativity for anti-HA IgM antibody.
(2) High serum levels of immunoglobulin G, over 25 g/l.
(3) Positivity for anti-nuclear antibody (ANA) by immunofluorescence or LE test, or positivity for LE cell phenomenon.
(4) Chronic or intermittent high serum level of aminotransferase.
(5) Histology showing chronic aggressive hepatitis, often with marked plasma cell infiltration in the portal area
(6) Systemic manifestations such as fever, joint pain and eruption, often complicated.
(7) Complication of other autoimmune disease.

Numbers 1, 2, 3 and 4 are essential for the diagnosis of AIH. Of course, alcoholic hepatitis and drug-induced hepatitis were strictly differentiated from the disease.

3.1.1. HLA analysis

HLA haplotypes in the diagnosis-confirmed cases, according to the above-mentioned criteria, were studied by the Japanese National Study Group supported by the Ministry of Health and Welfare in 1982. In this study, it became clear that Japanese cases of AIH had specific AIH-related HLA haplotypes different from Caucasians in whom HLA-B8 and -DR3 are apparently risky haplotypes in AIH (Mackay and Tait, 1980). Among the Japanese cases of AIH, the frequency of HLA-A26 and HLA-DR4 was significantly higher than in normal national controls, the P-value was 0.02 and 0.001, respectively. Furthermore, this study revealed that most of the cases had both HLA-A26 and -DR4. There were apparent clinical differences between HLA-A26- and/or -DR4-positive cases and both negative cases (Table 3). Clinical manifestations of HLA-A26- and/or -DR4-positive cases were more severe than both negative cases as shown in Table 3. The study concluded that the disease-susceptible gene-related HLA-DR4 and -A26 may restrict the pathogenesis of Japanese AIH. However, this nationwide survey was performed before the discovery of the hepatitis C virus (HCV)-related antibody assay system, indicating the cases' analyzed HLA phenotype may possibly include HCV-positive chronic hepatitis. After developing the assay system of HCV-related antibody, it became clear that most cases of non-A, non-B (NANB) hepatitis in Japan could be diagnosed as type C hepatitis by the positivity of the C-100 antibody. It is possible that some of the analyzed cases for the HLA phenotype who were first diagnosed as AIH might now be diagnosed as type C hepatitis. Recently, it was reported that more than 90% of

Table 3

Different clinical manifestations between HLA-A26- and/or HLA-DR4-positive
cases

	HLA-A26+, DR4+ HLA-A26+, DR4− HLA-A26−, DR4+	HLA-A26−, DR4−
Family history +	10%	9%
Other autoimmune disease +	37%	45%
AST (U/ml)	471 ± 448	425 ± 355
ALT (U/ml)	342 ± 294	294 ± 220
T. Bil. (mg/dl)	6.12 ± 7.70	2.29 ± 2.79
> 3 mg/dl	36%	13%
Cholinesterase (0.5δ pH)	0.37 ± 0.16	0.61 ± 0.35
< 0.5δ pH	67%	25%
γ-Globulin (g/dl)	3.47 ± 1.18	3.12 ± 1.78
> 3.0 g/dl	68%	38%
< 30% ICG R15	36%	40%

the Japanese cases of AIH who were negative for the HCV-antibody have
HLA-DR4 (Seki et al., 1990; Zeniya et al., 1991). Furthermore, these authors
pointed out that HLA-Bw54 was significantly more frequent in AIH than in
healthy subjects. They reported that the calculated relative risk of DR4-positive
Japanese AIH was 14.8 compared with that of healthy controls. Among the HLA-
DR4-positive AIH patients, there were no significant clinical and laboratory
differences between those positive or negative for HLA-Bw54. These data
suggested that AIH-associated HLA phenotype in Japan is different from the
Western countries where a strong association between HLA-A1-B8-DR3 and
AIH is well characterized. The cause of this difference may be explained by
geographical and racial differences. However, Donaldson (Donaldson et al.,
1991) reported in 1990, that there was a striking secondary association with DR4
in English as well as Japanese people. In his report, the frequency of DR4 was
clearly raised in Northern European AIH patients, though it was not significant
at the 5% level. However, 83 (90%) of 92 cases of AIH who were DR-typed had
either DR3 or DR4 compared with 53% of controls ($P < 0.0005$). Subtraction of
the DR3-positive individuals from the patient population revealed that there was
a significant secondary association with DR4: 35 (80%) of 44 remaining patients
were DR4-positive compared with 31 (39%) of 79 DR3-negative controls.
Interestingly, they also reported that patients with HLA-A1-B8-DR3 were seen
at a younger age than those without. In other words, the average age of
HLA-DR4-positive patients was older than those of HLA-A1- B8-DR3-positive
cases. In Japan, where most cases of AIH were positive for HLA-DR4, the
average age at onset of AIH was in middle age, suggesting there may be two
subsets of AIH, both of which have different genetic factors.

Recently, we re-analyzed the HLA haplotypes in 17 newly diagnosed cases of AIH who completely satisfied the above criteria and lived in the Tokyo metropolitan area. HLA phenotypes were analyzed by microcytotoxicity assay described by Terasaki and McClelland (1964) and compared to normal controls who lived in the same Tokyo metropolitan area where the patients lived. The clinical manifestations of the patients are shown in Table 4. The male:female ratio was 3:14, and the average age was 47.1 years (range 33–62 years). The serum levels of ALT and AST at initial diagnosis were 342 ± 294 and 471 ± 448 U/ml (mean $\pm$ S.E.M.), respectively, and the average titer of ANA was over $640 \times$ by immunofluorescent techniques using Hep-2 cells as a nuclear target. One case was complicated by chronic thyroiditis. All cases showed good response to corticosteroid treatment, at an initial dose of 30 mg/day, and showed rapid normalization of the serum aminotransferase level within 2 months of beginning corticosteroid administration. Comparing the reported cases in Western countries, the clinical data of the AIH patients studied here seemed to be mild. Furthermore, the average age of the patients was 47.1 years and was more than the Caucasian cases of AIH. We found a case who complained of symptoms and was diagnosed as AIH after 62 years of age. Most cases showed a mild clinical course. No case had hepatic failure during the observation period. The results of the HLA analysis are shown in Table 5. HLA-B35, -DR4, -DRw6 and -DQw4 had a high frequency in AIH patients, indicating these haplotypes had AIH susceptibility in Japan. The frequencies of these haplotypes were higher in the Japanese general population than the Caucasian population; however, the frequency of these haplotypes is higher in AIH than in the general Japanese population.

Furthermore, specific linkages of HLA haplotypes were clarified as shown in Table 5. Among them, HLA linkages such as HLA-A24-DR4, HLA-A24-B35, HLA-DR4-DQw4 showed a high value of relative risk. Furthermore, the linkages, HLA-A24-DR4-DQw4, -B35-DR4-DQw4, -A24-B35-DR4-DQw4, and -A24-B35-Cw3-DR4-DQw4 had significant high values of relative risk compared to normal Japanese controls. These linkages were not Japanese-specific linkages,

Table 4
Clinical manifestations of AIH
Serum AST, ALT and IgG values are means $\pm$ S.E.M.

Total number	17
Sex ratio (male:female)	3:14
Average age (years)	47.1
AST (U/ml)	496.6 ± 85.4
ALT (U/ml)	557.7 ± 117.0
IgG (g/dl)	3125.5 ± 165.2
ANA (%)	100

Table 5
HLA phenotype and haplotypes linkage in Japanese AIH

HLA	Control ($n = 340$)	AIH ($n = 15$)	HLA	Control ($n = 340$)	AIH ($n = 15$)
A2	42.6	46.7	Bw61	22.6	20
A11	14.7	13.3	Bw62	17.1	3.4
A24	57.7	66.7	Bw67	1.2	20
A26	21.8	26.7	Cw1	34.7	40
A31	15.9	6.7	Cw3	46.8	33.3
Aw33	14.7	13.3	Cw4	7.9	0
B7	12.4	0	Cw7	22.6	20
B17	0.3	0	Cw11	1.8	0
B35	10.6	26.7	DR1	14.1	6.7
B38	0.3	0	DR2	37.9	20
B39	7.4	13.3	DR4	40.6	100
B44	13.5	13.3	DR5	7.1	0
Bw46	11.8	6.7	DRw6	22.9	26.7
Bw48	4.7	13.3	DRw8	20.9	13.3
B51	13.2	0	DR9	25.6	13.3
Bw52	23.2	20	DQw1	73.5	73.3
Bw54	15.9	26.7	DQw3	53.5	33.3
Bw55	5.9	0	DQw4	14.4	73.3
Bw60	12.1	20			

HLA	n	%	χ^2	χ^2 (control)	P-value	Response rate
A24	10	66.7	0.48	0.181	—	1.47
B35	4	26.7	3.715	2.281	—	3.07
DR4	15	100	20.678	18.326	<0.01	∞
DQw4	11	73.3	35.51	31.441	<0.01	16.33
A24-DR4	10	66.7	14.732	12.481	<0.01	6.72
A24-B35	3	20	7.948	4.846	<0.01	5.82
DR4-DQw4	11	73.3	38.121	33.813	<0.01	17.58
A24-DR4-DQw4	8	53.3	28.721	24.378	<0.01	11.39
B35-DR4-DQw4	3	20	38.984	26.258	<0.01	42.25
A24-B35-DR4-DQw4	3	20	38.984	26.258	<0.01	42.25
A24-B35-Cw3DR4-DQw4	2	13.3	20.947	11.069	<0.01	26

suggesting these HLAs showed AIH susceptible linkages in Japan. In particular, the existence of HLA-DR4 was observed in all cases of AIH, and there was no case who had DR3, which is the main genetic factor in Europe, especially in Caucasians. Furthermore, our data revealed that all patients who had HLA-DR4 possessed HLA-DRw53 and DQw4.

3.1.2. DNA analysis of DR4
It has recently been reported that the specific sequences of polymorphic HLA class II have an important role in the immunopathogenesis of several autoim-

mune disorders, including rheumatoid arthritis (Gregersen et al., 1987; Nepom et al., 1987), insulin-dependent diabetes mellitus (Todd et al., 1988; Baisch et al., 1990), celiac disease (Sollid et al., 1989) and pemphigus vulgaris (Scharf et al., 1989). In particular, specific amino acid residues in HLA-DRB1 and -DQB1 molecules have been thought to contribute to the susceptibility to autoimmune

Table 6

Allelic differences in amino acid sequences from positions 6–16, 57 and 70 of the first domain of the HLA-DRB1 chain

Dash indicates identity with the 0101 sequence

DR	Allele	Dw	Position of amino acid		
			6 9 13 16	57	70
DR1	0101	Dw1	R F L W Q L K F E C H	D	R
	0102	Dw20	- - - - - - - - - - -	—	—
	0103	DBON	- - - - - - - - - - -	—	E
DR2	1501	Dw2	- - - - - - P - R - - -	—	A
	1502	Dw12	- - - - - - P - R - - -	—	A
	1601	Dw21	- - - - - - P - R - - -	—	—
	1602	Dw22	- - - - - - P - R - - -	—	—
DR3	0301	Dw3	- - - E Y S T S - - -	—	K
	0302	DwRSH	- - - E Y S T S - - -	—	K
DR4	0401	Dw4	- - - E - V - H - - -	—	K
	0402	Dw10	- - - E - V - H - - -	—	E
	0403	Dw13a	- - - E - V - H - - -	—	—
	0404	Dw14a	- - - E - V - H - - -	—	—
	0405	Dw15	- - - E - V - H - - -	S	—
	0406	DKT2	- - - E - V - H - - -	—	—
	0407	Dw13b	- - - E - V - H - -	—	—
	0408	Dw14b	- - - E - V - H - - -	—	—
DR5	1101	Dw5	- - - E Y S T S - - -	—	—
	1102	DwJVM	- - - E Y S T S - - -	—	E
	1103	?	- - - E Y S T S - - -	—	E
	1104	DwFS	- - - E Y S T S - - -	—	—
	1201	DwDB6	- - - E Y S T G - - Y	V	—
	1202	?	- - - E Y S T G - - Y	V	—
DR6	1301	Dw18	- - - E Y S T S - - -	—	E
	1302	Dw19	- - - E Y S T S - - -	—	E
	1401	Dw9	- - - E Y S T S - - -	A	—
	1402	Dw16	- - - E Y S T S - - -	—	—
DR7	0701	Dw17	- - - - - - G - Y K - -	V	—
	0702	DB1	- - - - - - G - Y K - -	V	—
DR8	0801	Dw8.1	- - - E Y S T G - - Y	S	—
	0802	Dw8.2	- - - E Y S T G - - Y	—	—
	0803	Dw8.3	- - - E Y S T G - - Y	S	—
DR9	0901	Dw23	- - - K - D - - - - -	V	—
DR10	1001	?	- - - E E V - - - - -	—	—
DRnew?	1403	?	- - - E Y S T S - - -	—	—

diseases including AIH. By the analysis using polymerase chain reaction-amplified DNA with allele-specific restriction endonucleases, Seki et al. (Seki et al., 1992) reported that the frequency of DRB1*0405, DQA1*0301 and DQB1*0401 alleles was significantly higher in Japanese AIH than in controls. However, they also reported that the association of DQA1*0301 and DQB1*0401 with Japanese AIH was weak compared to that of HLA-DR4, and the association of DQA1*0301 and DQB1*0401 with AIH was thought to be dependent on a linkage disequilibrium with HLA-DR4 in Japanese. We also observed that the incidence of HLA-DR4-associated Dw alleles was not different between HLA-DR4-positive AIH and the HLA-DR4-positive controls (unpublished data). These data indicated that HLA-DR4-specific amino acid sequences may be responsible for AIH in Japan. As shown in Table 6, HLA-DR4-specific amino acid residues may be key factors as the trigger for AIH.

4. Family studies

Family study is one of the analytical methods to solve the question of genetic factors in AIH. Though liver diseases only infrequently affect many members of one family, we have hypothesized that genetic factors may well regulate the course of liver disease in a family who are infected by HBV. Unfortunately, there are no reports in Japan to confirm this. Krawitt (Krawitt et al., 1987) reported that the positive rate of serum autoantibodies such as ANA, anti-actin antibody, anti-SMA and anti-liver–kidney microsomal (anti-LKM) antibody, was high in the family members of a patient with AIH.

Although the differential expression of autoantibodies as shown implies some specificity, these families also illustrate the fact that familial occurrences of autoantibody 'positivity' do not necessarily imply a genetic predisposition to autoantibody formation. The presence of autoantibodies in the spouses of family members suggests that environmental factors are also of importance. In this report, Krawitt concluded that despite the occurrence of autoantibody positivity in first-degree relatives of AIH patients, there was no evidence that this trait has a simple genetic basis, or that it is an alternative manifestation of a postulated disease-susceptible gene conferring a predisposition to AIH.

Considering the heterogeneity of AIH and the variation in published results of immunoregulatory function, it is possible that immunoregulatory dysfunction plays a role in the pathogenesis of the course of AIH in some families.

5. Non-A, non-B hepatitis

After discovering the assay system of HCV-related antibody (Kuo et al., 1989), most cases of NANB hepatitis, especially in Japan, can be diagnosed as type

C hepatitis. Interestingly, when we diagnosed the patients as NANB hepatitis because of the lack of a detection system for HCV infection, the frequency of autoantibodies in most cases of NANB hepatitis was thought to be much less than type B hepatitis. Until recently, the absence of autoantibodies was used as one of the diagnostic markers for differentiating chronic NANB hepatitis from AIH. However, the situation has been dramatically changed. It has been reported that a relatively high population of anti-HCV-positive patients tend to be positive for ANA or SMA and LKM (Lenzi et al., 1990; Manns, 1991), indicating that these autoantibodies are associated with some cases of HCV infection or that HCV infection may be one of the triggering factors in AIH (McFarlane et al., 1990).

However, our recent data showed that the HLA phenotypes of autoantibody-positive type C hepatitis, most of them ANA-positive in low titer, are different from prototype AIH cases who are negative for all virus markers. Even so, the clinical manifestation, including response to therapy to autoantibody-positive type C hepatitis is quite similar to AIH. It has been reported that AIH patients have high titers of antibodies against measles and rubella viruses and other pathogens (Haukenes et al., 1990), suggesting that in Japan and the Mediterranean area where the HCV-positive rate is high, some cases of AIH have persisting anti-HCV following an undocumented exposure to the virus without any clinical manifestation of chronic HCV infection or presuming that HCV infection has triggered their AIH. Recently, over 80% of NANB chronic hepatitis patients have circulating autoantibodies (anti-GOR) against a pentadecapeptide that is produced by normal liver and is HCV-specific (Mishiro et al., 1990), suggesting that an autoimmune response related to HCV infection may exist. This phenomenon is now understood to be the result of molecular mimicry between the HCV genome and the host genome. However, this fact may implicate that HCV infection can induce liver autoreaction during its course. Our HLA analysis of anti-HCV-positive AIH showed that there are differences of HLA phenotype frequencies between HCV-positive and -negative AIH (unpublished data). At this point, there is possible involvement of the MHC in virus infection, especially HCV infection. Further study is needed to clarify the relationship between HCV infection and liver autoreaction.

6. Conclusions

Recent developments in molecular biology have clarified the genetic background of AIH. Through these analyses, it has become apparent that there are obvious ethnic differences in AIH between Caucasian and Japanese patients. However, the immunopathogenetic mechanism of AIH is still unclear. Further immunological analysis at the molecular level is needed.

References

Baisch, J.M., Weeks, T., Giles, R., Hoover, M., Stastny, P. and Capra, J.D. (1990) Analysis of HLA-DQ genotypes and susceptibility in insulin-dependent diabetes mellitus. N. Engl. J. Med. 322, 1836–1841.

Bodmer, W.F., Batchelor, J.R., Bodmer, V.G. et al. (Eds.) (1978) Histocompatibility Testing 1977. Munksgaard, Copenhagen.

Donaldson, P.T., Deherty, D.G., Hayllar, K.M., McFarlane, I.G., Johnson, P.J. and Williams, R. (1991) Susceptibility to autoimmune chronic active hepatitis: human leukocyte antigens DR4 and A1-B8-DR3 are independent risk factors. Hepatology 13, 701–706.

Eddleston, A.L.W.F. and Williams, R. (1978) HLA and liver diseases. Br. Med. Bull. 34, 295–300.

Esteban, J.L., Esteban, R., Viadomiu, L. et al. (1990) Hepatitis C virus antibodies among risk group in Spain. Lancet 335, 258–259.

Freudenberg, J., Baumann, H., Arnold, W. et al. (1977) HLA in different forms of chronic active hepatitis. A comparison between adult patients and children. Digestion 15, 260–270.

Galbraith, R.M., Eddleston, A.L.W.F., Williams, R. et al. (1976) Enhanced antibody responses in active chronic hepatitis. Relation to HLA-B8 and HLA-B12 and porto-systemic shunting. Lancet I, 930–934.

Gregersen, P.K., Silver, J. and Winchester, R.J. (1987) The shared epitope hypothesis: an approach to understanding the molecular genetics of susceptibility to rheumatoid arthritis. Arthritis Rheum. 30, 1205–1213.

Haukenes, G., Martre, R., Toder, O. et al. (1990) Measles and rubella antibodies in patients with chronic liver diseases (Letter). J. Hepatol. 11, 386.

Krawitt, E.L., Kilby, A.E., Albertini, R.J. et al. (1987) Immunogenetic studies of autoimmune chronic active hepatitis: HLA, immunoglobulin allotype and autoantibodies. Hepatology 7, 1305–1310.

Kunkel, H.G., Ahrens, E.H., Jr., Eisenmenger, W.J. et al. (1951) Extreme hypergammaglobulinemia in a young woman with liver disease of unknown etiology, J. Clin. Invest. 30, 654.

Kuo, G., Choo, Q.-L., Alter, H.J. et al. (1989) An assay for circulating antibodies to a major etiologic agent of human non-A, non-B hepatitis. Science 244, 362–364.

Lenzi, M., Ballardini, G., Fusconi, M. et al. (1990) Type 2 autoimmune hepatitis and hepatitis C virus infection. Lancet 335, 258–259.

Lepage, V., Degos, F., Carella, G., De Lima, M., Giraud, M.C. and Degos, L. (1981) HLA-Cw7 and HBsAg negative chronic active hepatitis. Tissue Antigens 18, 105–107.

Mackay, I.R. and Tait, B.D. (1980) HLA association with autoimmune-type chronic active hepatitis: identification of B8-DRw3 haplotype by family studies. Gastroenterology 79, 95–98.

Mackay, I.R., Taft, L.T. and Cowling, D.C. (1956) Lupoid hepatitis. Lancet ii, 123–126.

Mackay, I.R. and Morris, P.J. (1976) Association of autoimmune active chronic hepatitis with HLA-A1, 8. Lancet 2, 793–795.

Manns, M.P. (1991) Cytoplasmic autoantigens in autoimmune hepatitis: molecular analysis and clinical relevance. Semin. Liver Dis. 11, 205–214.

McFarlane, I.G., Smith, H.M., Johnson, P.J. et al. (1990) Hepatitis C virus antibodies in chronic active hepatitis: pathogenesis factor of false-positive results? Lancet 335, 754–757.

Mishiro, S., Hoshi, Y., Takeda, K. et al. (1990) Non-A, Non-B hepatitis specific antibodies at host-derived epitope: implication for an autoimmune response. Lancet 336, 1400–1403.

Nepom, G.T., Hausen, J.A. and Nepom, B.S. (1987) The molecular basis for HLA class II associations with rheumatoid arthritis. J. Clin. Immunol. 7, 1–7.

Ohta, Y. (1993) Report of Research Subgroup of autoimmune hepatitis/primary biliary cirrhosis. Gastroenterol. Japon. 28 (Suppl. 4), 128–133.

Opelz, G., Vogten, A.J.M., Summerskill, W.H.J. et al. (1977) HLA determination in chronic active liver disease: possible relation of HLA-Dw3 to prognosis. Tissue Antigens 9, 36–40.

Seki, S., Kiyosawa, K., Iniko, H. and Ota, M. (1990) Association of autoimmune hepatitis with HLA-Bw54 and DR4 in Japanese patients. Hepatology 12, 1300–1304.

Seki, T., Ota, M., Furuta, S., Fukushma, H., Kondo, T., Hino, K., Mizuki, N., Ando, A., Tsuji, K., Inoko, H. and Kiyosawa, K. (1992) HLA class II molecules and autoimmune hepatitis susceptibility in Japanese patients. Gastroenterology 103, 1041–1047.

Sharf, S.J., Freidmann, A., Stenman, I., Brautbar, C. and Erlich, H.A. (1989) Specific HLA-DQB and HLA-DRB1 alleles confer susceptibility to pemphigus vulgaris. Proc. Natl. Acad. Sci. U.S.A. 86, 6215–6219.

Sollid, L.M., Markussen, G., Gjerde, H., Vartdal, F. and Thorsby, E. (1989) Evidence for a primary association of celiac disease to a particular HLA-DQ α/β heterodimer. J. Exp. Med. 169, 345–350.

Terasaki, P.I. and McClelland, J.O. (1964) Microdroplet assay of human serum cytotoxins. Nature 204, 998–1000.

Todd, J.A., Bell, J.I. and McDevitt, H.O. (1988) A molecular basis for genetic susceptibility to insulin-dependent diabetes mellitus. Immunol. Today 4, 129–134.

Waldenström, J. (1950) Liver Blutprotein und Nahrungseweiss. Dtsch. Z. Verdgs Stoffwechs. Krh. Sonderband XV Taung, Bad Kissingen, p. 8.

Whittingham, S., Irwin, J., Mackay, I.R. and Smalley, M. (1966) Smooth muscle autoantibody in 'autoimmune' hepatitis. Gastroenterology 51, 499–505.

Zeniya, M., Takahashi, H., Aoyama, N., Aizawa, Y. and Kameda, H. (1991) Revaluation of liver splenic protein and immunogenetic analysis on the pathogenesis of autoimmune hepatitis. In: M. Tsuchiya et al. (Eds.), Frontiers of Mucosal Immunology, Vol. 2, Excerpta Medica, Amsterdam, pp. 61–64.

Zeniya, M., Fumitoki, W., Aizawa, Y. and Toda, G. (1993) Immunogenetic background of hepatitis B virus infection and autoimmune hepatitis in Japan. Gastroenterol. Japon. 28 (Suppl. 4), 69–75.

Section VII

Treatment of Autoimmune Hepatitis

Autoimmune Hepatitis
Edited by M. Nishioka, G. Toda and M. Zeniya
© 1994, Elsevier Science B.V. All rights reserved

Chapter 17

Treatment of autoimmune hepatitis

Albert J. Czaja

*Hepatobiliary Unit, Division of Gastroenterology, Mayo Clinic and Mayo Medical School,
Rochester, MN 55905 (U.S.A.)*

1. Introduction

Multiple controlled clinical trials have demonstrated the efficacy of corticosteroid therapy in the management of patients with severe autoimmune hepatitis (Cook et al., 1971; Soloway et al., 1972; Murray-Lyon et al., 1973). Prednisone alone or in combination with azathioprine can ameliorate symptoms, improve biochemical and histologic abnormalities, and enhance immediate survival in most patients with severe disease. Treatment strategies, however, remain complex and in many instances, uncertain because the diagnostic criteria of autoimmune hepatitis are still evolving, results from controlled treatment trials apply only to a small subset of patients with autoimmune hepatitis, and not all patients who are treated with autoimmune hepatitis, and not all patients who are treated with corticosteroids respond satisfactorily (Czaja, 1981). Deterioration during therapy occurs in 9% of patients (Czaja, 1991); improvement that is insufficient to satisfy criteria for remission occurs in 13% (Czaja, 1991); relapse eventuates in the majority after drug withdrawal (Czaja et al., 1980, 1981a, 1987a; Hegarty et al., 1983); cirrhosis may develop despite adequate therapy (Davis et al., 1984); and prolonged treatment may be associated with side effects that include a low but probably increased risk of malignancy (Wang and Czaja, 1988; Wang et al., 1989).

   The requirements for an effective treatment strategy are an accurate diagnosis, a careful analysis of prognostic factors, institution of an appropriate treatment regimen, application of confident monitoring mechanisms, definition of realistic treatment end points and an understanding of alternative therapies for a suboptimal response (Czaja, 1991, 1984a). In each patient, the consequences of untreated disease must be balanced against the benefits and risks of long-term therapy and the decision of when and how to treat must be based on a highly individualized judgement that cannot be reduced to a simple or universally applicable formula.

2. Diagnosis

Autoimmune hepatitis is a diagnosis that requires the exclusion of virus-induced, drug-related, hereditary, and immunologic disorders of the liver that may have similar manifestations, but different pathogenic mechanisms, clinical and histologic expressions, and treatment options (Czaja, 1984b,c). The hallmarks of the diagnosis are the presence of periportal hepatitis ('piecemeal necrosis') on histologic examination and the recognition of an autoantibody in serum. These requisites may be shared by a variety of acute and chronic liver diseases of diverse etiologies and consequently, the differential diagnosis of autoimmune hepatitis is broad. It includes chronic hepatitis B virus (HBV) and hepatitis C virus (HCV) infections, chronic exposure to drugs such as oxyphenisatin, isoniazid, nitrofurantoin or α-methyldopa, Wilson's disease, α_1-antitrypsin deficiency, hemochromatosis, primary biliary cirrhosis, primary sclerosing cholangitis, alcoholic liver disease, and non-alcoholic steatohepatitis (Czaja, 1981, 1984b). Fortunately, a careful clinical and family history and specific laboratory and histologic findings are usually sufficient to exclude these conditions and establish the correct diagnosis.

Importantly, patients with autoimmune hepatitis may commonly have false seropositivity for antibodies to HCV and they may be misdiagnosed as having chronic HCV infection (McFarlane et al., 1990; Czaja et al., 1991b, 1992a). The spurious reactivity of their serum by enzyme immunoassay has been associated with the hypergammaglobulinemia that accompanies autoimmune hepatitis (McFarlane et al., 1990; Czaja et al., 1992a). This hypergammaglobulinemia represents a polyclonal antibody response that may cross-react with the HCV-encoded antigen used in the assay and thereby confound the interpretation of the result. The specificity of the antibodies detected by enzyme immunoassay for HCV-encoded antigens must be documented in all seropositive patients by recombinant immunoblot assay (RIBA) before the possibility of an HCV infection can be accepted (Czaja et al., 1991b, 1992a). Hepatitis C virus has not been established as a cause of autoimmune hepatitis (Esteban et al., 1989; Lenzi et al., 1990) and its presence precludes a definite diagnosis. Patients with autoimmune hepatitis must be distinguished from patients with chronic hepatitis C who have non-specific, typically low titer, immunoserologic markers (Sanchez-Tapias et al., 1990; Czaja et al., 1992b) since therapies are different and they may be deleterious if instituted in the wrong condition (Vento et al., 1989).

Chronic ulcerative colitis (CUC) has had a long and 'classical' association with autoimmune hepatitis, but recent studies have emphasized the high frequency of CUC in primary sclerosing cholangitis (PSC) and the difficulty in distinguishing

PSC from autoimmune hepatitis by clinical, biochemical, and histologic findings (Ludwig et al., 1984; Perdigoto et al., 1992). Consequently, it is important to exclude PSC by cholangiography in all patients with CUC and features of autoimmune hepatitis. The conditions may closely resemble each other or co-exist in the same patient and the presence of abnormal bile ducts by cholangiography may be associated with a suboptimal response to corticosteroid therapy (Perdigoto et al., 1992).

The diagnosis of autoimmune hepatitis requires the presence of at least one autoantibody in serum (Czaja et al., 1983). Failure to detect such a marker in a patient who has otherwise been fully screened and negative for viral and drug-related risk factors would justify the diagnosis of cryptogenic chronic hepatitis (Czaja et al., 1990a). Unfortunately, there is a plethora of organ- and non-organ-specific autoantibodies in serum that are each sufficient to establish the diagnosis of autoimmune hepatitis (Table 1). Consequently, the generic diagnosis of autoimmune hepatitis does not connote a particular clinical or immunoserologic profile. None of the autoantibodies has disease specificity and none has been shown to be pathogenic or associated with a specific immunogenic stimulus other than hepatocytic necrosis (Czaja, 1990a). A single species of autoantibody has not been regularly associated with the disease or required for its diagnosis and as yet the degree of seropositivity for any one marker has not

Table 1

Organ- and non-organ-specific autoantibodies in autoimmune hepatitis

Non-organ-specific antibodies	Organ-specific antibodies
Nuclear antigens	Liver membrane antigen
Double-stranded DNA	(Type 1 hepatitis)
Single-stranded DNA	Asialoglycoprotein receptor
Centromere	Hepatic lectin
Histone	Liver-specific protein
Smooth muscle antigens	Antigen complex
F-actin	Thyroid antigens
(Type 1 hepatitis)	Thyroglobulin
Liver/kidney microsomes	Microsomal
Type 1/P-450-IID6	Acetylcholine receptor
(Type 2 hepatitis)	Parietal cell
Mitochondrial antigens	Islets of langerhans
M4/pyruvate dehydrogenase	
complexes	
Liver soluble antigen	
Cytokeratins 8, 18	
(Type 3 hepatitis)	
Liver cytosol	
Soluble cytolic antigen type 1	
(Idiopathic and type 2 hepatitis)	

been standardized. Indeed, the serum titers of autoantibodies are continuous variables in any one patient and there are no objectively defined lower limits of significant reactivity. Consequently, the specificity of an autoantibody may depend not on its presence or absence, but rather on an arbitrarily selected cut-off value that may not have universal acceptance (Czaja, 1990a).

Importantly, the diagnostic criteria for autoimmune hepatitis are still evolving. Efforts are being made to identify disease-specific immunoserologic markers and eliminate dependence on a generic diagnosis that necessarily must encompass patients with diverse findings and prognoses. The proposal that patients with autoimmune hepatitis be divided into homogeneous subgroups with distinctive clinical, immunoserologic, and prognostic features is a result of these efforts (Maddrey, 1987). Subclassifications of this nature promise to facilitate investigations of pertinent pathogenic mechanisms, foster meaningful comparative analyses, and improve treatment outcomes. The validity of such subclassifications has not as yet been established, but efforts to institute them will improve diagnostic precision and promote a common language and understanding.

Three subclassifications of autoimmune hepatitis have been proposed. 'Type 1' autoimmune hepatitis ('classical', 'lupoid' or 'anti-actin' hepatitis) is characterized by the presence of smooth muscle antibodies (SMA) or anti-nuclear antibodies (ANA) in serum, human leukocyte antigen (HLA) positivity for A1, B8, DR3, or DR4, and responsiveness to corticosteroid therapy (Czaja et al., 1983; Czaja, 1984c). The presence of antibodies to F-actin (anti-actin) in serum increases the specificity of SMA-positivity for type 1 disease. Typically, this form of autoimmune hepatitis afflicts women (71%) of ages 40 years or less (48%), but it may involve individuals from 6 months to 81 years of age. 'Type 2' autoimmune hepatitis is characterized by the presence of antibodies to liver–kidney microsome type 1 (anti-LKM-1) and it involves predominately children (ages 2 to 14 years), but adults can also be afflicted (20–30%) (Homberg et al., 1987). Concurrent immunologic disorders are common (40%) and hypergammaglobulinemia is less pronounced than in type 1 disease. Non-organ-specific autoantibodies are rare while organ-specific autoantibodies, such as anti-thyroid microsome, anti-thyroglobulin, and anti-parietal cell antibodies (Table 1), are frequently demonstrated (30%). Importantly, anti-LKM-1 reactivity by indirect immunofluorescence may be misinterpreted as anti-mitochondrial antibody (AMA) positivity and as many as 27% of patients with features of chronic active hepatitis and AMA may be re-classifiable as anti-LKM-1 positive by repeat testing (Czaja et al., 1991a). Serum from patients with anti-LKM-1 must produce staining of the distal tubules of the murine kidney and uniform staining of the cytoplasm of murine hepatocytes by indirect immunofluorescence to be established as anti-LKM-1 positive. This pattern of indirect immunofluorescence is distinctive from that of AMA which is characterized by staining of the distal tubules of the murine kidney and the gastric parietal cells of the murine stomach. 'Type 3' autoimmune hepatitis is characterized by the presence of antibodies to soluble liver antigen (anti-SLA) in serum (Manns et al., 1987). These patients are mostly women (91%) with a mean age of 37 years (range, 17–67 years) and they lack antibodies to nuclear antigens, LKM-1, and thryoglobulin, but they may have SMA, antibodies to liver membrane antigen, and AMA (74%). Because these patients share clinical and immunoserologic features with patients with type 1 autoimmune hepatitis, it is still uncertain if anti-SLA is the hallmark of a unique disease with a variety of non-specific immunoserologic manifestations or an unusual but non-specific marker of type 1 hepatitis. Importantly, a disciplined diagnostic process that excludes similar but different diseases and characterizes the immunoserologic nature of the patients as fully as possible, as indicated above, will ensure that the first step in developing a treatment strategy is on solid ground.

3. Prognostic factors

The major determinant of prognosis is the severity of inflammatory activity at the time of presentation as assessed by biochemical indices and histologic features (Geall et al., 1968). Sustained elevation of the serum aspartate aminotransferase (AST) level to at least 10-fold normal or 5-fold normal in conjuction with at least a 2-fold elevation of the serum γ-globulin level has been associated with a 3-year mortality of 50% and 10-year mortality of 90% (Geall et al., 1968). When these same biochemical criteria have been assessed prospectively in controlled clinical trials, the mortality has been as high as 40% within 6 months (Soloway et al., 1972).

Histologic features of bridging necrosis or multilobular mecrosis are associated with an 82% frequency of cirrhosis within 5 years and a mortality of 45% (Schalm et al., 1977). Patients with bridging necrosis between portal tracts and central veins may more commonly develop cirrhosis than those with bridging necrosis between portal tracts and portal tracts (29 vs 10%) (Cooksley et al., 1986). These distinctions, however, are often difficult to make with certainty and mixed features are frequently present. Cirrhosis at presentation is associated with a 5-year mortality of 58% (Schalm et al., 1977) and death from hemorrhage may occur in 20% of those with esophageal varices within 2 years (Murray-Lyon et al., 1973).

Patients with less severe biochemical and histologic findings have better prognoses. The 15-year survival of such patients exceeds 80% and the probability of progression to cirrhosis is 49% (Czaja, 1986). Patients with periportal hepatitis have a 17% frequency of cirrhosis within 5 years and a normal life expectancy during this interval (Schalm et al., 1977). Clearly, in these latter patients, the benefit:risk ratio of treatment may be so low that therapy is unjustified. Additionally, autoimmune hepatitis may improve or resolve spontaneously in 13–20% of patients regardless of disease activity (Czaja, 1986). Mortality is highest during the early, most active stages of the disease and if survival beyond

2 years can be achieved, inactivity may eventuate in as many as 40% of survivors (Czaja, 1986). These patients, however, typically develop cirrhosis and they are at risk for the late complications of portal hypertension and hepatocellular cancer.

The HLA phenotype also has prognostic significance in patients with autoimmune hepatitis (Czaja et al., 1990b; Donaldson et al., 1991; Sanchez-Urdazpal et al., 1992). HLA-B8 has been found in from 34 to 82% of patients with autoimmune hepatitis depending on the stringency of the diagnostic criteria (Czaja et al., 1990b). HLA-A1 has been found with similar frequency and the co-occurrence HLA-A1,-B8 and -DR3 in 94% of patients testing positive for either antigen has indicated a strong linkage disequilibrium between these alleles (Czaja et al., 1990b). Patients with HLA-B8 or -DR3 are younger, have higher serum levels of AST and bilirubin, and more commonly have histologic features of bridging necrosis, multilobular necrosis, and cirrhosis at presentation than counterparts without HLA-B8 or -DR3 (Czaja et al., 1990b). These patients also respond more slowly to therapy, relapse after drug withdrawal more frequently, deteriorate during treatment more commonly, and require liver transplantation more frequently than patients with other phenotypes (Czaja et al., 1990b; Donaldson et al., 1991; Sanchez-Urdazpal et al., 1992). The nature of the HLA phenotype does not dissuade therapy, but it may well identify patients that require closer monitoring and individuals who are earlier candidates for alternative therapies.

Other factors that have been associated with a poor prognosis include abrupt onset of disease, encephalopathy, cholestasis, ascites, and ulcerative colitis. PSC has the same HLA phenotype as autoimmune hepatitis and it may commonly resemble or co-exist with autoimmune hepatitis in patients with CUC (Perdigoto et al., 1992). In such patients, cholangiography is required to establish the diagnosis since the presence of PSC and not CUC is the important prognostic determinant (Perdigoto et al., 1992).

4. Indications for treatment

Patients with severe, rapidly progressive, potentially life-threatening disease have been well studied by controlled clinical trial and the benefit:risk ratio of treatment has been well defined for these patients (Cook et al., 1971. Soloway et al., 1972; Murray-Lyon et al., 1973). The absolute indications for corticosteroid therapy in these individuals are sustained severe biochemical abnormalities and/or the presence of bridging or confluent necrosis on histologic examination (Table 2). Relative indications for treatment are incapacitating symptoms that can be attributed to hepatocellular inflammation or evidence of relentless disease progression (Table 2).

Patients with less than severe disease have not been studied by controlled clinical trial and they lack confident treatment guidelines. These patients are best

Table 2
Indications for treatment of autoimmune hepatitis
AST, serum aspartate aminotransferase level; GG, serum γ-globulin level.

Objective indications	Subjective indications
AST > 10-fold normal	Incapacitating symptoms
AST > 5-fold normal and	Fatigue
GG > 2-fold normal	Myalgias
Bridging necrosis	Arthralgias
Multilobular necrosis	Disease progression
	Ascites
	Encephalopathy

managed expectantly or enrolled in a prospective clinical trial, such as the one ongoing at the Mayo Clinic, which is evaluating the benefit:risk ratio of therapy in patients with mild to moderate disease activity and few or no symptoms (Hay et al., 1989). The frequency that asymptomatic patients with mild to moderate autoimmune hepatitis become severe is unknown, but such transitions undoubtedly occur and this possibility justifies regular follow-up assessments (Hay et al., 1989).

5. *Treatment regimens*

Two treatment regimens are of equal efficacy in the management of severe autoimmune hepatitis (Table 3) (Czaja, 1983, 1984c). Prednisone alone or a smaller dose of prednisone in conjunction with a low dose of azathioprine (Table 3) is each able to induce clinical, biochemical, and histologic remission with comparable frequency in patients with severe type 1 or 'classical' autoimmune hepatitis and each has been shown to be superior to placebo and non-steroidal regimens in this regard. Although these regimens have been studied only in patients with type 1 autoimmune hepatitis and the frequencies of response may differ in type 2 or 3 disease, there is as yet no reason to prefer other therapies for these other types.

Prednisone in combination with azathioprine is the preferred treatment since it is associated with a lower frequency of corticosteroid-induced side effects than the regimen using a higher dose of prednisone alone (10 vs 44%). It is ideal in postmenopausal patients and others who have osteoporosis, cushingoid features, emotional lability, diabetes, or hypertension (Table 3). Prednisone alone is warranted in those patients with cytopenia, pre-existent malignancy, pregnancy or the contemplation of pregnancy in whom there is a reluctance to administer azathioprine (Table 3). Additionally, therapy with prednisone alone is suited for patients in whom only a short (3–6 month) treatment trial is proposed since the

Table 3
Treatment regimens for severe autoimmune hepatitis

Time interval	Combination treatment (mg/day)		Prednisone treatment (mg/day)
	Prednisone	Azathioprine	Prednisone
1 week	30	50	60
1 week	20	59	40
2 weeks	15	50	30
Until end point	10	50	20
Indications	Postmenopausal		Cytopenia
	Osteoporosis		Pregnancy
	Cushingoid		Malignancy
	Hypertension		Short-term trial
	Diabetes		
	Emotional liability		

steroid-sparing advantages of combination therapy become apparent only after 12 or more months of continuous therapy (Table 3).

Cosmetic changes develop in 80% of patients after 2 years of corticosteroid therapy regardless of the regimen while severe debilitating complications (osteoporosis, diabetes, hypertension, cataracts, and psychosis) usually develop in from 10 to 44% of patients after 18 months of treatment and at doses of prednisone that exceed 10 mg daily (Czaja, 1981). Complications of azathioprine include cholestatic hepatitis, nausea, emesis, rash, and cytopenia. Side effects develop in fewer than 10% of patients receiving 50 mg daily of azathioprine and all toxicities can be reversed by reduction of the dose or discontinuation of the drug (Czaja, 1981). Importantly, the complications of the medication are frequently indistinguishable from the side effects of the liver disease. As a result, they may not resolve after drug withdrawal or be a reliable indication for the termination of therapy. In fact, the side effects of the medication are generally well tolerated and although they may commonly develop in patients on long-term treatment, they necessitate dose reduction or drug withdrawal in only 13% of patients (Czaja et al., 1984).

Surprisingly, postmenopausal women are able to tolerate initial corticosteroid therapy as well as premenopausal counterparts and the response of their liver disease to such treatment is as satisfactory (Wang and Czaja, 1989). The risk for these patients increases with subsequent treatments after relapse and the majority will develop some complication under these circumstances. Consequently, postmenopausal women who have never received cortiocosteroid therapy previously should be treated in a conventional fashion at presentation. Relapse after drug withdrawal, however, justifies less aggressive management using a long-term, low-dose prednisone or azathioprine regimen. Since osteoporosis with vertebral compression can develop regardless of age or hormonal status, adjunctive therapy with calcium supplement (1–1.5 g/day) and vitamin D (50,000 units/week) is recommended for all patients undergoing therapy. Estrogens should be avoided as prophylactic therapy if the liver disease is active or unstable. They can be used judiciously, however, if manifestations of osteoporosis are present.

The long-term complications of immunosuppressive therapy include the theoretical possibilities of teratogenicity and oncogenicity (Czaja, 1981, 1991). Skeletal anomalies, cleft palate, reduction in thymic size, hydrops fetalis, anemia, and hematopoietic suppression have been described in mice treated experimentally with higher than pharmacologic doses of azathioprine (Czaja, 1981, 1991). Such effects undoubtedly reflect the experimental conditions, excessive dose schedules, and animal species tested, but they generate sufficient concern to limit the use of azathioprine in pregnant women. Similar concerns have not been justified in corticosteroid-treated patients.

The oncogenicity of immunosuppressive therapy has been suggested mainly by the development of lymphomas in patients undergoing transplantation. In the Mayo experience, the incidence of extra-hepatic malignancy in corticosteroid-treated patients with autoimmune hepatitis is 1 per 194 patient-years of surveillance and the probability of tumor occurrence is 3% after 10 years (Wang et al., 1989). The risk is 1.4-fold greater than that in an age- and sex-matched normal population and no specific neoplastic cell type predominates (Wang et al., 1989). The low but probably increased risk of malignancy in these patients does not contraindicate the use of these medications in patients with autoimmune hepatitis, but it does underscore the importance of carefully selecting patients for such therapy.

6. *Treatment end points*

Therapy is continued until the criteria for remission, treatment failure, arrested or incomplete response, or drug toxicity are satisfied. Remission connotes disappearance of symptoms, resolution of biochemical abnormalities (except for a less than 2-fold elevation of AST), and improvement of the histologic findings to those of non-specific hepatitis, portal hepatitis, inactive cirrhosis or normal. Biochemical improvement should be evident within 2 weeks after institution of therapy and 65% will satisfy all criteria for remission within 3 years. The average duration of treatment until remission is 22 months (Czaja et al., 1983).

Importantly, histologic improvement lags behind clinical and biochemical improvement by 3–6 months and active histologic disease can be found in 55% of patients who undergo liver biopsy when serum AST and γ-globulin levels reach remission range (Czaja et al., 1981a). Consequently, it is essential to treat long enough to realize the maximum benefit from corticosteroid therapy and to eliminate premature drug withdrawal as a cause of relapse. This is best done by using histologic resolution as a treatment end point. Treatment until there is complete reversion of the hepatic architecture to normal is associated with only a 20% frequency of relapse after drug withdrawal (Czaja et al., 1984). Treatment until improvement to the features of non-specific or portal hepatitis is associated with 50% frequency of relapse within 6 months and 70% frequency of relapse within 3 years of drug withdrawal (Czaja et al., 1980, 1981a). Treatment until inactive cirrhosis is associated with an 87–100% likelihood of relapse depending on whether the cirrhosis was present prior to therapy (87%) or developed during treatment (100%) (Czaja et al., 1984; Davis et al., 1984). Patients with cirrhosis deserve one opportunity to sustain their remission without medication, but the vast majority will relapse and require long-term, continuous, low-dose maintenance therapy.

'Cure' of autoimmune hepatitis is possible, but it occurs infrequently, slowly, and unpredictably (Czaja et al., 1984). It is not, therefore, a primary goal of treatment. Although patients may lose all manifestations of their disease and sustain this improvement indefinitely after initial treatment, permanent disappearance of the disease ('cure') usually occurs spontaneously after discontinuation of therapy or eventuates after additional therapy following relapse (Czaja et al., 1984). Since the presence of cirrhosis precludes reversion of the hepatic architecture to normal, these patients are not eligible for 'cure' by strict definition. In the Mayo experience, only 18 of 83 patients without cirrhosis prior to therapy (22%) had reversion of their liver tissue to normal during 91 ± 5 months of follow-up (Czaja et al., 1984). Of these, only 13 patients had no manifestations of disease after 71 ± 11 months of observation, including 8 who had been followed up for the requisite period of 5 years to justify a 'cure'. Although 'cure' was possible, it was achieveable in only 16% of patients without cirrhosis at presentation and it was not clearly a direct result of treatment (Czaja et al., 1984).

Treatment failure connotes worsening of the disease despite compliance with the treatment regimen. Failure to improve or improvement that is insufficient to satisfy remission criteria is not treatment failure but rather an incomplete or arrested response. Deterioration during therapy occurs in only 9% of patients with type 1 autoimmune hepatitis and it is usually apparent within 2 months after institution of treatment (Czaja, 1991). Patients failing treatment can be managed on higher doses of prednisone alone (60 mg daily) or prednisone (30 mg daily) in conjunction with azathioprine (150 mg daily) (Czaja, 1991). During high-dose therapy, patients should be monitored each month and attempts made to reduce the dose of medication if clinical and biochemical improvements can be demonstrated. Seventy-five percent of patients will respond to this regimen, but histologic remission can be achieved in only 20% (Schalm et al., 1976). Long-term, higher than conventional, doses of medication are usually required to control inflammatory activity and these patients are at risk for liver failure and drug toxicity. Such patients are candidates for orthotopic liver transplantation and they should be monitored and evaluated with this expectation.

Importantly, there are no features before therapy that predict treatment failure and patients with severe inflammatory activity, encephalopathy, ascites, co-agulopathy, and depressed synthetic and detoxification functions can be resurrected during treatment (Czaja et al., 1988; Sanchez-Urdazpal et al., 1992). Consequently, orthotopic liver transplantation should be deferred, if possible, until the reponse to corticosteroid therapy can be evaluated. Typically, a 2-week interval of treatment is sufficient to identify patients with a poor immediate prognosis in whom the evaluation for transplantation should be expedited (Czaja et al., 1988). Patients with multilobular necrosis at presentation who fail to improve a pretreatment hyperbilirubinemia, have worsening of other laboratory parameters, or fail to correct at least one laboratory abnormality during 2 weeks of therapy die within 4 months and they are ideal candidates for consideration of early transplantation after just 2 weeks of treatment (Czaja et al., 1988). In contrast, patients who do not demonstrate these deficiencies in treatment response after 2 weeks have a high (98%) frequency of survival beyond 6 months. The liver transplantation decision can be deferred in such individuals.

Failure to induce remission after 3 years of continuous conventional therapy connotes an incomplete or arrested response and it occurs in 13% of patients (Czaja, 1991). These patients have not deteriorated, but they have not improved or fully realized the expectations of treatment. The majority of patients with type 1 autoimmune hepatitis who enter remission (87%) do so within 3 years, and the probability of entering remission during this interval exceeds that of developing major drug-related side effects, thereby maintaining a favorable benefit:risk ratio. This ratio decreases thereafter for each year of treatment without remission and these patients should be considered for empiric low-dose indefinite prednisone therapy rather than the standard fixed daily dose regimens (Czaja, 1990b). Importantly, of patients still requiring continuous standard therapy after 4 years, 69% ultimately deteriorate and satisfy criteria for treatment failure (Sanchez-Urdazpal et al., 1992). Indeed, failure to achieve remission within 4 years and the HLA-A1-B8-DR3 phenotype augur a poor prognosis and these patients should be monitored for possible transplantation (Sanchez-Urdazpal et al., 1992).

Drug toxicity compels premature discontinuation of therapy in 13% of patients (Czaja et al., 1984). Most commonly, intolerable obesity or cosmetic changes (47%) justify this action. Osteoporosis with vertebral compression (27%), brittle diabetes (20%), and peptic ulceration (6%) limit therapy less frequently (Czaja et al., 1984). In the presence of drug-related complications, the management of the liver disease becomes improvisional as efforts are made to control inflammatory manifestations with the lowest dose of medication possible.

7. *Indices of response*

Treatment strategies are based on accurate determinations of response. The serum AST and γ-globulin levels remain the most practical and useful indices to follow (Czaja et al., 1981b). In patients with histologic features of moderate to severe periportal hepatitis prior to therapy, an abnormal AST or gamma globulin level during treatment correctly predicts the presence of residual histologic activity that still warrants treatment in 91–98% of instances (Czaja et al., 1981b). The absence of biochemical abnormality, however, predicts the absence of histologic disease in only 36–44% of instances and histologic examination is still required to confirm the disappearance of inflammatory activity (Czaja et al., 1981b). In monitoring patients after induction of remission and drug withdrawal, an abnormal serum AST level predicts histologic recrudescence in 79% of instances and an abnormal γ-globulin concentration connotes histologic relapse in 93% (Czaja et al., 1981b). Normal serum AST and γ-globulin levels after drug withdrawal indicate the absence of histologic disease in 81% of instances and of those patients with active disease and normal laboratory findings, only 7% have severe potentially aggressive histologic findings (Czaja et al., 1981b). To date, no other laboratory tests have been as well studied or as successful as the serum AST and γ-globulin levels in predicting histologic activity.

Serum procollagen type III peptide concentrations are elevated to the same extent in patients with type 1 autoimmune hepatitis with and without cirrhosis at presentation and during therapy these abnormally increased levels improve to normal as histologic remission is achieved (McCullough et al., 1987a, 1987b). The procollagen type III levels, however, change in concert with standard AST and γ-globulin determinations and they do not quantitatively reflect inflammation or static measurements of hepatic fibrosis. Consequently, their determination does not offer a distinct advantage over conventional testing.

Initial studies indicated that fasting serum bile acid concentrations (cholic acid conjugates) were more sensitive than conventional laboratory tests in reflecting histologic activity and in predicting sustained remission or relapse after drug withdrawal (McCullough, 1986). Unfortunately, these early observations were not confirmed by other studies which indicated only a 56% sensitivity of serum bile acid abnormalities for chronic active hepatitis and only a weak correlation with periportal hepatitis (McCullough, 1986). Similarly, improvements in the molar ratio of plasma branched to aromatic amino acids were initially associated with reductions in inflammatory activity and the likelihood of a sustained remission after drug withdrawal (McCullough et al., 1981). Prospective studies, however, failed to confirm the value of these assessments in monitoring disease activity or in predicting a treatment end point, and they were subsequently abandoned as a clinical aid in the management of type 1 autoimmune hepatitis (Shiels et al., 1985). The aminopyrine breath test suffered a similar fate because of discrepant reports and its inability to distinguish mild chronic active hepatitis from chronic persistent hepatitis (McCullough, 1986).

Perhaps the best measure of response will be by assay systems not now available that reflect changes in the immunopathogenic mechanisms of the disease. Studies have indicated that treatment until disappearance of antibodies to liver-specific protein is associated with sustained remission after drug withdrawal (McFarlane et al., 1984) and this concept may well be extended if assays become available by which blood levels of cytokines can be measured or suppressor T-cell function can be monitored.

Histologic examination assesses the degree and pattern of inflammatory activity in patients with type 1 autoimmune hepatitis with 90% consistency (Soloway et al., 1975). Reproducibility of the morphologic interpretation by the same observer is 94% and sampling error is trivial. Unfortunately, the sampling error for cirrhosis may exceed 60% and intra-observer variability in diagnosing cirrhosis may approach 50% unless the definition of cirrhosis as fibrosis with an encapsulated regenerative nodule is strictly enforced (Soloway et al., 1975). Liver biopsy examination, therefore, while excellent for evaluating inflammatory changes, cannot confidently exclude cirrhosis and it cannot be used as a reliable monitoring mechanism to assess progression to cirrhosis or the effect of drugs on the prevention of cirrhosis. Peritoneoscopy allows examination of the surface configuration of the liver and it permits visually directed sampling of the most representative abnormalities, but it also suffers from intra-observer variation as well as a failure rate that relates to postoperative changes that limit examination of the right upper quadrant (Czaja et al., 1973). Until reliable non-invasive quantitative liver function tests become available and the absence of disease can be established by demonstrating the absence of perpetuating mechanisms, the clinician must continue to depend on the basic laboratory menu and the biopsy needle to assess the response to treatment.

8. Treatment results

Remission is achieved in 65% of patients with severe type 1 autoimmune hepatitis after 22 ± 2 months of corticosteroid therapy (Czaja, 1984c). Patients without cirrhosis prior to therapy have 5- and 10-year life expectancies after treatment that exceed 90%, while patients with cirrhosis at presentation have a 5-year life expectancy of 80% and 10-year life expectancy of 65% (Czaja, 1984c). Although patients with cirrhosis have shorter survivals than counterparts without cirrhosis at presentation, they live significantly longer than untreated patients with disease of comparable severity (Soloway et al., 1972).

Unfortunately, corticosteroid therapy does not prevent eventual progression to cirrhosis and up to 40% of patients will have this consequence within 10 years, despite compliance with the treatment regimen (Davis et al., 1984). The mean annual incidence of cirrhosis is 11% during the first 3 years and 1% thereafter. Progression to cirrhosis reflects the infrequency that corticosteroids permanently induce a completely inactive disease. Its development, however, does not alter immediate survival and the 5-year life expectancy after cirrhosis is 93% (Davis et al., 1984). Longevity after the development of histologic cirrhosis undoubtedly depends on the stage of the disease and the degree of inflammatory activity that accompanies the lesion and corticosteroid therapy may modify these factors. Preliminary studies indicate that patients with type 2 (anti-LKM-1 positive) autoimmune hepatitis progress more rapidly to cirrhosis than patients with type 1 disease (82 vs 43%) (Homberg et al., 1987). This difference in behavior may reflect differences in the intrinsic aggressiveness of each subtype which in turn influences their responsiveness to treatment.

Treatment failure (9%), incomplete or arrested improvement (13%), and drug toxicity which warrants premature discontinuation of medication (13%) occur infrequently and their eventuation cannot be reliably predicted (Czaja, 1991). Each consequence, however, compels a deviation from conventional therapy and it frequently requires the implementation of a strategy that may be novel, unproven, or empiric.

Relapse after induction of remission and cessation of therapy is the most common and challenging problem in the management of type 1 autoimmune hepatitis (Czaja et al., 1980, 1981a, 1987a; Hegarty et al., 1983). Premature withdrawal of medication is one cause of relapse, but treatment to normal laboratory tests and hepatic tissue does not prevent its occurrence (Czaja et al., 1984), suggesting that the pathogenic mechanisms which perpetuate the disease cannot be permanently disrupted by corticosteroid therapy. Interestingly, relapse occurs more commonly in patients who are HLA-A1-B8-positive (Czaja et al., 1990b) and it is possible that this phenotype identifies patients with a genetically acquired predisposition for enhanced immunoreactivity to an autoantigen that limits their ability to sustain a remission. Although patients who relapse progress to cirrhosis and die of liver failure more frequently than counterparts who sustain their remission, these differences have not been shown to be statistically significant (Czaja et al., 1987a). Indeed, the major consequence of relapse and treatment is a higher frequency of drug-related complications in the patients who relapse (70 vs 30%) (Czaja et al., 1987a). Individuals who relapse multiply have such a high likelihood of developing complications from additional standard therapies that alternative approaches are warranted.

The enhanced survival of patients with cirrhosis and their frequent requirement for prolonged or repeated courses of immunosuppressive therapy may explain the frequency of hepatocellular cancer which is now being recognized (Wang and Czaja, 1988). The incidence of hepatocellular cancer in patients with type 1 autoimmune hepatitis is 1 per 350 patient-years of follow-up and the frequency of liver neoplasm in patients with cirrhosis of at least 5 years' duration is 7% (Wang and Czaja, 1988). The incidence of hepatocellular cancer in these patients with long-standing cirrhosis is 1 per 182 patient-years of follow-up and the probability of liver tumor is 29% after 13 years (Wang and Czaja, 1988). Indeed, when compared to an age- and sex-matched normal population, the risk of hepatocellular cancer in these patients is increased by 311-fold (Wang and Czaja, 1988). The late propensity for hepatocellular cancer may reflect the risk of neoplasm associated with cirrhosis regardless of etiology, unrecognized infection with potentially oncogenic viruses, or alterations in immunologically mediated host defense mechanisms by the long-term administration of immunosuppressive medication. This risk is sufficient to justify the prospective evaluation of surveillance protocols that might include systematic screening with serum α-fetoprotein determinations, hepatic ultrasonography, or other combinations of tumor markers and imaging studies. Importantly, the serum α-fetoprotein level is abnormally elevated in 35% of patients with severe autoimmune hepatitis (Czaja et al., 1987b) and the significance of the elevation must be carefully evaluated in each patient since it may be a non-specific feature of hepatocellular necrosis and regeneration. The abnormality typically resolves after corticosteroid therapy and it does not have prognostic significance (Czaja et al., 1987b). An elevation that persists after therapy, especially in the absence of disease activity, suggests primary hepatocellular carcinoma.

Extra-hepatic neoplasms may also complicate long-term immunosuppressive therapy (Wang et al., 1989). Patients who develop extra-hepatic malignancies cannot be distinguished by age, sex, treatment regimen, cumulative duration of treatment, or individual features of the liver disease. No specific cell type predominates as neoplasms of the breast, bladder, soft tissue, cervix, and lymphatic tissue have been reported. Additionally, they may occur unpredictably, developing after 18–164 months of treatment and follow-up. The relative risk for extra-hepatic cancer is estimated as being 1.4-fold greater than that in an age- and sex-matched normal population (95% confidence interval, 0.6–2.9-fold normal) (Wang et al., 1989).

9. Alternative treatments

Failure of conventional corticosteroid regimens to induce a sustained remission after drug withdrawal connotes a suboptimal response to treatment and such patients are candidates for alternative therapies. Since relatively few patients achieve the ideal result of permanent remission, the majority of patients with type 1 autoimmune hepatitis are theoretically eligible for a treatment change at some point during their management. Clearly, the threshold for a treatment change can vary greatly since it depends on the assessment (and acceptance) of the actual treatment response and the availability of suitable alternative strategies.

298   *A.J. Czaja*

9.1. Alternative therapies at presentation

Several novel therapies are available for the decompensated patient at the time of
presentation, but there is no justification to institute alternative non-steroidal
regimens or unconventional corticosteroid protocols for the previously untreated patient. As many as 20% of patients with severe type 1 autoimmune
hepatitis will improve spontaneously, but the consistency of the response to
conventional corticosteroid treatment, its safety and inexpensiveness justify
prompt institution of corticosteroid therapy in all patients regardless of the
possibility of spontaneous improvement.

Liver transplantation is extremely successful in managing the decompensated
patient as evidenced by a 5-year survival after transplantation of 96% and the
absence of disease recurrence in the implant (Sanchez-Urdazpal et al., 1992). The
transplantation decision, however, should be deferred, if possible, for at least
2 weeks in the untreated decompensated patient so that the response to corticosteroids can be assessed (Czaja et al., 1988). Liver transplantation is best justified
if conventional corticosteroid regimens fail to improve the disease. Indeed, in
some patients liver transplantation can be avoided or deferred by the 'treat-first'
approach.

High-dose prednisone administered as 90 mg doses daily for 5 days each month
is intended to improve impaired non-antigen-specific suppressor T-cell function,
selectively inhibit immunoglobulin G synthesis, and avoid cumulative corticosteroid-related toxicities (Chase et al., 1982). This regimen has had anecdotal
success, but a controlled treatment trial in patients who had relapsed multiply
indicated the inferiority of this regimen to conventional protocols (Czaja et al.,
1991c). Consequently, it is not recommended in lieu of or after standard therapy.
Similarly, alternate-day corticosteroid therapy is less effective than fixed
daily dose regimens in inducing histologic remission (Summerskill et al.,
1975). Therefore, its use is considered improvisational and it should be reserved
for individuals who have manifested significant toxicity to the standard regimens.

Polyunsaturated phosphatidylcholine has been used successfully in conjunction with prednisone as the initial management of autoimmune hepatitis, but its
role in such treatment has not been established. A double-blind controlled trial
has indicated that this combination can reduce histologic activity better than
prednisone alone, presumably by modifying the hepatocyte membrane and
blocking or altering the cytotoxic attack on the liver cell (Jenkins et al., 1982). The
early reported success of this regimen has not been confirmed and the combination cannot as yet be recommended as the first approach to therapy.

9.2. Alternative therapies after treatment failure

The administration of higher than conventional doses of prednisone alone or in
combination with azathioprine improves the clinical and biochemical manifesta-

tions of the disease in 75% of instances (Schalm et al., 1976). Only 25% of patients, however, achieve histologic resolution and consequently, most remain at risk for drug-related complications and death from liver failure. The preferred treatment for such patients is liver transplantation. Patients who continue to deteriorate on high-dose regimens are candidates for immediate transplantation (Czaja et al., 1988) while those who improve, but fail to satisfy criteria for remission, can be monitored expectantly. These latter patients have a frequency of decompensation that increases with the duration of continuous disease activity such that 69% of patients who are still on continuous therapy for more than 4 years die of liver failure (Sanchez-Urdazpal et al., 1992). Liver transplantation should be instituted in these patients at the first clinical sign of decompensation (i.e., ascites formation during therapy).

Cyclosporine (5–6 mg/day) has been used anecdotally in patients who have been intolerant of corticosteroid therapy (Mistilis et al., 1985; Hyams et al., 1987) and theoretically it might be of advantage in patients who are deteriorating despite administration of high-dose corticosteroid regimens. Cyclosporine suppresses clonal expansion of activated T-helper cells, blocks the release of lymphokines such as interleukin-2 from antigen-primed T-helper cells, prevents activation and expansion of cytotoxic T-cells, and decreases antibody production by B-cells dependent on T-cell interaction (Canfax and Ascher, 1983). These actions should interfere with an antibody-dependent, cell-mediated form of cytotoxicity and ameliorate the condition. Cyclosporine therapy, however, is investigational and its benefits must be measured against its potential for immediate (hypertension, renal insufficiency) and long-term consequences (neoplasia) before any recommendation for its standard use can be made.

Fk-506 is a neutral macrolide antibiotic which has been extracted from a soil fungus (*Streptomyces tsukubaensis*) and found to have immunosuppressive properties that exceed those of cyclosporine (Thomson, 1990). It inhibits the expression of helper T-cell activation genes and thereby prevents lymphokine production, proliferation of activated T-lymphocytes, and the generation of cytotoxic T-cells. Its immunosuppressive actions have been purported to occur with few or no complications and it is currently being evaluated in prospective treatment trials as a means of rescuing liver transplantation recipients with acute and chronic rejection. If FK-506 can be shown to be safe and effective in inhibiting allograft rejection, its further evaluation in the management of immunologically mediated chronic liver diseases can be justified.

9.3. Alternative therapies after relapse

Conventional fixed daily dose regimens can reliably induce remission after relapse. The probability of a subsequent relapse after drug withdrawal, however, increases and in the patient who has relapsed at least twice the risks of conventional therapy exceed the benefits. In these patients, low-dose, indefinite prednisone therapy is preferred. The dose of prednisone should be reduced by 2.5 mg each month as long as there are no symptoms and serum AST levels remain at or below 5-fold normal. The lowest effective dose is then determined on an individual basis and maintained thereafter (Czaja, 1990b). Eighty-seven percent of patients who have relapsed multiply can be maintained in this fashion long-term (up to 149 months) on 10 mg or less of prednisone daily (median dose, 7.5 mg daily) (Czaja, 1990b). Corticosteroid-related side effects that had accrued during conventional therapy improve in 85% of patients and mortality from liver-related complications is comparable to that in patients who are treated repeatedly with conventional regimens (9 vs 10%) (Czaja, 1990b).

Indefinite azathioprine therapy (2 mg/kg) can also sustain a remission induced by prednisone and facilitate resolution of cushingoid features and corticosteroid-related side effects (Stellon et al., 1988). Unfortunately, these patients may experience severe myalgias and arthralgias associated with corticosteroid withdrawal and they are at an uncertain long-term risk for the theoretical complications associated with teratogenicity and oncogenicity.

Thymic hormone extracts have been shown to stimulate suppressor T-cell activity and inhibit immunoglobulin production (Hegarty et al., 1984). Consequently, there is a rationale for their use in autoimmune hepatitis. Unfortunately, an early controlled treatment trial failed to demonstrate a difference in the frequency of relapse after conventional drug withdrawal in patients receiving the extract or no therapy during the tapering process (Hegarty et al., 1984). Optimal doses, duration of treatment, and mode of administration, however, were uncertain and the promise of such therapy cannot as yet be discounted. Indeed, recent studies using thymosin in patients with chronic hepatitis B have suggested that it may promote disease remission and inhibit virus replication (Mutchnick et al., 1991).

9.4. *Alternative therapies for the incomplete response*

Long-term, low-dose prednisone therapy is the most intuitively appealing approach to the patient with an incomplete or arrested response on protracted conventional therapy. There are no controlled treatment trials, however, which have established the efficacy of such therapy in this situation and alternative regimens such as alternate day prednisone or azathioprine alone cannot be disregarded. Treatment, in fact, is improvisational and based on the premise that disease control at minimal risk is desirable.

Ursodeoxycholic acid has recently been shown to reduce serum aminotransferase and γ-glutamyltranspeptidase levels in patients with chronic active hepatitis (Crosignani et al., 1991). This pilot study was uncontrolled, included patients with mainly chronic hepatitis B and C virus infections, and failed to correlate the biochemical changes with the clinical and histologic findings. Nevertheless, the experience is promising since biochemical improvement was realized with a low dose of ursodeoxycholic acid (250 mg daily) (Crosignani et al., 1991). Future studies assessing ursodeoxycholic acid in conjunction with low-dose prednisone in the management of patients with protracted disease would be of interest.

Acknowledgement

Linda Grande is acknowledged for her secretarial assistance.

References

Canafax, D.M. and Ascher, N.L. (1983) Cyclosporine immunosuppression. Clin. Pharm. 2, 515–524.

Chase, W.F., Winn, R.E. and Mayes, G.R. (1982) Oral pulse prednisone therapy in the treatment of HBsAg negative chronic active hepatitis. Gastroenterology 83, 1292–1296.

Cook, G.C., Mulligan, R. and Sherlock, S. (1971) Controlled prospective trial of corticosteroid therapy in active chronic hepatitis. Q. J. Med. 40, 159–185.

Cooksley, W.G.E., Bradbear, R.A., Robinson, W., Harrison, M., Halliday, J.W., Powell, L.W., Ng, H.-S., Seah, C.-S., Okuda, K., Scheuer, P.J. and Sherlock, S. (1986) The prognosis of chronic active hepatitis without cirrhosis in relation to bridging necrosis. Hepatology 6, 345–348.

Crosignani, A., Battezzati, P.M., Setchell, K.D.R., Camisaca, M., Bertolini, E., Roda, A., Zuin, M. and Podda, M. (1991) Effects of ursodeoxycholic acid on serum liver enzymes and bile acid metabolism in chronic active hepatitis: a dose–response study. Hepatology 13, 339–344.

Czaja, A.J. (1981) Current problems in the diagnosis and management of chronic active hepatitis. Mayo Clin. Proc. 56, 311–323.

Czaja, A.J. (1983) Chronic active hepatitis. In: L.M. Lichtenstein and A.S. Fauci (Eds.), Current Therapy in Allergy and Immunology 1983–1984, Decker, Burlington, Ont., pp. 239–244.

Czaja, A.J. (1984a) Strategies in the management of chronic active hepatitis. Surv. Dig. Dis. 2, 233–243.

Czaja, A.J. (1984b) Diagnosis and treatment of chronic hepatitis. Compr. Ther. 10, 58–63.

Czaja, A.J. (1984c) Natural history, clinical features, and treatment of autoimmune hepatitis. Semin. Liver Dis. 4, 1–12.

Czaja A.J. (1986) Natural history of chronic active hepatitis. In: A.J. Czaja and E.R. Dickson (Eds.), Chronic Active Hepatitis. The Mayo Clinic Experience, Marcel Dekker, New York, pp. 9–24.

Czaja, A.J. (1990a) Autoimmune chronic active hepatitis – a specific entity? The negative argument. J. Gastrol. Hepatol. 5, 343–351.

Czaja, A.J. (1990b) Low dose corticosteroid therapy after multiple relapses of severe HBsAg-negative chronic active hepatitis. Hepatology 11, 1044–1049.

Czaja, A.J. (1991) Diagnosis, prognosis, and treatment of classical autoimmune chronic active hepatitis. In: E.L. Krawitt and R.H. Wiesner (Eds.), Autoimmune Liver Disease, Raven, New York, pp. 143–166.

Czaja, A.J., Steinberg, A.S., Saldana, M. and Marin, G.A. (1973) Peritoneoscopy: its value in the diagnosis of liver disease. Gastrointest. Endosc. 20, 23–25.

Czaja, A.J., Ammon, H.V. and Summerskill, W.H.J. (1980) Clinical features and prognosis of severe chronic active liver disease (CALD) after corticosteroid-induced remission. Gastroenterology 78, 518–523.

Czaja, A.J., Ludwig, J., Baggenstoss, A.H. and Wolf, A.M. (1981a) Corticosteroid-treated chronic active hepatitis in remission: uncertain prognosis of chronic persistent hepatitis. N. Engl. J. Med. 304, 5–9.

Czaja, A.J., Wolf, A.M. and Baggenstoss, A.H. (1981b) Laboratory assessment of severe chronic active liver disease (CALD): correlation of serum transaminase and gamma globulin levels with histologic features. Gastroenterology 80, 687–692.

Czaja, A.J., Davis, G.L., Ludwig, J., Baggenstoss, A.H. and Taswell, H.F. (1983) Autoimmune features as determinants of prognosis in steroid-treated chronic active hepatitis of uncertain etiology. Gastroenterology 85, 713–717.

Czaja, A.J., Davis, G.L., Ludwig, J. and Taswell, H.F. (1984) Complete resolution of inflammatory activity following corticosteroid treatment of HBsAg-negative chronic active hepatitis. Hepatology 4, 622–627.

Czaja, A.J., Beaver, S.J. and Shiels, M.T. (1987a) Sustained remission following corticosteroid therapy of severe HBsAg-negative chronic active hepatitis. Gastroenterology 92, 215–219.

Czaja, A.J., Beaver, S.J., Wood, J.R., Klee, G.G. and Go, V.L.W. (1987b) Frequency and significance of serum alpha-fetoprotein elevation in severe hepatitis B surface antigen-negative chronic active hepatitis. Gastroenterology 93, 687–692.

Czaja, A.J., Rakela, J. and Ludwig, J. (1988) Features reflective of early prognosis in corticosteroid-treated severe autoimmune chronic active hepatitis. Gastroenterology 95, 448–453.

Czaja, A.J., Hay, J.E. and Rakela, J. (1990a) Clinical features and prognostic implications of severe corticosteroid-treated cryptogenic chronic active hepatitis. Mayo Clin. Proc. 65, 23–30.

Czaja, A.J., Rakela, J., Hay, J.E. and Moore, S.B. (1990b) Clinical and prognostic implications of human leukocyte antigen B8 in corticosteroid-treated severe autoimmune chronic active hepatitis. Gastroenterology 98, 1587–1593.

Czaja, A.J., Manns, M.P. and Homburger, H.A. (1991a) Specificity of antibodies to liver/kidney microsome type 1 for type 2 autoimmune chronic active hepatitis: evidence against overlapping syndromes and hepatitis B and C viruses as important immunogenic stimuli. Hepatology 14, 134A.

Czaja, A.J., Taswell, H.F., Rakela, J. and Schimek, C. (1991b) Frequency and significance of antibody to hepatitis C virus in severe corticosteroid-treated autoimmune chronic active hepatitis. Mayo Clin. Proc. 66, 572–582.

Czaja, A.J., Wang, K.K. and Katzamann, J.A. (1991c) Cellular and humoral immune responses after relapse of severe autoimmune chronic active hepatitis: effects of different corticosteroid regimens. Hepatology 14, 192A.

Czaja, A.J., Taswell, H.F., Rakela, J. and Rabe, D. (1992a) Duration and specificity of antibodies to hepatitis C virus in corticosteroid-treated HBsAg-negative chronic active hepatitis. Gastroenterology 102, 1675–1679.

Czaja, A.J., Taswell, H.F., Rakela, J. and Schimek, C. (1992b) Frequency of antibody to hepatitis C virus in asymptomatic HBsAg-negative chronic active hepatitis. J. Hepatol., in press.

Davis, G.L., Czaja, A.J. and Ludwig, J. (1984) Development and prognosis of histologic cirrhosis in corticosteroid-treated HBsAg-negative chronic active hepatitis. Gastroenterology 87, 1222–1227.

Donaldson, P.T., Doherty, D.G., Hayllar, K.M., McFarlane, I.G., Johnson, P.J. and Williams, R. (1991) Susceptibility to autoimmune chronic active hepatitis: human leukocyte antigens DR4 and A1-B8-DR3 are independent risk factors. Hepatology 13, 701–706.

Esteban, J.I., Esteban, R., Viladomiu, L., Lopez-Talavera, J.C., Gonzalez, A., Hernandez, J.M., Roget, M., Vargas, V., Genesca, J., Buti, M. and Guardia, J. (1989) Hepatitis C virus among risk groups in Spain. Lancet 2, 294–297.

Geall, M.G., Schoenfield, L.J. and Summerskill, W.H.J. (1968) Classification and treatment of chronic active liver disease. Gastroenterology 55, 724–729.

Hay, J.E., Czaja, A.J., Rakela, J. and Ludwig, J. (1989) The nature of unexplained chronic aminotransferase elevations of a mild to moderate degree in asymptomatic patients. Hepatology 9, 193–197.

Hegarty, J.E., Nouri-Aria, K.T., Portmann, B., Eddleston, A.L.W.F. and Williams, R. (1983) Relapse following treatment withdrawal in patients with autoimmune chronic active hepatitis. Hepatology 3, 685–689.

Hegarty, J.E., Nouri-Aria, K.T., Eddleston. A.L.W.F. and Williams, R. (1984) Controlled trial of a thymic hormone extract (Thymostimulin) in 'autoimmune' chronic active hepatitis. Gut 25, 279–283.

Homberg, J.-C., Abuaf, N., Bernard, O., Islam, S., Alvarez, F., Khalil, S.H., Poupon, R., Darnis, F., Levy, V.-G., Grippon, P., Opolon, P., Bernuau, J., Benhamou, J.-P. and Alagille, D. (1987) Chronic active hepatitis associated with antiliver/kidney microsome antibody type 1: a second type of 'autoimmune' hepatitis. Hepatology 7, 1333–1339.

Hyams, J.S., Ballow, M. and Leichtner, A.M. (1987) Cyclosporine treatment of autoimmune chronic active hepatitis. Gastroenterology 93, 890–893.

Jenkins, P.J., Portmann, B.P., Eddleston, A.L.W.F. and Williams, R. (1982) Use of polyunsaturated phosphatidyl choline in HBsAg negative chronic active hepatitis: results of prospective double-blind controlled trial. Liver 2, 77–81.

Lenzi, M., Ballardini, G., Fusconi, M., Cassani, F., Selleri, L., Volta, U., Zauli, D. and Bianchi, F.B. (1990) Type 2 autoimmune hepatitis and hepatitis C virus infection. Lancet 335, 258–259.

Ludwig, J., Czaja, A.J., Dickson, E.R., LaRusso, N.F. and Wiesner, R.H. (1984) Manifestations of nonsuppurative cholangitis in chronic hepatobiliary diseases: morphologic spectrum, clinical correlations and terminology. Liver 4, 105–116.

Maddrey, W.C. (1987) Subdivisions of idiopathic autoimmune chronic active hepatitis. Hepatology 7, 1372–1375.

Manns, M., Gerken, G., Kyriatsoulis A., Staritz, M. and Meyer zum Büschenfelde, K.-H. (1987) Characterization of a new subgroup of autoimmune chronic active hepatitis by autoantibodies against a soluble liver antigen. Lancet 1, 292–294.

McCullough, A.J. (1986) Laboratory assessment of liver function and inflammatory activity in chronic active hepatitis. In: A.J. Czaja and E.R. Dickson (Eds.), Chronic Active Hepatitis. The Mayo Clinic Experience, Marcel Dekker, New York, pp. 205–246.

McCullough, A.J., Czaja, A.J., Jones, J.D. and Go, V.L.W. (1981) The nature and prognostic significance of serial amino acid determinations in severe chronic active liver disease. Gastroenterology 81, 645–652.

McCullough, A.J., Stassen, W.N., Wiesner, R.H. and Czaja, A.J. (1987a) Serial determinations of the amino-terminal peptide of type III procollagen in severe chronic active hepatitis. J. Lab. Clin. Med. 109, 55–61.

McCullough, A.J., Stassen, W.N., Wiesner, R.H. and Czaja, A.J. (1987b) Serum type III procollagen peptide concentrations in severe chronic active hepatitis: relationship to cirrhosis and disease activity. Hepatology 7, 49–54.

McFarlane, I.G., Hegarty, J.E., McSorley, C.G., McFarlane, B.M. and Williams, R. (1984) Antibodies to liver-specific protein predict outcome of treatment withdrawal in autoimmune chronic active hepatitis. Lancet 2, 954–956.

McFarlane, I.G., Smith, H.M., Johnson, P.J., Bray, G.P., Vergani, D. and Williams, R. (1990) Hepatitis C virus antibodies in chronic active hepatitis: pathogenetic factor or false-positive result? Lancet 335, 754–757.

Mistilis, S.P., Vickers, C.R., Darroch, M.H. and McCarthy, S.W. (1985) Cyclosporin, a new treatment for autoimmune chronic active hepatitis. Med. J. Aust. 143, 463–465.

Murray-Lyon, I.M., Stern, R.B. and Williams, R. (1973) Controlled trial of prednisone and azathioprine in active chronic hepatitis. Lancet 1, 735–737.

Mutchnick, M.G., Appleman, H.D., Chung, H.T., Aragona, E., Gupta, T.P., Cummings, G.D., Waggoner, J.G., Hoofnagle, J.H. and Shafritz, D.A. (1991) Thymosin treatment of chronic hepatitis B: a placebo-controlled pilot trial. Hepatology 14, 409–415.

Perdigoto, R., Carpenter, H.A. and Czaja, A.J. (1992) Frequency and significance of chronic ulcerative colitis in severe corticosteroid-treated autoimmune hepatitis. J. Hepatol. 14, 325–331.

Sanchez-Tapias, J.M., Barrera, J.M., Costa, J., Ercilla, M.G., Pares, A., Comalrrena, L., Soley, F., Bruix, J., Calvet, X., Gil, M.P., Mas, A., Bruguera, M., Castillo, R. and Rodes, J. (1990) Hepatitis

C virus infection in patients with nonalcoholic chronic liver disease. Ann. Intern. Med. 112, 921–924.

Sanchez-Udrazpal, L., Czaja, A.J., Van Hoek, B., Krom, R.A.F. and Wiesner, R.H. (1992) Prognostic features and role of liver transplantation in severe corticosteroid-treated autoimmune chronic active hepatitis. Hepatology 15, 215–221.

Schalm, S.W., Ammon, H.V. and Summerskill, W.H.J. (1976) Failure of customary treatment in chronic active liver disease: causes and management. Ann. Clin. Res. 8, 221–227.

Schalm, S.W., Korman, M.G., Summerskill, W.H.J., Czaja, A.J. and Baggenstoss, A.H. (1977) Severe chronic active liver disease: prognostic significance of initial morphologic patterns. Am. J. Dig. Dis. 22, 973–980.

Shiels, M.T., Czaja, A.J., Ludwig, J., McCullough, A.J., Jones, J.D. and Go, V.L.W. (1985) Diagnostic and prognostic implications of plasma amino acid determinations in chronic active hepatitis. Dig. Dis. Sci. 30, 819–823.

Soloway. R.D., Summerskill, W.H.J., Baggenstoss. A.H., Geall, M.G., Gitnick, G.L., Elveback, L.R. and Schoenfield, L.J. (1972) Clinical, biochemical, and histological remission of severe chronic active liver disease: a controlled study of treatments and early prognosis. Gastroenterology 63, 820–833.

Soloway, R.D., Baggenstoss, A.H., Schoenfield, L.J. and Summerskill, W.H.J. (1975) Observer error and sampling variability tested in evaluation of hepatitis and cirrhosis by liver biopsy. Am. J. Dig. Dis. 20, 1087–1090.

Stellon, A.J., Keating, J.J., Johnson, P.J., McFarlane, I.G., Williams, R. (1988) Maintenance of remission in autoimmune chronic active hepatitis with azathioprine after corticosteroid withdrawal. Hepatology 8, 781–784.

Summerskill, W.H.J., Korman, M.G., Ammon, H.V. and Baggenstoss, A.H. (1975) Prednisone for chronic active liver disease: dose titration, standard dose, and combination with azathioprine compared. Gut 16, 876–883.

Thomson, A.W. (1990) FK-506: profile of an important new immunosuppressant. Transplant. Rev. 4, 1–13.

Vento, S., DiPerri, G., Garofano, T., Cosco, L., Concia, E., Ferraro, T. and Bassetti, D. (1989) Hazards of interferon therapy for HBV-seronegative chronic hepatitis. Lancet 2, 926.

Wang, K.K. and Czaja, A.J. (1988) Hepatocellular cancer in corticosteroid-treated severe autoimmune chronic active hepatitis. Hepatology 8, 1679–1683.

Wang, K.K. and Czaja, A.J. (1989) Prognosis of corticosteroid-treated hepatitis B surface antigen-negative chronic active hepatitis in postmenopausal women: a retrospective analysis. Gastroenterology 97, 1288–1293.

Wang, K.K., Czaja, A.J., Beaver, S.J. and Go, V.L.W. (1989) Extra-hepatic malignancy following long-term immunosuppressive therapy of severe hepatitis B surface antigen-negative chronic active hepatitis. Hepatology 10, 39–43.

Autoimmune Hepatitis
Edited by M. Nishioka, G. Toda and M. Zeniya
© *1994, Elsevier Science B.V. All rights reserved*

Chapter 18

Treatment of autoimmune hepatitis in Japan

Tetsuo Kuroki, Takeyuki Monna and Sukeo Yamamoto

Third Department of Internal Medicine and Department of Public Health, Osaka City University Medical School, and Naniwa Hepatitis Research Center, Osaka (Japan)

1. Introduction

The pathogenesis of autoimmune hepatitis (AIH) is unknown, but the concept of lupoid hepatitis or AIH originally proposed by Mackay et al. (1956, 1965) pointed to the possibility that an autoimmune mechanism is inseparably involved in the onset and progression of this active disorder of the liver, and its clinical findings are unique, even within the disease category of chronic active hepatitis (CAH). In Japan, it was believed for years that AIH is a very rare disease, but the nationwide survey from 1975 to 1984 by the Study Group of Autoimmune Hepatitis (Table 1) under the auspices of the Ministry of Health and Welfare has revealed that it is by no means a rare disease (Monna et al., 1985).

Patients with CAH with hypergammaglobulinemia (≥ 20 g/l) included in the survey were classified by the following diagnostic criteria.

(1) AIH type 1 (314 cases):
    (a) positive for anti-nuclear antibody (ANA), lupus erythematosus (LE) cell test or anti-DNA antibody;
    (b) negative for HBs antigen (HBsAg);
    (c) histologically proven CAH accompanied by marked infiltrations of lymphocytes and plasma cells in the liver;
    (d) systemic manifestations in regions other than the liver;
    (e) responsive to corticosteroid therapy.
(2) CAH type B (125 cases).
(3) CAH type non-A, non-B (159 cases). These patients were negative for autoantibodies and HBsAg.

Table 1

Study Group's members and institutes concerning hepatitis organized under the auspices of the Ministry of Health and Welfare of Japan

Hasumaura, Y.	Int. Med., Tokyo Medical and Dental University School of Medicine
Hattori, N.	Int. Med., School of Medicine, Kanazawa University
Ichida, F.	Int. Med., Niigata University School of Medicine
Ito, K.	Int. Med., Kochi Medical School
Juji, T.	Blood Transfusion Service, Tokyo Women's Medical College
Kakumu, S.	Int. Med., Nagoya University School of Medicine
Kameda, H.	Int. Med., The Jikei University School of Medicine
Matsushita, H.	Public Health, Hamamatsu University School of Medicine
Nagashima, H.	Int. Med., Okayama University Medical School
Namihisa, T.	Int. Med., Junterndo University School of Medicine
Nishioka, M.	Int. Med., Kagawa Medical School
Oda, T.	National Medical Center of Japan
Ohkochi, K.	Central Laboratory, Faculty of Medicine, Kyushu University
Ohta, G.	Pathology, School of Medicine, Kanazawa University
Ohta, Y.	Int. Med., Ehime University School of Medicine
Oka, H.	Int. Med., Faculty of Medicine, University of Tokyo
Sasaki, H.	Int. Med., Toyama Medical and Pharmaceutical University Faculty of Medicine
Suzuki, H.	Int. Med., Yamanashi Medical College
Tsuji, T.	Okayama University Health Research Center
Others	157 institutes and hospitals in Japan

In this survey, the average γ-globulin level was 33.6 g/l in autoimmune hepatitis type 1, 24.1 g/l in CAH type non-A, non-B (NANB) and 23.0 g/l in CAH type B.

In 115 (37%) of 314 cases with AIH type 1, the LE cell phenomenon was positive. ANA was positive in 90%, the LE test was positive in 45%, anti-DNA antibody was positive in 74%, anti-smooth muscle antibody (anti-SMA) was positive in 67% and anti-mitochondrial antibody (AMA) was positive in 11% of cases of AIH type 1.

2. Therapeutic effect of immunosuppressants

About 80% of patients with AIH type 1 were treated with immunosuppressants. The present survey was carried out during the period when immunosuppression for CAH type B was not widely accepted. In spite of this fact, 40% of patients with CAH type B underwent immunosuppression therapy (Table 2).

Of patients with AIH treated with immunosuppressants, 86% were treated with corticosteroids alone, 12 were treated with corticosteroids and azathioprine and several cases were treated with azathioprine alone or corticosteroids and D-penicillamine. Thus, corticosteroid monotherapy predominated.

It was judged that immunosuppressants were effective in 85% of cases with AIH, 71% of cases with chronic active NANB hepatitis and 59% of cases

Table 2
Kinds of treatment with immunosuppressants for patients with autoimmune hepatitis type 1

Treatment	Autoimmune hepatitis type 1	Non-A, non-B chronic hepatitis	Type-B chronic hepatitis
Immunosuppressants	196/253 (77%)	49/154 (32%)	44/110 (40%)
Glucocorticoid	169/196 (86%)	41/49 (84%)	37/44 (84%)
Azathioprine	3/196 (2%)	2/49 (4%)	3/44 (7%)
Glucocorticoid + azathioprine	23/196 (12%)	6/49 (12%)	4/44 (9%)
Others	1/196	0/49	0/41

Table 3
Efficacy of treatment with immunosuppressants for patients with autoimmune hepatitis type 1

Treatment	Autoimmune hepatitis type 1	Non-A, non-B chronic hepatitis	Type-B chronic hepatitis
Immunosuppressants	102/120 (85%)	17/24 (71%)	10/17 (59%)
Glucocorticoid	86/100 (86%)	14/21 (67%)	8/14 (57%)
Azathioprine	1/2	–	1/1
Glucocorticoid + azathioprine	14/17 (82%)	3/3	1/2
Others	1/1	–	–

with CAH type B. In conclusion, immunosuppressants were of high value specifically for the management of patients with AIH type 1 (Table 3).

3. The cumulative survival after treatment

3.1. Cumulative survival after corticosteroid therapy

On the basis of the cumulative survival rate determined according to the life table method, factors affecting the prognosis and therapeutic effects in AIH type 1 were studied.

                                    T. Kuroki et al.

AIH is treated mainly with immunosuppressants, particularly corticosteroids. Approximately 80% of the patients surveyed received steroids. The replies to the questionnaires showed that short-term corticosteroid therapy was effective in approximately 90% of the cases. Furthermore, the cumulative survival was studied in each individual type of CAH treated with corticosteroids (Fig. 1). The 5-year survival was no more than 84%, which was fairly low compared with the corresponding ratios in chronic active NANB hepatitis (97%) and type B CAH (91%). It may be concluded from the above that AIH type 1 shows a good response to short-term steroid therapy, but long-term prognosis is not necessarily favorable, even if steroid therapy is continued. Such being the case, it is desirable to find a better regimen for the long-term management of patients with AIH type 1 using corticosteroids.

3.2. *Duration of treatment and cumulative survival*

Patients with AIH type 1 treated with corticosteroids were classified into two groups according to the treatment period. In the group treated with corticosteroids for more than 6 months, survival rates 1, 2 and 3 years after the first examination were 97%, 91% and 89%, respectively. The corresponding rates

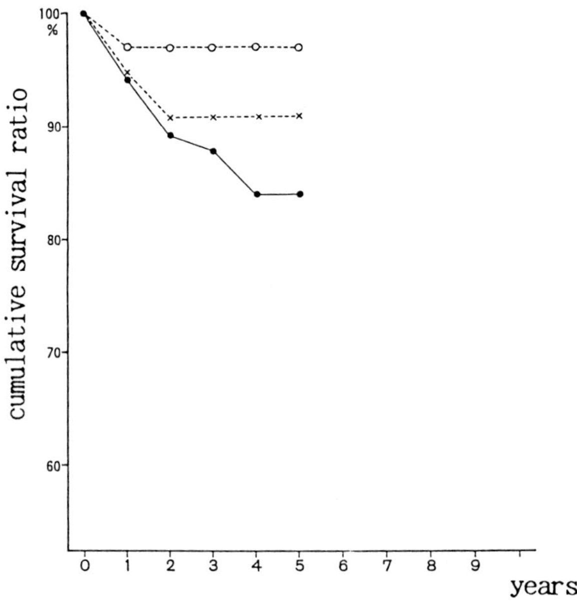

Fig. 1. Cumulative survival of autoimmune hepatitis type 1, chronic hepatitis type B and type non-A, non-B. ●, autoimmune hepatitis type 1; ○, chronic hepatitis type non-A, non-B; X, chronic hepatitis type B.

were lower (89%, 80% and 80%, respectively) in the group treated for less than 6 months.

The patients were classified by the total dosage which the individuals received. The 1-, 2- and 3-year survival rates in the group that received less than 3000 mg of prednisolone, were lower than the respective rates in the group that received more than 3000 mg.

These observations suggest that in the therapy for AIH type 1, the administration period and dosage of corticosteroids are decisive factors regulating therapeutic performance. Particularly in view of the fact that the mortality rate was high in the group treated for less than 6 months, it is of vital importance to initiate an adequate treatment as early as possible.

3.3. Age at onset and cumulative survival

The relationship of the prognosis after the treatment in autoimmune disease with the age at onset was investigated.

When the population was divided by the age at onset into a group of young patients under 40 years and a group of middle-aged and elderly patients aged 40 years and over, the survival rate in the group of young patients was definitely lower, suggesting the relatively poor prognosis of autoimmune disease in young patients (Fig. 2). The low survival rate among young patients was mostly

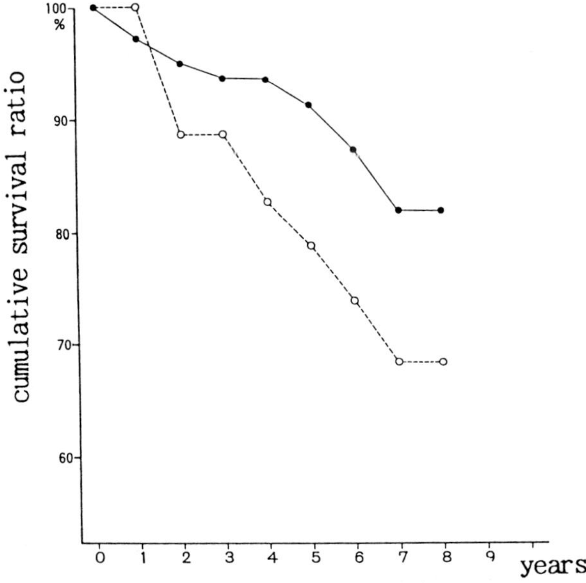

Fig. 2. Cumulative survival of autoimmune hepatitis type 1, in older and younger patients. ●, ≥ 40 years old; ○, < 40 years old.

attributable to the higher incidence of death within 1–2 years of onset and indicated the paramount importance of an early treatment of AIH type 1.

3.4. *Immunological features and cumulative survival*

3.4.1. *Associated autoimmune disease*
The investigation as to whether the complication of another autoimmune disease in AIH type 1 has any bearing on cumulative survival rate showed no difference at all between complicated and non-complicated cases.

3.4.2. *LE cell phenomenon*
When AIH was classified into an LE cell-positive group and an LE cell-negative group and the cumulative survival rates in these groups were compared, the LE cell-positive group showed slightly lower rates than the LE cell-negative group, but no significant difference was found, indicating that the two groups were very much alike, not only in clinical features, but also in prognosis.

3.4.3. *Serum γ-globulin value*
When the patients were divided by serum γ-globulin level into a group with severe hypergammaglobulinemia ($\geq 30\,\text{g/l}$) and group with moderate hypergamma-globulinemia ($< 30\,\text{g/l}$), there was no significant difference between the groups.

3.4.4. *ANA titer*
When the patients were divided by ANA titer into a group with high titer ($\geq 1:320$) and a group with low titer ($1 < 1:320$), there was no significant difference in cumulative survival rate that might be associated with ANA titer.

4. *Prognosis*

The predominant therapy of AIH type 1 is the administration of immunosuppressive drugs, especially glucocorticoids. The nationwide survey has shown that steroid therapy was attempted in more than 80% of cases of this disease. The short-term therapeutic efficacy of treatment with corticosteroids was effective in approximately 90% of cases, but in the long-term the incidence of death was never low. These results indicate that while AIH type 1 responds well to corticosteroid treatment on a short-term basis, it is not rare that the prognosis is poor in the long run, and suggests that a more effective therapeutic regimen must be explored.

Hepatic failure with or without gastrointestinal hemorrhage was the most frequent cause of death in AIH type 1 and several patients died due to primary liver cancer. The finding of note was that several cases were fatal due to agranulocytosis, pneumonia or disseminated intra-vascular coagulation (DIC), each apparently associated with side effects of the respective immunosuppressants, implying a serious problem with immunosuppressant therapy.

5. *Recurrence of AIH*

A recurrence of AIH was found in 44 (25%) of 179 cases who had achieved remission after the administration of corticosteroids. In 87 patients who did not receive maintenance therapy with corticosteroids after the remission, 34 patients (39%) relapsed within 6 years. The relapses were frequently recognized within 1 year after the discontinuation of therapy. These recurrences were serious and 9 (26%) of 34 cases of AIH ended with death from hepatic failure or gastrointestinal hemorrhage. On the other hand, in 92 patients who received maintenance therapy with corticosteroids after the remission, 10 patients (11%) relapsed within 6 years. However, these recurrences were not serious and there were no fatalities (Table 4).

The results so far obtained may be summarized as follows. For the treatment of AIH, early diagnosis, early treatment and long-term corticosteroid therapy (including combination therapies with other immunosuppressants) appear to be important. For the future, a sophisticated therapeutic guideline for 'maximal effect with minimal adverse drug reaction' has to be established.

6. *Infection with HCV in AIH*

The causes of AIH are not well established, but something seems to trigger this disorder — possibly the measles virus or hepatitis virus (HCV). Many patients with several types of AIH have antibodies to HCV (Esteban et al., 1989; Lenzi et al., 1990). However, McFarlane et al. (1990) suggested that serum from patients with AIH type 1 contains a component that gives false-positive results in the HCV ELISA assay (Ortho). In this study, we examined the titer of HCV antibodies in the serum of patients with AIH type 1 using 4 kinds of assay kits,

Table 4

Recurrence in patients with autoimmune hepatitis type 1 treated with glucocorticoid

Treatment with glucocorticoid	No. of patients	Relapses	Death due to relapses
Short-term treatment	87	34/87 (39%)	9/34 (26%)
Long-term maintenance therapy	92	10/92 (11%)	0/10 (0%)

and checked the serum for HCV-RNA by the polymerase chain reaction (PCR) (Weiner et al., 1990) to find whether the antibodies detected by the kits were actually antibodies to HCV. We also analyzed the relationship between a therapeutic efficacy of corticosteroid and HCV infection in AIH type 1.

6.1. Anti-HCV in AIH type 1

We measured anti-HCV in serum from 26 patients with AIH type 1 treated in our department.

The patients studied had AIH type 1, were hospitalized in our hepatic care unit, and fulfilled the following criteria: the diagnosis of autoimmune hepatitis was histologically confirmed after liver biopsy; the concentration of serum γ-globulin was at least 20 g/l, and ANA and anti-SMA were present. Results of tests for HBsAg were negative. We selected 26 patients for study: 23 women and 3 men, ranging in age from 27 to 69 years (mean 52 years). Of these 26 patients, 13 had LE cell phenomenon and 5 had had blood transfusions.

Table 5 shows patient profiles. A larger proportion of women were categorized as having AIH type 1, and this group had high serum γ-globulin levels.

Serum samples obtained from patients with AIH during the active period of liver damage were stored frozen before being tested for anti-HCV and HCV-RNA.

6.1.1. HCV antibody testing

6.1.1.1. ELISA-I.
HCV antibodies were measured with ELISA-I kits (ELISA-I Ortho Diagnostics KK, Japan). The C100-3 antigen used in this kit is a sequence of 363 amino acids in the non-structural (NS) region 4: the antigen was identified

Table 5

Clinical findings of patients with autoimmune hepatitis type 1 and controls with chronic hepatitis type non-A, non-B

ALT, alanine aminotransferase.

Variable	Autoimmune hepatitis type 1 ($n = 26$)	Non-A, non-B chronic hepatitis ($n = 52$)	P-value
Mean age (years)	52 ± 11	48 ± 13	0.13[a]
Sex			
Female	23	16	< 0.01[b]
Male	3	36	
Serum ALT (U/l)	5.5 ± 4.5	3.4 ± 2.5	0.08[a]
Serum γ-globulin			
concentration (g/l)	35 ± 11	19 ± 3	< 0.01

[a] By Wilcoxon rank-sum test.
[b] By Fisher exact test.

in the genome of HCV by Choo et al. (1989). In ELISA-I, the C100-3 antigen and superoxide dismutase (SOD) are fused and are used to coat the wells of a microplate.

6.1.1.2. RIA-I. HCV antibodies were also measured with C100-3 radioimmunoassay (Ortho RIA-I, Ortho and Ohtsuka Assay, Japan) that also used the C100-3 antigen and SOD as a single fusion protein. The Ortho RIA-I was a modification of the method of Kuo and colleagues (1989).

6.1.1.3. ELISA-II. HCV antibodies were also measured with a second-generation ELISA kit (ELISA-II, Ortho). The kit combines the expression peptide C22-3 from the core region and the expression peptide C33c from the NS-3 region with the C100-3 antigen and detects antibodies for these 3 antigens (Bassetti et al., 1991).

6.1.1.4. RIBA-II. Test results with ELISA-I, RIA-I and ELISA-II were checked with a second-generation recombinant immunoblot assay (RIBA-II: Chiron Co. U.S.A., and Ortho, Japan). The RIBA-II, recommended as a confirmatory test for anti-HCV, was used to check the specificity of the results from the other tests. This method uses 4 peptides with sequences of 5-1-1, C100-3, C33c and C22-3, coded for by HCV, and fixed to a strip. Antibodies to SOD are also detectable with this assay (Van der Poel et al., 1991) (Table 6). All positive results were checked by retesting on two subsequent occasions.

6.1.2. Test results for anti-HCV

Of the 26 patients with AIH, 23 (88%) were anti-HCV-positive by ELISA-I; of these, 10 patients had a high titer (cut-off index of 6.0 or more). Twelve patients (46%) had anti-HCV detected by RIA-I and 20 patients (77%) by ELISA-II. Of these 26 patients, however, 9 (35%) had anti-HCV confirmed by RIBA-II (Table 6).

6.2. HCV-RNA in AIH type 1

6.2.1. HCV-RNA testing

We extracted RNA using the method of Chomczynski and Sacchi (1987), and complementary DNA (cDNA) was prepared with reverse transcriptase. Primers and a probe were constructed for the 5′-non-coding region based on sequence data for HCV (Okamoto et al., 1990).

The outer primers used were 5′-ACTCCACCATAGATCACTCCC-3′ (sense) and 5′-CCCAACACTACTCGGCTAGCA-3′ (anti-sense). The cDNA was amplified by 30 cycles of the PCR. One portion of the products of this reaction was sampled and used with another pair of primers designed to be inside those named above. Another 30 cycles of the PCR were done. We used a sense primer of

Table 6

Antibodies to hepatitis C virus (HCV) and HCV-RNA in patients with autoimmune hepatitis type 1
The antigen band intensities were compared with weakly positive (1 +) and moderately positive (3 +)
control bands, and were graded from negative (–) to 4 + for each antigen. A response of 1 + or greater
to any one HCV antigen was considered an indeterminate result (I), and a response to two or more
HCV antigens was considered a positive result (+). The result for HCV-RNA was considered positive
if staining was detected by Southern blotting. Minus (–) = negative result.

No. of cases	ELISA-I (C100-3)	RIA-I (C100-3)	ELISA-II	RIBA-II						HCV-RNA
				5-1-1	C100-3	C33	C22-3	SOD	Decision	
4	+	+	+	+	+	+	+	−	+	−
1	+	+	+	−	+	+	+	−	+	−
1	+	+	+	+	−	+	−	−	+	−
1	−	−	+	−	−	−	+	−	I	−
3	+	+	+	−	−	−	−	−	−	−
6	+	−	+	−	−	−	−	−	−	−
3	+	−	−	−	−	−	−	−	−	−
2	−	−	−	−	−	−	−	−	−	−
3	+	+	+	+	+	+	+	−	+	+
1	+	−	+	−	+	−	−	−	I	+
1	+	−	−	−	−	−	−	−	−	+
26	23/26 (88%)	12/26 (46%)	20/26 (77%)	8/26 (31%)	9/26 (35%)	9/26 (35%)	9/26 (35%)	0	9/26 (35%)	5/26 (19%)

5′-TTAGTATGAGTGTCGTGCAGC-3′. The product obtained was treated by
electrophoresis and then by Southern blotting using a probe, 5′-GCAAT-
TCCGGTGTACTCACC-3′, labeled with ^{32}P.

All PCR were initially done in duplicate. This reaction was done a third time
with the same serum sample after 1 week. Each PCR included 3 negative controls
and 3 positive controls. Using this method, we were able to check for false-
positive results caused by contamination and for false-negative results, Taq
polymerase activity or similar reactions.

6.2.2. Test results for HCV-RNA

Only 5 (19%) had HCV-RNA in their serum by PCR in 26 patients with AIH type
1. Of 20 patients with AIH type 1 positive for anti-HCV by ELISA-II, 4 (20%) had
HCV-RNA in their serum. Of 11 patients with autoimmune hepatitis who were
positive or indeterminate for anti-HCV by RIBA-II, 4 (36%) had HCV-RNA in
their serum and 9 were positive for anti-C100-3 by RIBA-II, 4 (44%) had
HCV-RNA in their serum. Therefore, 'real' HCV antibodies co-existed with
HCV-RNA in 20% to 45% of such patients, depending on the test. None of
these patients had antibodies to SOD.

The sensitivities of the assay kits for the patients with AIH type 1 were 5 of 5 (100%) by ELISA-I, 3 of 5 (60%) by RIA-I, 4 of 5 (80%) by ELISA-II and 3 of 5 (60%) by RIBA-II.

The specificities of the assay kits in patients with AIH type 1 were 3 of 21 (14%) by ELISA-I, 12 of 21 (57%) by RIA-I, 5 of 21 (24%) by ELISA-II, and 15 of 21 (71%) by RIBA-II. The specificities of the ELISA-I and -II assays were lower than those of the other assays in patients with AIH type 1.

6.3. Therapeutic efficacy in AIH type 1 with HCV-RNA

All patients with AIH received treatment with corticosteroid after serum samples were obtained. Twenty-one (81%) had a complete response as shown by normalization of serum alanine aminotransferase (ALT) and serum γ-globulin levels. The ALT levels of the remaining 5 patients decreased after the treatment, but did not attain normal values. Of the 21 patients who responded completely to therapy, 18 had anti-HCV (86%) by ELISA-I. Of these 18 patients, only 5 had anti-HCV confirmed by RIBA-II. These 5 patients, however, did not have HCV-RNA. The titer of anti-HCV detected by ELISA-II decreased in these patients during the treatment with corticosteroids when the serum γ-globulin level decreased to normal. Three of these 5 patients, however, remained anti-HCV-positive. We detected HCV-RNA before and during the treatment in two patients who responded completely to the therapy. One had indeterminate results by RIBA-II; and the other had negative results by this assay. One patient had a history of blood transfusion. Their serologic profiles were typical of AIH type 1 and their clinical courses did not differ from those of the 19 patients who did not have HCV-RNA.

Of the 5 patients who did not respond completely to the treatment with corticosteroids, all had anti-HCV detected by ELISA-I, RIA-I and ELISA-II: 4 patients had anti-HCV detected by RIBA-II and 3 had HCV-RNA (Table 7), these patients had severe hypergammaglobulinemia and a high titer of ANA: two patients had LE cells. One patient had a history of blood transfusion. During the treatment with corticosteroids, the anti-HCV titer decreased but remained. Based solely on pretreatment clinical data, these patients could not have been distinguished from those who had a complete response to therapy.

Table 7

Efficacy of treatment with glucocorticoid for autoimmune hepatitis type 1 with or without HCV-RNA in serum by PCR

HCV-RNA in serum by PCR	No. of patients	Complete response to treatment
Negative	21	19/21 (90%)
Positive	5	2/5 (40%)

References

Bassetti, D., Cutrupi, V., Dallago, B. et al. (1991) Second-generation RIBA to confirm diagnosis of HCV infection (Letter). Lancet 337, 317–319.

Comczynski, P. and Sacchi, N. (1987) Single-step method of RNA isolation by acid guanidinium thiocyanate-phenol-chloroform extraction. Anal. Biochem. 162, 156–159.

Choo, Q.L., Kuo, G., Weiner, A.J. et al. (1989) Isolation of a cDNA clone derived from a blood-borne non-A, non-B viral hepatitis genome. Science 244, 359–362.

Esteban, J.I., Esteban, R., Viadomiu, L. et al. (1989) Hepatitis C virus antibodies among risk groups in Spain. Lancet 2, 294–297.

Kuo, G., Choo, Q.L., Alter, H.J. et al. (1989) An assay for circulating antibodies to a major etiologic virus of human non-A, non-B hepatitis. Science 244, 362–364.

Lenzi, M., Ballardini, G., Fusconi, M. et al. (1990) Type 2 autoimmune hepatitis and hepatitis C virus infection. Lancet 335, 258–259.

Mackay, I.R., Taft, L.T. and Cowling, D.C. (1956) Lupoid hepatitis. Lancet 2, 13–23.

Mackay, I.R. et al. (1965) Autoimmune hepatitis. Ann. NY Acad. Sci 124, 767.

McFarlane, I.G., Smith, H.M., Johnson, P.J. et al. (1990) Hepatitis C virus antibodies in chronic active hepatitis: pathogenetic factor or false-positive result? Lancet 335, 754–757.

Monna, T., Kuroki, T. and Yamamoto, S. (1985) Autoimmune hepatitis: the present status in Japan. Gastroenterol. Jap. 20, 260–271.

Okamoto, H., Okada, S., Sugiyama, Y. et al. (1990) The 5′-terminal sequence of the hepatitis C virus genome. Jap. J. Exp. Med. 60, 167–177.

Van der Poel, C.L., Cuipers, H.T.M., Reesink, H.W. et al. (1991) confirmation of hepatitis C infection by new four-antigen recombinant immunoblot assay. Lancet 337, 317–319.

Weiner, A.J., Kuo, G., Bradley, D.W. et al. (1990) Detection of hepatitis C viral sequences in non-A, non-B hepatitis. Lancet 335, 1–3.

Section VIII

Recent Aspects of Autoimmune Hepatitis

Autoimmune Hepatitis
Edited by M. Nishioka, G. Toda and M. Zeniya
© *1994, Elsevier Science B.V. All rights reserved*

Chapter 19

Recent aspects of autoimmune hepatitis

Mikio Nishioka and Syed Ahmed Morshed

Third Department of Internal Medicine, Kagawa Medical School, 1750-1, Ikenobe,
Miki-cho, Kita-gun, Kagawa, 761-07 (Japan)

1. Introduction

Autoimmune hepatitis (AIH) is a self-perpetuating inflammation of the liver that is characterized by hypergammaglobulinemia, the presence of autoantibody and histological feature of periportal hepatitis (Czaja et al., 1983; Czaja, 1984). The etiology of the autoimmune response and the pathophysiology of chronic inflammation in this syndrome are not clear (Meyer zum Büschenfelde et al., 1990). AIH is frequently associated with other autoimmune disorders. Association with HLA-A1-B8, -DR3 and -DW3, increase of the peripheral CD4:CD8 ratio and a suppressor T-cell defect reversible by prednisolone in vitro have been described. Epidemiologic and virologic studies suggest that autoimmune hepatitis is not the result of an ongoing viral infection with hepatitis B virus, hepatitis D virus or hepatitis C virus. Some drugs are also implicated in the development of this disorder that are similar to those described in other autoimmune disorders.

Previous observations of the natural course of AIH stressed the severity of the disease and a poor prognosis (Bearn et al., 1956; Wilcox and Isselbacher, 1961; Mackay and Wood, 1962). Results of controlled trials confirmed these observations (Copenhagen Study Group, 1969; Cook et al., 1971) and supported the view that AIH is an etiologically and clinically distinct subgroup of acute and chronic active hepatitis that benefits from immunosuppressive therapy (Kirk et al., 1980; Czaja et al., 1983). During the past 10 years, lymphocyte subsets and epitopes relevant for T-cell activation were identified. It was shown that CD8-positive lymphocytes are the predominant population of the inflammatory infiltrate in chronic viral hepatitis, as well as AIH (Autschbach et al., 1991), with a substantial proportion of lymphocytes expressing activation antigens like T11/3 (CD2) and IL2-R (CD25). LFA-3 (CD58), the natural ligand of the CD2/T11 lymphocyte surface receptor could be demonstrated on Kupffer cells, endothelial cells and hepatocytes. These data indicate that along with antigen-specific mechanisms, effector target cell interactions between hepatocytes and lymphocytes, mediated via an alternative pathway, may play a role in chronic autoimmune liver disease.

2. Deviation of age at onset among Japanese AIH patients

Since the initial report by Waldenström (1950), it is now known that the majority of patients with AIH are females between the ages of 10 and 30 years. However, the disease occurs in some postmenopausal women and in men as well.

In Japan, AIH seemed to be a rare disease 20 years ago. With the advent of diagnostic techniques such as detection of autoantibodies by immunofluorescence, the number of AIH patients is increasing (Monna et al., 1985). Presently, AIH patients, although seen in the past, are not so common in Japan. In addition, the age at onset of AIH seems to be increasing. A retrospective analysis by Nishioka et al. (1988) of 300 cases of AIH over 19 years starting in 1966 and ending in 1985 demonstrated that the peak incidence in terms of age at onset was 50–59 years (108 cases among 300 cases), whereas in the period 1966–1975 the peak was 40–49 years. It is clear that in Japan the age at onset of AIH has shifted to 50–59 years from 40–49 years, particularly in postmenopausal females (Table 1).

The reason for the increase in number of AIH patients in old people is unknown, but the rare incidence of the patients under 20 years of age in recent years may be one of the causes. Recently in Japan, the elderly population is rapidly increasing. It was also found that this increasing tendency of age at onset of AIH is shifting to 60–70 years.

Table 1

Number of patients with autoimmune hepatitis of different ages and time periods

	Age (years)							Total
	10–19	20–29	30–39	40–49	50–59	60–69	70–79	
1966–1970	0	2	2	3	1	0	0	8
1971–1975	4	6	11	21	20	8	.0	70
1976–1980	1	7	31	31	58	22	0	150
1981–1985	1	4	7	18	29	10	3	72
Total	6	19	51	73	108	40	3	300

3. Autoantibody patterns in AIH

Circulating autoantibodies are an important marker for the diagnosis of autoimmune chronic active hepatitis (CAH) and also for the classification of AIH patients (Manns, 1989). The so-called 'lupoid' hepatitis, which can be considered as classical autoimmune CAH, was first distinguished by the presence of hyper-gammaglobulinemia (Waldenström, 1950) and lupus erythematosus (LE) cells (Joske and King, 1955; Mackay et al., 1956), and later by antibodies to nuclei, smooth muscle (Johnson et al., 1965), and actin (Gabbiani et al., 1973). A second type of autoimmune CAH, referred to as AIH type 2 or anti-liver–kidney microsomes (anti-LKM-1)-positive CAH, because of the presence of circulating antibodies to LKM, may also be associated with anti-cytosol antibodies (Rizzetto et al., 1973; Homberg et al., 1974, 1987; Martini et al., 1988). Additional classification of autoimmune CAH has been proposed based on the presence of anti-'soluble liver-antigen' antibodies (Manns et al., 1987), antibodies to the liver-pancreas protein (Teufel et al., 1983) and to nuclear envelope proteins (lamins A and C) (Wesiersk-Gadek et al., 1988).

3.1. Antibodies to DNA and nuclear antigens

The anti-nuclear antibody (ANA), responsible for LE cell formation and homogeneously staining reactions by immunofluorescence, attributed to determinants on nuclear histones (Tan, 1989), was described in autoimmune CAH patients. The actual nuclear antigenic specificity for ANA reactions in AIH is still not fully defined and may be multiple. Among the reactants are antibodies to nuclear histones as well as antibodies to some saline-extractable nuclear antigens designated XR and XH, which are found in 25% and 10% of patients, respectively (Bernstein et al., 1984). Antibodies to nuclear lamins are found in 70% of patients (Lassoued et al., 1988; Wesiersk-Gadek et al., 1988). Few patients with AIH are also positive for antibodies to nucleolar constituents (Kenneally et al., 1984).

Extractable nuclear antigens (ENAs) are molecules now identified as ribonucleoproteins, of which there are two major groups (Whittingham and McNeilage, 1988; Van Venrooij and Sellekens, 1989; Tan, 1989). These are the U-RNPs, particularly U1-RNP and the Sm antigen, and the Ro (SS-A) and La (SS-B) antigens that are constituted of various RNA species which are associated with polypeptides of cytoplasmic (Ro) or nuclear origin (La). These antibodies occur in a number of cases of systemic lupus erythematosus (SLE) and related diseases, but seldom in CAH.

In our recent studies (Terada et al., 1991), anti-SS-A was seen in 23% of our AIH patients. Only one patient with AIH, complicated with Sjögren's syndrome (SjS), had anti-SS-B (Table 2). This antibody seems very rare in AIH patients and may be more specific for SjS patients. Two out of 35 AIH patients also had anti-RNP antibodies in their sera, and one of the patients was complicated with

Table 2
Incidence of anti-nuclear antibodies (ANA) in autoimmune diseases (%)
AIH, autoimmune hepatitis; SLE, systemic lupus erythematosus; MCTD, mixed connective tissue
disorder; PSS, progressive systemic sclerosis; SjS, Sjögren's syndrome; RA, rheumatoid arthritis

Antibodies	AIH	SLE	MCTD	PSS	SjS	RA
ANA[a]	94	75	100	89	79	75
Anti-SS-A[b]	23	61	38	47	86	75
Anti-SS-B[b]	6	8	0	0	50	0
Anti-RNP[b]	6	33	100	21	14	21
Anti-ds-DNA[c]	19	38	36	90	50	75
Anti-ss-DNA[c]	97	94	94	32	7	75

[a] Immunofluorescence; [b] Ouchterlony; [c] ELISA (IgG).

another autoimmune disorder, such as progressive systemic sclerosis (PSS). Anti-ss-DNA was found in almost all AIH patients, but anti-ds-DNA was detected in only 19% of these patients.

In the current study, ANA were studied on the basis of immunofluorescent and Western blot analysis. In our study of 35 Japanese patients with AIH, the homogeneous pattern of ANA was found to be common (55%). Other patterns such as speckled (17%), centromers (10%) and diffuse perinuclear (6%) were also detected. Among the speckled, the fine pattern was usually seen in 12% of AIH patients. No nucleolar dot pattern was detected in any case of AIH (Nishioka, 1993).

There was a heterogeneity among the antigens specific for ANA as detected by Western blot. Apparent target peptides of: 33, 36, 50, 55, 60, 62, 64, 80 and 100 kDa in the homogeneous pattern; 12, 29, 33, 50, 60, 70 and 80 kDa in the speckled pattern; 17, 25, 30, 80, 100, 120 and 140 kDa in the centromere pattern; and 70, 90 and 100 kDa in the peripheral pattern were found in the sera of these AIH patients (Nishioka, 1993).

Recent advances of recombinant DNA technology have made it possible to synthesize recombinant proteins. Detection of ANA subtypes will be replaced by more reliable enzyme-linked immunosorbent assay (ELISA) using recombinant

Table 3
Incidence of antibodies to recombinant proteins in autoimmune liver diseases

	No. of Cases	Antibodies to				
		U1-RNP-A	U1-RNP-70	SS-A-60	SS-A-52	Cenp-B
AIH	35	5 (14%)	6 (17%)	4 (11%)	7 (20%)	5 (14%)
PBC	10	0 (0%)	1 (10%)	2 (20%)	7 (70%)	4 (40%)
Normal	20	0 (0%)	0 (0%)	0 (0%)	0 (0%)	0 (0%)

proteins. We synthesized RNP-70 and RNP-A which are autoantigens of anti U1-RNP, 52K- and 60K-SS-A/Ro which are recognized by anti-SS-A/Ro and Cenp-B which is an 80 kDa centromere antigen. Antibodies to recombinant peptides such as RNP-70 (17%), RNP-A (14%), 52K-SS-A/Ro (20%), 60K-SS-A/Ro (11%) and Cenp-B (14%) were detected in sera from AIH patients by ELISA (Nishioka, 1993) (Table 3). They were frequently found in AIH patients with complications of autoimmune-related diseases such as SjS, PSS and Raynaud's phenomenon (Terada et al., 1991).

3.2. Antibodies to smooth muscle antigens

Antibody reactivities to smooth muscle antigen (SMA) of vascular (glomerular) endothelium indicated that the reactant was not limited to smooth muscle (Whittingham et al., 1966a). It was then ascertained that the antibody reacted with a submembranous constituent of cultured cells (Mackay, 1985), which was identified as actin. Various other reactants for SMA were found, with the common property as elements of the cellular cytoskeleton. Actin, vimentin, and tubulin were found to be the 3 main reactants for SMA.

The antibodies to native actin-containing microfilaments are also a marker for AIH (Toh, 1979). The main autoantigen appears to be actin itself, but antibodies to troponin, tropomyosin, and α-actinin can be demonstrated as well. However, antibodies in CAH associated with a viral infection react mainly with intermediate-sized filaments. The main subunit protein was found to be vimentin (Toh, 1979). These antibodies are frequently found together with ANA in lupoid hepatitis or may represent their own serologic subgroup when no other autoantibodies are detectable (Odievre et al., 1983). Anti-actin is helpful in distinguishing autoimmune CAH from presumed virally induced types in which anti-vimentin accounts for SMA reactivity (Gerken et al., 1987). Since the anti-actin type of SMA is a marker for autoimmune CAH and does not occur in SLE, it serves for serologic differentiation between these two diseases (Pedersen et al., 1982). Anti-actin autoantibodies may, in part, be responsible for the in vitro binding of immunoglobulin G (IgG) to the surface of mechanically isolated hepatocytes (Whittingham et al., 1966b).

SMA, such as antibodies to microfilament, intermediate filament and microtubules, can be detected at variable rates in liver diseases including AIH (Table 4) (Kurki and Virtanen, 1984; Nishioka et al., 1985; Zauli et al., 1985). However, 78% of AIH patients in this study were positive for antibody to SMA and most sera reacted with both microfilaments and intermediate filaments.

3.3. Antibodies to liver–kidney microsomal antigens

Antibodies to liver–kidney microsome (LKM) were differentiated from anti-mitochondrial antibodies (AMA) independently by Rizzetto et al. (1973, 1974)

                    M. Nishioka and S.A. Morshed

Table 4
Autoantibodies to cytoskeleton in sera from patients with liver diseases
CAH, chronic active hepatitis; PBC, primary biliary cirrhosis; ALD, autoimmune liver diseases;
NC, normal control; CLD, chronic liver disease; AIH, autoimmune hepatitis; MF, microfilaments;
IMF, intermediate filaments; MT, microtubules.

Reference	Patients and controls	Antibodies to cytoskeleton (%)		
		MF	IMF	MT
Kurki et al. (1984)	CAH	55–67	88	15
	PBC	53	93	7
	ALD	25	50	50
	NC	3	14–63	3–9
Zauli et al. (1985)	CLD			
	HBV (+)	3	32	15
	HBV (−)	66	66	10
	PBC	18	81	0
	ALD	33	69	22
	NC	0	10	0
Nishioka et al. (1985)	Acute hepatitis			
	Hepatitis A	0	100	0
	Hepatitis B	12	12	0
	Non-A, non-B	0	0	0
	CAH			
	HBs (+)	21	7	0
	HBs (−)	22	22	11
	AIH	100	100	0
	Liver cirrhosis	25	25	25
	PBC	33	33	0
	NC	0	0	0

and Homberg et al. (1974) using immunofluorescence of tissues obtained from the liver, kidney and stomach. This type of antibody has been described in patients who commonly have associated immunologic disorders, and absence of both SMA and ANA (Maggiore et al., 1986; Homberg et al., 1987; Manns and Meyer zum Büschenfelde, 1990). They have often been diagnosed as AIH type 2 because of anti-LKM-1 seropositivity (Maddrey, 1987; Homberg et al., 1987). Preliminary studies have suggested that these subclassifications are important because individuals with type 2 disease may progress more rapidly to cirrhosis than their counterparts with type 1 disease (classical or lupoid hepatitis) (Homberg et al., 1987). However, AIH type 2 is a disease described mainly in Europe (Maggiore et al., 1986; Homberg et al., 1987; Manns and Meyer zum Büschenfelde, 1990; Manns, 1991), and infrequently in the United States (Czaja et al., 1992) and Japan (Monna et al., 1985; Miyachi et al., 1991).

Table 5
Incidence of anti-liver–kidney microsomal (LKM) antibodies in patients
with chronic active hepatitis

CAH	No. of cases	Anti-LKM antibodies[a]	Anti-LKM-1 (P-450-IID6) antibodies[b]
B virus	56	0 (0%)	0 (0%)
C virus	95	3 (3.2%)	0 (0%)
δ Virus	10	0 (0%)	0 (0%)
Non-A, non-B	25	0 (0%)	0 (0%)
AIH	35	2 (5.7%)	1 (2.8%)
Total	221	5 (2.2%)	1 (0.4%)

[a] Detected by immunofluorescence using mouse liver and kidney section.
[b] Detected by Western blot using recombinant P-450-IID6 antigen.

We have analyzed sera from 221 patients with CAH including hepatitis B virus, hepatitis C virus (HCV), non-A, non-B, non-C, hepatitis D virus, and AIH by immunofluorescence assay using frozen sections from a mouse kidney–liver block. The presence of anti-LKM-1 antibody was confirmed by immunoblot assay using recombinant P-450-IID6 (Gift from Dr. M.P. Manns, Hannover, Germany) as a target antigen (50 kDa). Anti-LKM antibodies were found in 5.7% of patients with AIH, 3.2% of patients with CAH-HCV, and in none of the other patients by immunofluorescence test (Table 5). Using immunoblot assay, anti-LKM-1 antibodies were detected in only one patient with AIH. Anti-LKM antibodies were positive in 2.2% of CAH patients and anti-LKM-1 antibodies were found in 0.5% of these patients, suggesting the low incidence of anti-LKM and anti-LKM-1 antibodies in Japanese CAH patients.

4. Human CYP2D6 gene in AIH patients

Cytochrome P-450 enzymes are components of the microsomal multisubstrate mono-oxygenase system responsible for the oxidative metabolism of a large number of endobiotic and xenobiotic substances (Boobis et al., 1985; Ortiz de Montellano, 1986; Nebert and Gonzalez, 1987). In recent years, several genetically determined polymorphisms of P-450-mediated drug oxidation have been discovered. The term genetic polymorphism refers to a Mendelian or monogenic trait that exists in the population in at least two phenotypes, neither of which is rare, i.e. occurs at a frequency of more than 1–2% (Vogel and Motulsky, 1979). Genetic polymorphisms of drug oxidation show impaired biotransformation of certain drugs in subjects who are called 'poor metabolizers' (PM). Because of their frequency of occurrence, genetic polymorphisms of drug oxidation are major determinants of inter-individual differences in the therapeutic and toxic responses to numerous clinically important drugs (Evans, 1986; Meyer et al., 1990). One of the most extensively studied examples of a genetically determined variation in drug metabolism is the debrisoquine genetic polymorphism (Mahgoub et al., 1977; Eichelbaum et al., 1979; Evans, 1986; Meyer et al., 1986, 1990) which occurs in 5–10% of individuals in Caucasian populations and which affects the metabolism of >20 drugs, including the prototype drugs such as debrisoquine, sparteine, dextromethorphan, and bufuralol and also β-adrenergic blocking agents, anti-depressants, anti-arrhythmics, and other drugs widely used in clinical medicine (Mahgoub et al., 1977; Eichelbaum et al., 1979; Evans, 1986). Pedigree studies suggest that this defect is monogenically inherited as an autosomal recessive trait (Evans et al., 1980).

The metabolic defect usually reflects an absence of CYP2D6 (the gene coding for P-450-IID6) protein caused by mutations in the CYP2D6 gene in affected individuals, which results in PM phenotype, as comapred to the wild type 'extensive metabolizer' (EM). Those two phenotypes are found to differ in their ability to oxidize drugs (Gough et al., 1990; Hanioka et al., 1990; Kagimoto et al., 1990; Gaedigk et al., 1991). Because of the high frequency of mutations in CYP2D gene (Gonzalez et al., 1988; Skoda et al., 1988), one may speculate that a mutation in a critical region of the P-450-IID6 gene could result in an alteration of the structure of the protein, and in the generation of autoantibodies against this protein as found in patients with AIH. Cytochrome P-450-IID6 is also the target antigen of LKM-1 antibody in AIH type 2 patients. It was recently shown, however, that all patients with AIH and anti-LKM-1 antibody, so far tested, are EM, and that the P-450-IID6 is normally present in their liver (Jacqz-Aigrain et al., 1990; Manns et al., 1990; Yamamoto et al., 1992). However, these results do not exclude the possibility of a mutation in one of the alleles, the other coding for a normal protein.

In our study on the phenotypes, DNA from peripheral blood mononuclear cell (PBMC) taken from various liver diseases and healthy volunteers was studied by polymerase chain reaction (PCR) amplification of two regions, i.e., fragment A with a frameshift mutation in the exon 5 and fragment B with a mutation in the splice site, of the CYP2D6 gene, that was introduced by Heim and Meyer (1990). In the first step, the 1123bp fragment A, containing both exons 5 and 6, was amplified by PCR and the product was re-amplified either with mutant or wild-type primers. Similarly, the 739bp fragment B, which includes both exons 3 and 4, was amplified and re-amplified either with mutant or wild-type primers (Heim and Meyer, 1990; Smith et al., 1992; Orishki et al., 1992).

All patients including AIH were found to be extensive metabolizers in the study (Orishki et al., 1992). One of 60 healthy volunteers showed a mutant type, but the frequency of the mutant type was very low in the Japanese population. There was no significant difference in the frequency of PM in the patients studied, suggesting no association of cytochrome P-450-IID6 phenotypes and liver diseases. However, our results do not completely exclude the possibility of mutations in a critical region of the protein which modifies its cellular location, triggering the autoimmune response in AIH type 2 patients. If ever the CYP2D6 gene is involved in autoimmune response in such patients, it could be only through subtle changes such as microdeletion, insertion or point substitutions which warrant sequencing of the gene.

5. *Cytokine expression in the liver of AIH patients*

Regulation of the immune response and host defense involves cytokines as effector molecules. Cytokines are pleomorphic proteins which are produced by cells of both hematopoetic and non-hematopoetic cell lineage. They act locally at sites of immune response and/or inflammation and are usually rapidly degraded. There is interacting cascade of cytokines which can synergize with or antagonize each other. Cytokines in the liver include those of the acute phase response, specific and non-specific responses to viral infection and autoimmune diseases. Cytokines are produced by, at or upon components of liver parenchyma such as hepatocytes, Kupffer cells, endothelial cells, Ito cells and synosoidal lining cells (Shiratori et al., 1988; Decker, 1989). Inflammation and tissue damage lead to the acute phase response with changes in levels of liver-derived proteins. These responses are mediated by interleukin (IL)-1, IL-6 and tumor necrosis factor (TNF) (Thiele, 1989; Andus et al., 1991). Viral infection stimulates various cytokines including interferons which in turn can induce other cytokines (Welsh, 1986; Janeway, 1988, 1989).

The mechanisms required to propagate autoimmune phenomena have not been well defined in autoimmune diseases, and even the role of specific cytokines is unclear. One of the key functional parameters determining the outcome of immune responses in autoimmune lesions is the patterns of the cytokine produced locally by immune cells, yet they are unknown for autoimmune liver diseases. There has been accumulating evidence that cytokines/lymphokines play an important role in the pathogenesis of AIH. Lymphokine-mediated events may occur during the initiation and effector stages of immune response in AIH. Our studies showed that levels of IL-6, and TNF-α are increased in sera from AIH patients (Fig. 1) when compared with non-autoimmune liver disease patients.

It is well known that unstimulated lymphocytes from patients with AIH and other hepatobiliary diseases such as CAH-B, CAH-C and chronic active non-A, non-B, non-C hepatitis and healthy controls do not produce detectable amounts of TNF-α, IL-1β, IL-6, IL-2 and interferon-γ (INF-γ). In an attempt to study the role of cytokines in the liver, IL-1β, IL-2, IL-6, IL-10, TNF-α and INF-γ genes have been investigated in situ using a reverse transcription-polymerase chain reaction (RT-PCR) technique (Wang et al., 1989; Gilliland et al., 1990;

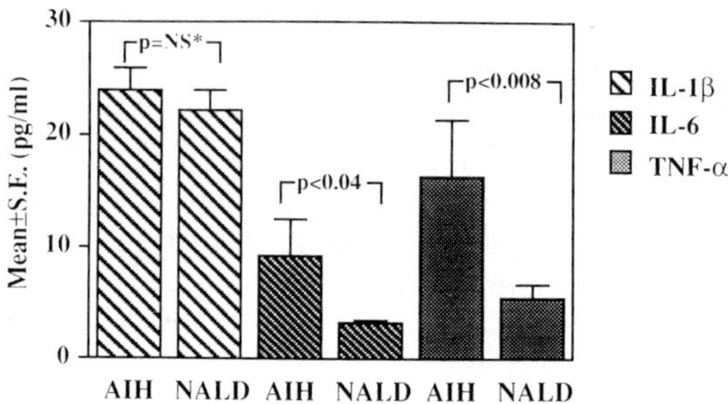

Fig. 1. Serum concentration of IL-1β, IL-6 and TNF-α in liver diseases. The concentration (pg/ml; mean $\pm$ S.E.) was measured by enzyme-linked immunosorbent assay (ELISA) kit. AIH, autoimmune hepatitis; NALD, non-autoimmune liver diseases; IL, interleukin; TNF, tumor necrosis factor. Wilcoxon-signed-Rank test for paired data was used to examine the significance of differences, with $P = 0.05$ as the minimum level of significance. NS*, not significant.

Yamamura et al., 1991; Morshed and Nishioka, 1992). In our studies, total RNA from the frozen tissues of biopsy specimens from AIH patients was purified by acid guanidium-thiocyanade-phenol-chloroform extraction. Ten to 100 ng mRNA was reverse transcribed to cDNA by the random priming method with hexanucleotide. Ten microliters of cDNA was specifically amplified with each cytokine specific 5' and 3' primers in 50 µl PCR reaction mixture by a DNA Thermal Cycler (Perkin Elmer Cetus). The amplified products of each sample were visualized by 1.7% agarose gel electrophoresis stained with ethidium bromide under ultraviolet light. Sensitivity and specificity of cytokines RT-PCR was also performed in a 10-fold serial dilutional assay of cytoplasmic RNA (100, 10, 1 ng, etc.) from lipopolysaccharide (LPS)-stimulated PBMC of healthy individuals. The specificity of the amplified products was validated by their predicted sizes an agarose gels (Yamamura et al., 1991; Morshed and Nishioka, 1992), and by slot-blot hybridization with [γ-^{32}P] ATP-end-labeled oligonucleotide probes internal to the primers.

The results in the RT-PCR study were semi-quantitatively analyzed by the densitometric tracing of slot-blot hybridization. IFN-γ and IL-6 were detected in all liver tissues of AIH patients at variable degrees of signal intensities (Fig. 2). IL-1β, IL-10 and TNF-α were detected in some AIH patients (Fig. 3). IL-2 gene was undetectable in all liver specimens of AIH patients while all cytokine RNA transcripts were detected in LPS-stimulated PBMC. In contrast, the expression of the cytokines was undetectable in normal human liver taken at autopsy. The results may indicate a possible link between reduced IFN-γ and increased IL-10 expressions judging by the presence of IL-10 that is produced by Th2-like lymphocytes in the liver of AIH patients (Yamamura et al., 1991). There is increasing evidence that human CD4 + T-cells involved in certain inflammatory

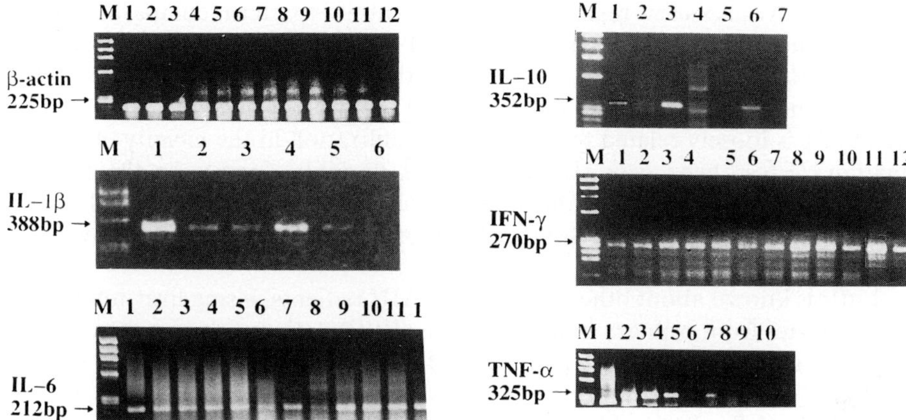

Fig. 2. Examples of reverse transcribed-polymerase chain reaction (RT-PCR) amplified products of β-actin and cytokines in the liver of autoimmune hepatitis (AIH) patients. As an internal control, β-actin primers were used for cytoplasmic actin gene in each sample of liver mRNA (10 ng) analyzed. Amplified products were electrophoresed in 1.7% agarose gel stained with ethidium bromide. Cytokine genes were detected according to their predicted sizes at variable staining intensities under UV-light. Lane M, ϕX174/Hae II digest as a size marker; lanes 1–12, β-actin, IL-6, IFN-γ; 1–6, IL-1β; and 1–7, IL-10. In TNF-α (325 bp), lane 1 is a β-actin product (225 bp). IL-2 gene was undetectable in all samples from AIH liver.

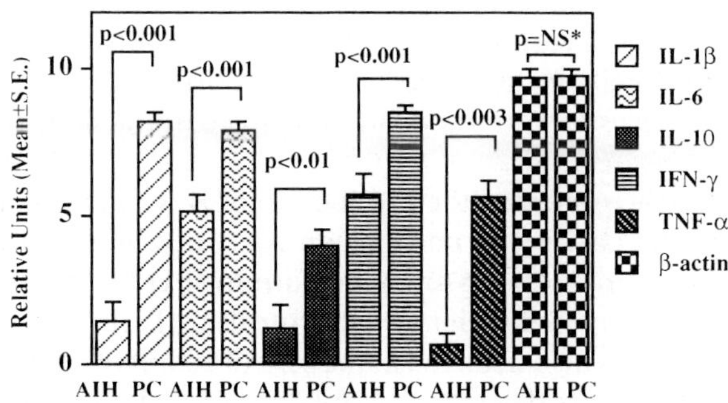

Fig. 3. Semi-quantitative analysis of RT-PCR cytokines produced in the liver of autoimmune hepatitis patients. Aliquots were removed after 35 cycles of PCR, transferred to nylon membranes for slot blots, hybridized with ^{32}P-labeled internal probes specific for cytokines and β-actin, and quantitated by densitometry tracing of the autoradiograph of slot-blot hybridization. Peak areas are given as relative units. RT-PCR, reverse transcribed-polymerase chain reaction; AIH, mRNA from liver of autoimmune hepatitis; PC, positive controls from lipopolysaccharide-induced peripheral blood mononuclear cells mRNA; IL, interleukin; IFN, interferon; TNF, tumor necrosis factor. β-Actin primers were used as an internal control for each RT-PCR sample examined. Wilcoxon signed-Rank test for paired data was used to examine the significance of differences, with $P = 0.05$ as the minimum level of significance. NS*, not significant.

or allergic diseases show restricted cytokine synthesis patterns comparable to the murine Th1 and Th2 subsets (Haanen et al., 1991; Del Prete et al., 1991; Wierenga et al., 1991; Yssel et al., 1991). However, in this study, IL-1β, IL-10 and TNF-α expression may be related to the severity of the disease since the expression of cytokines is loosely related to lymphocytic infiltration in the vicinity of inflammation. IFN-γ gene was also detected at variable degrees in the liver of HCV-infected patients at various stages (Morshed and Nishioka, 1992). It seems that IFN-γ is an important cytokine playing a key role in the cytokine network of the liver.

Little is known about other cytokines in AIH patients. Using liver-infiltrating lymphocytes from primary biliary cirrhosis (PBC) patients, the cytokine profile has been described (Pape et al., 1991). Reduced lymphokine production such as TNF-α, TNF-β and IFN-γ in PBC patients was reported by Pape et al. (1991). Using cloned T-cells from liver infiltrates, Schlaak et al., described an increased production of IL-4 in AIH patients when compared with non-autoimmune liver diseases (Schlaak et al., 1992). IFN-γ production was found to be at variable degrees, resulting in Th2- or Th0-like profiles in their study. They stressed that studies on liver-infiltrating T-cells obtained from patients with AIH and non-autoimmune liver diseases were associated with different cytokine profiles. However, this evidence seems problematic since these cells may not reflect the functional state of lymphocytes in the liver, as they require a rigorous in vitro manipulation. Our findings of IL-10 and IFN-γ in the liver of AIH patients as shown in Fig. 3 indicate similar phenomena to those described by Schlaak et al. (1992). Since we have used total RNA from liver tissues, the findings, in fact, represented the in vivo cytokine status. Further studies, such as localization of cytokine-producing cells in the liver by immunohistochemistry and by in situ hybridization, are necessary for understanding the pathogenetic role of cytokines in AIH.

In another study, we detected the production of IL-6, TNF-α and IFN-γ from PBMC of either AIH patients or normal controls. Increased production of these cytokines was found in 24-h phytohemagglutinin (PHA)-stimulated PBMC of AIH patients when compared with normal controls by ELISA (Schumacher et al., 1988) (Fig. 4). IL-1β was also detected in the sera of 10 out of 12 AIH patients, and both IL-6 and TNF-α were detected in 6 of 12 patients. A slight increase of IFN-γ in the sera was also found in 5 of 12 AIH patients (Fig. 4). Four of 12 patients showed a simultaneous increase of IL-1β, IL-6, TNF-α and IFN-γ in their sera, suggesting the in vivo activation of these cytokines and the production of IFN-γ may be associated with the cytokines of the acute-phase response.

Cytokine function seems to provide an interactive communication network to coordinate the immune response in the development of inflammation and specific immune reaction. Transient production of picomolar concentrations of these cytokines is limited to a discrete local area. Recent investigations suggest that local lymphokine production is also necessary for the induction of anti-self

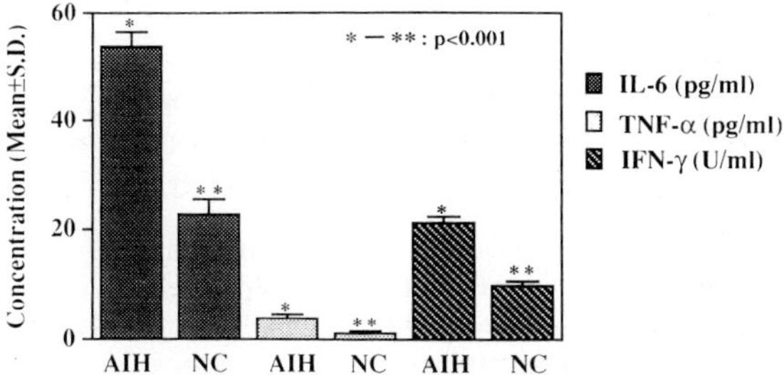

Fig. 4. Production of IL-6, TNF-α and IFN-γ in culture medium of peripheral blood mononuclear cells (PBMC). The PBMCs were stimulated with phytohemagglutinin for 24 h from patients with autoimmune hepatitis (AIH) and from healthy controls (NC). The concentration (mean ± S.D.) of cytokines was measured by enzyme-linked immunosorbent assay (ELISA) kit. IL, interleukin; TNF, tumor necrosis factor; IFN, interferon. Wilcoxon signed-Rank test for paired data was used to examine the significance of differences, with $P = 0.05$ as the minimum level of significance.

T-cells (Sarvetnick et al., 1988). Because of their importance in coordinating the immune response and the interwoven nature of their effector function, it is clear that an abnormality in regulation of their production or the reception of their signal could contribute to the development of autoimmunity (Pujol-Borrel et al., 1987; Paul and Ruddle, 1988; Taniguchi, 1988; Balkwill and Burke, 1989; Beutler and Cerami, 1989; Jacob et al., 1990; Sinha et al., 1990).

Previous studies have suggested that anergic T-cells are best characterized in vitro by their inability to produce certain cytokines such as IL-2 (Schwartz et al., 1989). It has also been demonstrated that in vivo administration of IL-2 turns on anergic self-reactive T-cells and leads to autoimmune disease in athymic nude mice (Andreu-Sanchez et al., 1991; Gutierrez-Ramos et al., 1992). We provide further evidence to support the fact that the inability of lymphocytes in the liver to produce detectable IL-2 gene and the simultaneous high expression of IFN-γ, IL-6 and possibly other cytokines (i.e., IL-1β, TNF-α and IL-10) may activate T-cell expansion and alter their function in vivo (Sarvetnick et al., 1988). It appears, therefore, that aberrant delivery of co-stimulatory signals in this case provided by certain cytokines may lead to the generation of aggressive autoreactive T-cells. This may be considered as a possible mechanism for the breakdown of tolerance in AIH patients as it is thought that the failure to achieve tolerance or the breakdown of tolerance can lead to the development of autoimmune diseases (Schwartz, 1989; Von Boehmer et al., 1989). Taken together, our findings of in vivo and in vitro studies suggest that cytokines produced at the site of inflammation as signal molecules may have a distinct role in the immunoregulatory circuit of the liver, and may be associated with autoimmune phenomenon seen in AIH patients.

References

Andreu-Sanchez, J.L., Moreno de Alboran, I.M., Marcos, M.A., Sanchez-Movilla, A., Martinez, A.C. and Kroemer, G. (1991) Interleukin 2 abrogates the nonresponsive state of T cells expressing a forbidden T cell receptor repertoire and induces autoimmune disease in neonatally thymectomized mice. J. Exp. Med. 173, 1323–1329.

Andus, T., Bauer, J., Gerok, W. (1991) Effects of cytokines on the liver. Hepatology 13, 364–375.

Autschbach, F., Meuer, S.C., Moebius, U. et al. (1991) Hepatocellular expression of lymphocyte function-associated antigen 3 in chronic hepatitis. Hepatology 14, 223–230.

Balkwill, F.R. and Burke, F. (1989) The cytokine network. Immunol. Today 10, 299–304.

Bearn, A.G., Kunkel, H.G., and Slater, R.J. (1956) The problem of chronic liver disease in young women. Am. J. Med. 21, 3–15.

Bernstein, R.M., Neuberger, J.M., Bunn, C.C., Callender, M.E., Hughes, G.R.V. and Williams, R. (1984) Diversity of autoantibodies in primary biliary cirrhosis and chronic active hepatitis. Clin. Exp. Immunol. 55, 553–560.

Beutler, B. and Cerami, A. (1989) The biology of cachectin/TNF – a primary mediator of the host response. Annu. Rev. Immunol. 7, 625–655.

Boobis, A., Caldwell, J., DeMatteis, F. and Elcombe, C.R. (Eds.) (1985) Microsomes and Drug Oxidations. Taylor and Francis, London, pp. 1–428.

Cook, G.C., Mulligan, R. and Sherlock, S. (1971) Controlled prospective trial of corticosteroid therapy in active chronic hepatitis. Q. J. Med. 40, 159–185.

Copenhagen Study Group for Liver Diseases (1969) Effect of prednisone on the survival of patients with cirrhosis of the liver. Lancet 1, 119–121.

Czaja, A.J. (1984) Natural history, clinical features, and treatment of autoimmune hepatitis. Semin. Liver Dis. 4, 1–12.

Czaja, A.J., Davis, G.L., Ludwig, J., Baggenstoss, A.H. and Taswell, H.F. (1983) Autoimmune features as determinants of prognosis in steroid-treated chronic active hepatitis of uncertain etiology. Gastroenterology 85, 713–717.

Czaja, A.J., Manns, M.P. and Homberger, H.A. (1992) Frequency and significance of antibodies to liver/kidney microsome type I in adults with chronic active hepatitis. Gastroenterology 103, 1290–1295.

Decker, K. (1989) Hepatic mediators of inflammation. In: E. Wisse, D.L. Knook and K. Decker (Eds.), Cells of the Hepatic Sinusoid. The Kupffer Cell Foundation, Rijswijk, Vol. 2, 86, 171–175.

Del Prete, G.F., De Carli, M., Mastromauro, C. et al. (1991) Purified protein derivative of mycobacterium tuberculosis and excretory–secretory antigen(s) of Toxacara canis expand in vitro human T cells with stable and opposite (type 1 helper or type 2 T helper) profile of cytokine production. J. Clin. Invest. 88, 346–350.

Eichelbaum, M., Sannbrucker, N., Steincke, B. and Dengler, H.J. (1979) Defective N-oxidation of sperteine in man: a new pharmacogenetic defect. Eur. J. Clin. Pharmacol. 16, 183–187.

Evans, D.A.P. (1986) Ethnic differences in reactions to drugs and xenobiotics: In: W. Kalow, H.W. Goedde and D.P. Agarwal (Eds.) Progress in Clinical and Biological Research. Liss, New York, 214, 491–526.

Evans, D.A., Mahgoub, A., Sloan, T.P., Idle, J.R. and Smith, R.L. (1980) A family and population study of the genetic polymorphism of debrisoquine oxidation in a white British population. J. Med. Genet. 17, 102–105.

Gabbiani, G., Ryan, G.B., Lamelin, J.P. et al. (1973) Human smooth muscle autoantibody. Its identification as antiactin antibody and a study of its binding to 'nonmuscular' cells. Am. J. Pathol. 72, 473–484.

Gaedigk, A., Blum, M., Gaedigk, R., Eichelbaum, M. and Meyer, U.A. (1991) Deletion of the entire CYP2D6 gene as a cause of impaired drug metabolism in poor metabolizers of the debrisoquine/sperteine polymorphism. Am. J. Hum. Genet. 48, 943–950.

Gerken, G., Manns, M., Ramadori, G. et al. (1987) Liver membrane autoantibodies in chronic active hepatitis: studies on mechanically and enzymatically isolated rabbit hepatocytes. J. Hepatol. 5, 65–74.

Gilliland, G., Perrin, S., Blanchard, K. and Bunn, H.F. (1990) Analysis of cytokine mRNA and DNA: detection and quantitation by competitive polymerase chain reaction. Proc. Natl. Acad. Sci. U.S.A. 87, 2725–2729.

Gonzalez, F.J., Skoda, R.C. and Kimura, S. et al. (1988) Characterization of the common genetic defect in humans deficient in debrisoquine metabolism. Nature 331, 442–446.

Gough, A.C., Miles, J.S., Spurr, N.K. et al. (1990) Identification of the primary gene defect at the cytochrome P450 CYP2D6 locus. Nature 347, 773–776.

Gutierrez-Ramos, J.C., Moreno de Alboran, I.M. and Martinez, A.C. (1992) In vivo administration of interleukin-2 turns on anergic self-reactive T cells and leads to autoimmune disease. Eur. J. Immunol. 22, 2867–2872.

Haanen, J.B., De Waal Malefizt, R., Res, P.C. et al. (1991) Selection of a human T helper type 1-like T cell subset by mycobacteria. J. Exp. Med. 174, 583–592.

Hanioka, N., Kimura, S., Meyer, U.A. and Gonzalez, F.J. (1990) The human CYP2D6 locus associated with a common genetic defect in drug oxidation: a G1943 to A base change in intron 3 of a mutant CYP2D6 allele results in an aberrant 3′ splice recognition site. Am. J. Hum. Genet. 47, 994–1001.

Heim, M. and Meyer, U.A. (1990) Genotyping of poor metabolizers of debrisoquine by allele-specific PCR amplification. Lancet 336, 529–530.

Homberg, J.C., Micouin, C., Peltier, A., Salmon, C. and Caroli, J. (1974) Un nouvel anticorps non specifique d'organe au cours d'hepatite chronique. Med. Chir. Dij. 3, 82–85.

Homberg, J., Abuaf, N., Bernard, O. et al. (1987) Chronic active hepatitis associated with anti-liver/ kidney microsome antibody type I: a second type of 'autoimmune' hepatitis. Hepatology 7, 1333–1339.

Jacob, C.O., Aiso, S., Michie, S.A., McDevitt, H.O. and Acha-Orbea, H. (1990) Prevention of diabetes in non-obese diabetic mice by tumor necrosis factor (TNF): similarities between TNF α and interleukin 1. Proc. Natl Acad. Sci. U.S.A. 87, 968–972.

Jacqz-Aigrain, E., Laurent, J. and Alvarez, F. (1990) Dextromethorphan phenotypes in pediatric patients with autoimmune hepatitis. Br. J. Clin. Pharmacol. 30, 153–154.

Janeway, C.A. (1988) Frontiers of immune system. Nature 333, 804–806.

Janeway, C.A. (1989) Natural killer cells. A primitive immune system. Nature 341, 108.

Johnson, G.D., Holborow, E.J. and Glynn, L.E. (1965) Antibody to smooth muscle in patients with liver disease. Lancet 2, 878–879.

Joske, R.A. and King, W.E. (1955) The L.E.-cell phenomenon in active chronic viral hepatitis. Lancet 2, 477–480.

Kagimoto, M., Heim, M., Kagimoto, K., Zeugin, T. and Meyer, U.A. (1990) Multiple mutations of the human cytochrome P450 IID6 gene (CYP2D6) in poor metabolizers of debrisoquine. J. Biol. Chem, 265, 17209–17214.

Kenneally, D., Mackay, I.R. and Toh, B.H. (1984) Antinucleolar antibodies demonstrated by monolayers of human fibroblast in sera from patients with systemic lupus erythematosus, progressive systemic sclerosis and chronic active hepatitis. J. Clin. Lab. Immunol. 14, 13–16.

Kirk, A.P., Jain, S., Pocock, S. et al. (1980) Late results of the Royal Free Hospital prospective controlled trial of prednisolone therapy in hepatitis B surface antigen negative chronic active hepatitis. Gut 21, 78–83.

Kurki, P. and Virtanen, I. (1984) The detection of human antibodies against cytoskeletal components. J. Immunol. Meth. 67, 209–223.

Lassoued, K., Guilly, M.-N., Danon, F. et al. (1988) Antinuclear autoantibodies specific for lamins. Ann. Intern. Med. 108, 829–833.

Mackay, I.R. (1985) Autoimmune diseases of the liver. In: N.R. Rose and I.R. Mackay (Eds.) The Autoimmune Diseases, Academic, Orlando, FL, pp. 291–337.

Mackay, I.R. and Wood, I.J. (1962) Lupoid hepatitis: a comparison of 22 cases with other types of chronic liver disease. Q. J. Med. 31, 485–507.

Mackay, I.R., Taft, L.I. and Cowling, D.C. (1956) Lupoid hepatitis. Lancet 2, 1323–1326.

Maddrey, W.C. (1987) Subdivisions of idiopathic autoimmune chronic active hepatitis. Hepatology 7, 1372–1375.

Maggiore, G., Bernard, O., Homberg, J.-C., et al. (1974) Characterization of the microsomal antigen related to a subclass of active chronic hepatitis. Immunology 26, 589–590.

Maggiore, G., Bernard, O., Homberg, J.C. et al. (1986) Liver disease associated with anti-liver–kidney microsome antibody in children. J. Pediatr. 108, 399–404.

Mahgoub, A., Idle, J.R., Dring, G.L., Lancaster, R. and Smith, R.L. (1977) Polymorphagic hydroxylation of debrisoquine in man. Lancet ii, 584–586.

Manns, M. (1989) Autoantibodies and antigens in liver diseases – updated. J. Hepatol. 9, 272–280.

Manns, M.P. (1991) Cytoplasmic autoantigens in autoimmune hepatitis: molecular analysis and clinical relevance. Semin. Liver Dis. 11, 205–214.

Manns, M.P. and Meyer zum Büschenfelde, K.-H. (1990) Nature of autoantigens and autoantibodies in autoimmune hepatitis. Springer Semin. Immunopathol. 12, 57–65.

Manns, M., Gerken, G., Kyriatsoulis, A. et al. (1987) Characterization of a new subgroup of autoimmune chronic hepatitis by autoantibodies against a soluble liver antigen. Lancet 1, 292–294.

Manns, M., Zanger, U., Gerken, G., et al. (1990) Patients with type II autoimmune hepatitis express functionally intact cytochrome P450 db1 that is inhibited by LKM-1 autoantibodies in vitro but not in vivo. Hepatology 12, 127–132.

Martini, E., Abuaf, N., Cavalli, F., Durand, V., Johanet, C. and Homberg, J.C. (1988) Antibody to liver cytosol (anti-LC1) in patients with autoimmune chronic active hepatitis type 2. Hepatology, 8, 1662–1666.

Meyer, U.A., Gut, J., Kronbach, T. et al. (1986) The molecular mechanisms of two common polymorphisms of drug oxidation – evidence for functional changes in cytochrome P-450 isozymes catalysing bufuralol and mephenytoin oxidation. Xenobiotica 16, 449–464.

Meyer, U.A., Skoda, R.C. and Zanger, U.N. (1990) The genetic polymorphism of debrisoquine/sperteine metabolism – molecular mechanisms. Pharmacol. Ther. 46, 297–308.

Meyer zum Büschenfelde, K.-H., Lohse, A.W., Manns, M. and Poralla, T. (1990) Autoimmunity and liver disease. Hepatology 12, 354–363.

Miyachi, K., Matsushima, H., Takano, S. et al. (1991) A case of chronic active hepatitis presenting with anti-liver/kidney microsome antibody. Acta Hepatol. Jap. 32, 175–179.

Monna, T., Kuroki, T. and Yamamoto, S. (1985) Autoimmune hepatitis: the present status in Japan. Gastroenterol. Jap. 20, 260–272.

Morshed, S.A., Nishioka, M. (1992) Interferon-γ gene in liver from patients with hepatitis C virus (HCV) infection. Gastroenterol. Jap. 27, 562.

Nebert, D.W. and Gonzalez, F.J. (1987) P450 genes: structure, evolution, and regulation. Annu. Rev. Biochem. 56, 945–993.

Nishioka, M. (1993) Nuclear antigens in autoimmune hepatitis. In: K.-H. Meyer zum Büschenfelde, J. Hoofnagle and M. Manns (Eds.), Immunology and Liver, Proc. Falk Symposium 70, Kluwer, pp. 193–205.

Nishioka, M., Aibiki, T. and Izumi, K. (1985) Smooth muscle antibody. Kan Tan Sui (Japan) 11, 591–597.

Nishioka, M., Kagawa, H., Yamamoto, S. and Kuroki, T. (1988) A study of the increasing age of occurrence of autoimmune hepatitis. Acta Hepatol. Jap. 29, 1274–1275.

Odievre, A.M., Maggiore, G., Homberg, J.-C. et al. (1983) Seroimmunologic classification of chronic hepatitis in 57 children. Hepatology 3, 407–409.

Orishki, M., Nishioka, M., Tsuneoka, Y., Matsuo, Y. and Ichikawa, Y. (1992) Human CYP2D6 gene in chronic liver diseases. In: Immunology and Liver, Falk Symposium No. 70. B. 161.

Ortiz de Montellano, P.R. (Ed.) (1986) Cytochrome P-450 Structure, Mechanism and Biochemistry. Plenum, New York, pp. 1–556.

Pape, G.R., Spengler, U., Hoffmann, R.M. and Jung, M.-C. (1991) Pathogenesis of primary biliary cirrhosis. In: E.L. Krawitt and R.H. Wiesner (Eds.) Autoimmune Liver Diseases. Raven, New York, pp. 43–62.

Paul, N.L. and Ruddle, N.H. (1988) Lymphotoxin. Annu. Rev. Immunol. 6, 407–438.

Pedersen, J.S., Toh, B.H., Mackay, I.R. et al. (1982) Segregation of autoantibody to cytoskeletal filaments, actin and intermediate filaments, with two types of chronic active hepatitis. Clin. Exp. Immunol. 48, 527–532.

Pujol-Borrel, R., Todd, I., Doshi, M. et al. (1987) HLA class II induction in human Islet cells by interferon-γ plus tumor necrosis factor or lymphotoxin. Nature 326, 304–306.

Rizzetto, M., Swana, G. and Doniach, D. (1973) Microsomal antibodies in active chronic hepatitis and other disorders. Clin. Exp. Immunol. 15, 331–344.

Rizzetto, M., Bianchi, F.B. and Doniach, D. (1974) Characterization of the microsomal antigen related to a subclass of active chronic hepatitis. Immunology 26, 589–590.

Sarvetnick, N., Liggitt, D., Pitts, S.L., Hansen, S.E. and Stewart, A. (1988) Insulin-dependent diabetes induced in transgenic mice by ectopic expression of class II MHC and interferon-γ. Cell 52, 773–782.

Schlaak, J., Lohr, H., Gallati, H., Meyer zum Büschenfelde, K.-H. and Fleischer, B. (1992) Elevated IL-4 production of liver infiltrating T cells in autoimmune hepatitis. Hepatology 16, 64A.

Schumacher, J.H., O'Garra, A., Shrader, B. et al. (1988) The characterization of four monoclonal antibodies specific for mouse IL-5 and development of mouse and human IL-5 enzyme-linked immunosorbent. J. Immunol. 141, 1576–1581.

Schwartz, R.H. (1989) Acquisition of immunologic self-tolerance. Cell 57, 1073–1081.

Schwartz, R.H., Mueller, D.L., Jenkins, M.K. and Quill, H.T. (1989) T cell clonal anergy. Cold Spring Harbor Symp. Quant. Biol. 54, 605–610.

Shiratori, Y., Kawase, T., Shiina, S. et al. (1988) Modulation of hepatotoxicity by macrophages in the liver. Hepatology 8, 815–821.

Sinha, A.A., Lopez, M.T. and McDevitt, H.O. (1990) Autoimmune diseases: the failure of self-tolerance. Science 248, 1380–1388.

Skoda, R.C., Gonzalez, F.J., Demierr, A. and Meyer, U.A. (1988) Two mutant alleles of the human cytochrome P-450db1 gene (P450CD1) associated with genetically deficient metabolism of debrisoquine and other drugs. Proc. Natl. Acad. Sci. U.S.A. 85, 5240–5243.

Smith, C.A.D., Gough, A.C., Leigh, P.N. et al. (1992) Debrisoquine hydroxylase gene polymorphism and susceptibility to Parkinson's disease. Lancet 339, 1375–1377.

Tan, E.M. (1989) Antinuclear antibodies: diagnostic markers for autoimmune diseases and probes for cell biology. Adv. Immunol. 44, 93–151.

Taniguchi, T. (1988) Regulation of cytokine gene expression. Annu. Rev. Immunol. 6, 439–464.

Terada, S., Hong, S.H., Watanabe, Y., Morshed, S.A. and Nishioka, M. (1991) Analysis of antinuclear antibodies (ANA) in autoimmune hepatitis. In: M. Tsuchiya, T. Hibi and I. Moro (Eds.) Frontiers of Mucosal Immunology, Proc. Sixth Int. Congr. Mucosal Immunology, Vol. 2, Elsevier, Amsterdam, pp. 39–42.

Teufel, M., Niessen, K.H. and Berg, P.A. (1983) Chronic active hepatitis in childhood with detection of liver–pancreas-specific autoantibodies. Eur. J. Pediatr. 140, 30–33.

Thiele, D.L. (1989) Tumor necrosis factor, the acute phase response and the pathogenesis of alcoholic liver disease. Hepatology 9, 497–499.

Toh, B.H. (1979) Smooth muscle autoantibodies and autoantigens. Clin. Exp. Immunol. 38, 621–628.

Van Venrooij, W.J. and Sellekens, P.T.G. (1989) Small nuclear RNA associated proteins: autoantigens in connective tissue diseases. Clin. Exp. Rheumatol. 7, 635–645.

Vogel, F. and Motulsky, A.G. (Eds.) (1979) Human Genetics. Springer, New York.

von Boehmer, H., Teh, H.S. and Kisielow, P. (1989) The thymus selects the useful, neglects the useless and destroys the harmful. Immunol. Today 10, 57–61.

Waldenström, J. (1950) Leber, Blutproteine and Nahrungeiweiss. Dtsch. Z. Verdau. Stoffwechselkz 2, 113–119.

Wang, A.M., Doyle, M.V. and Mark, D.F. (1989) Quantitation of mRNA by the polymerase chain reaction. Proc. Natl. Acad. Sci. U.S.A. 86, 9717–9721.

Welsh, R.M. (1986) Regulation of virus infections by natural killer cells. A review. Nat. Immun. Cell Growth Regul. 5, 169–199.

Wesiersk-Gadek, J., Penner, E., Hitchman, E. and Sauermann, G. (1988) Antibodies to nuclear lamins in autoimmune liver disease. Clin. Immunol. Immunopathol. 49, 107–115.

Whittingham, S. and McNeilage, L.J. (1988) Antinuclear antibody as molecular and diagnostic probes. Mol. Cell. Probes 2, 169–179.

Whittingham, S., Mackay, I.R. and Irwin, J. (1966a) Autoimmune hepatitis: immunofluorescent reactions with cytoplasm of smooth muscle and renal glomerular cells. Lancet 1, 1333–1336.

Whittingham, S., Irwin, J., Mackay, I.R. and Smalley, M. (1966b) Smooth muscle autoantibody in 'autoimmune' hepatitis. Gastroenterology 51, 499–505.

Wierenga, E.A., Snoek, M., Jansen, H.M. et al. (1991) Human atopen-specific types 1 and 2 T helper cell clones. J. Immunol. 147, 2942–2949.

Wilcox, R.G. and Isselbacher, K.J. (1961) Chronic liver disease in young people. Clinical features and course of thirty-three patients. Am. J. Med. 30, 185–195.

Yamamoto, A.M., Mura, C., Morales, M.G., Bernard, O., Krishnamoorthy, R. and Alvarez, F. (1992) Study of CYP2D6 gene in children with autoimmune hepatitis and P450 IID6 autoantibodies. Clin. Exp. Immunol. 87, 251–255.

Yamamura, M., Uyemura, K., Deans, R. et al. (1991) Defining protective responses to pathogens: cytokine profiles in leprosy lesions. Science, 254, 277–279.

Yssel, H., Shanafelt, M.C., Soderberg, C. et al. (1991) Borrelia burgdorferi activaties a T helper type 1-like T cell subset in lyme arthritis. J. Exp. Med. 174, 593–601.

Zauli, D., Crespi, C., Amore, P.D. et al. (1985) Relationship between cytoskeleton and smooth muscle antibodies (SMA) in chronic liver disease (CLD). J. Hepatol. 1 (Suppl.), 155.

<h1 style="text-align:center">Subject Index</h1>